Engaging with Climate Change

How can we help and support people to face climate change?

Engaging with Climate Change is the first book of its kind to explore in depth what climate change actually means to people. It is the first to bring members of a wide range of different disciplines in the social sciences together in discussion and to introduce a psychoanalytic perspective. The important insights that result have real implications for policy, particularly with regard to how to relate to people when discussing the issue. Topics covered include:

- what lies beneath the current widespread denial of climate change
- how do we manage our feelings about climate change
- our great difficulty in acknowledging our true dependence on nature
- our conflicting identifications
- the effects of living within cultures that have perverse aspects
- the need to mourn before we can engage in a positive way with the new conditions we find ourselves in.

Through understanding these issues and adopting policies that recognize their implications humanity can hope to develop a response to climate change of the nature and scale necessary. Aimed at the general reader as well as psychoanalysts, psychotherapists and climate scientists, this book will deepen our understanding of the human response to climate change.

Sally Weintrobe, a practising psychoanalyst, is a Fellow of the Institute of Psychoanalysis in London. She sees a psychoanalytic perspective as a vital part of understanding how to engage people about the seriousness of climate change and how to understand current levels of denial. She has written and lectured widely on these subjects and on our relationship with nature. Her commitment to fostering interdisciplinary exchange with other human scientists has led to this remarkable book.

The New Library of Psychoanalysis
General Editor: Alessandra Lemma

The New Library of Psychoanalysis was launched in 1987 in association with the Institute of Psychoanalysis, London. It took over from the International Psychoanalytical Library which published many of the early translations of the works of Freud and the writings of most of the leading British and Continental psychoanalysts.

The purpose of the New Library of Psychoanalysis is to facilitate a greater and more widespread appreciation of psychoanalysis and to provide a forum for increasing mutual understanding between psychoanalysts and those working in other disciplines such as the social sciences, medicine, philosophy, history, linguistics, literature and the arts. It aims to represent different trends both in British psychoanalysis and in psychoanalysis generally. The New Library of Psychoanalysis is well placed to make available to the English-speaking world psychoanalytic writings from other European countries and to increase the inter-change of ideas between British and American psychoanalysts. Through the *Teaching Series*, the New Library of Psychoanalysis now also publishes books that provide comprehensive, yet accessible, overviews of selected subject areas aimed at those studying psychoanalysis and related fields such as the social sciences, philosophy, literature and the arts.

The Institute, together with the British Psychoanalytical Society, runs a low-fee psychoanalytic clinic, organizes lectures and scientific events concerned with psychoanalysis and publishes the *International Journal of Psychoanalysis*. It runs a training course in psychoanalysis which leads to membership of the International Psychoanalytical Association – the body which preserves internationally agreed standards of training, of professional entry, and of professional ethics and practice for psychoanalysis as initiated and developed by Sigmund Freud. Distinguished members of the Institute have included Michael Balint, Wilfred Bion, Ronald Fairbairn, Anna Freud, Ernest Jones, Melanie Klein, John Rickman and Donald Winnicott.

Previous general editors have included David Tuckett, who played a very active role in the establishment of the New Library. He was followed as general editor by Elizabeth Bott Spillius, who was in turn followed by Susan Budd and then by Dana Birksted-Breen.

Current members of the Advisory Board include Liz Allison, Giovanna di Ceglie, Rosemary Davies and Richard Rusbridger.

Previous Members of the Advisory Board include Christopher Bollas, Ronald Britton, Catalina Bronstein, Donald Campbell, Sara Flanders, Stephen Grosz, John Keene, Eglé Laufer, Alessandra Lemma, Juliet Mitchell, Michael Parsons, Rosine Jozef Perelberg, Mary Target and David Taylor.

ALSO IN THIS SERIES

The Theory and Technique of Psychoanalytic Supervision: The Sao Paulo Clinical Seminars Antonino Ferro

TITLES IN THE NEW LIBRARY OF PSYCHOANALYSIS
TEACHING SERIES
Reading Freud: A Chronological Exploration of Freud's Writings Jean-Michel Quinodoz
Listening to Hanna Segal: Her Contribution to Psychoanalysis Jean-Michel Quinodoz
Reading French Psychoanalysis Edited by Dana Birksted-Breen, Sara Flanders and Alain Gibeault
Reading Winnicott Lesley Caldwell and Angela Joyce
Initiating Psychoanalysis: Perspectives Bernard Reith, Sven Lagerlöf, Penelope Crick, Mette Møller and Elisabeth Skale
Infant Observation Frances Salo
Reading Anna Freud Nick Midgley

TITLES IN THE NEW LIBRARY OF PSYCHOANALYSIS
'BEYOND THE COUCH' SERIES
Under the Skin: A Psychoanalytic Study of Body Modification Alessandra Lemma
Engaging with Climate Change: Psychoanalytic and Interdisciplinary Perspectives Edited and introduced by Sally Weintrobe

Engaging with Climate Change

Psychoanalytic and interdisciplinary
perspectives

Edited by Sally Weintrobe

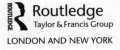

Routledge
Taylor & Francis Group

LONDON AND NEW YORK

First published 2013
by Routledge
27 Church Road, Hove, E Sussex BN3 2FA

Simultaneously published in the USA and Canada
by Routledge
711 Third Avenue, New York, NY 10017

Routledge is an imprint of the Taylor & Francis Group, an informa business

British Library Cataloguing in Publication Data
A catalogue record for this book is available from the British Library

Library of Congress Cataloging in Publication Data
Engaging with climate change: psychoanalytic and interdisciplinary
perspectives / edited by Sally Weintrobe.
  p. cm. — (The new library of psychoanalysis)
ISBN 978–0–415–66760–9 (hbk.) — ISBN 978–0–415–66762–3
(pbk.) 1. Climatic changes—Psychological aspects.
2. Environmental psychology. I. Weintrobe, Sally.
BF353.5.C55E55 2012
363.738'74019—dc23

                                                              2012005624

ISBN: 978–0–415–66760–9 (hbk)
ISBN: 978–0–415–66762–3 (pbk)
ISBN: 978–0–203–09440–2 (ebk)

Typeset in Times New Roman
by RefineCatch Limited, Bungay, Suffolk

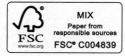

MIX
Paper from
responsible sources
FSC® C004839
www.fsc.org

Printed and bound in Great Britain by
TJ International Ltd, Padstow, Cornwall

For my grandparents Elsie and Colin, who nurtured
my love of nature, with gratitude

Contents

Acknowledgements

I would like to thank the following people who helped this book come to fruition. First, the 22 authors without whom there would be no book. They also offered me considerable help and encouragement. Then Alessandra Lemma, Editor of the New Library of Psychoanalysis, for all her editorial support, and Kate Hawes, General Editor at Routledge, for her support and faith in the project. Then Judith Anderson, Lothar Bayer, David Bell, Lucy Anne Bishop, Jill Boswell, Chris Close, Penny Crick, Dennis Duncan, Mary Eckert, Jeremy Gaines, Nicky Gavron, Michael Hathorn, Liam Humphreys, Tim Kasser, Kannan Navaratnem, Sheelagh Neuling, Vanessa Neuling, Anton Obholzer, Daniel Pick, David Riley, Ben Rometsch, Anne-Marie Sandler, Wilhelm Skogstad, Philip Stander, Adrian Tait, Mary Target, Lisa Weintrobe, Tanya Weintrobe, Sandra White, Jan Woolf and Paul Zeal, who all helped me in different ways. Then Lez Weintrobe for his ongoing encouragement, help and support.

Finally, I want to thank the psychoanalyst Hanna Segal, who died in July 2011, for her inspiration as well as her personal support for the book. At her funeral her grandson, Paul Segal, said:

> For Granny the take-home message was that however dark the circumstances, it is essential 'to keep a little fire burning'. In that conversation she said how important it was for psychoanalysts to keep a little fire burning in the face of what she called the 'anti-mind' approach.

Special permissions have been granted for various quotations to be used in Chapter 2 'What History can Teach Us About Climate Change Denial' by Clive Hamilton. For kind permission to quote from a paper by Rowe (1986) on page 29 thanks to Chicago University Press, from Rowe (2006) on page 22 thanks to Springer Science+Media BV, from D. Buchwald et al. (2006) 'The Collected Papers of Albert Einstein, Vol. 10' on page 20 thanks to Princeton University Press and from Albert Camus' 'The Plague' on pages 26–8 thanks to Penguin UK, Random House USA and Gallimard Press.

Contributors

Jon Alexander, MSc, a former advertising executive, currently works for the National Trust as well as consulting to several other organizations on how they can generate and embody hope for the future. His projects include MyFarm, which sees the National Trust hand over the running of Wimpole Farm to 10,000 people through the Internet, and Eurostar's Culture Connect partnership. He won the inaugural Ashridge Sustainable Innovation Award in 2009. Blog available at: www.conservation-economy.org and tweets @jonjalex.

Ted Benton is Professor of Sociology at the University of Essex. He has written extensively on philosophy of social science, history of the life sciences, social theory and Marxism. Since the 1980s, his main focus has been on re-working the heritage of left theory in response to 'green' thought and practice, and since 1992 this has been taken further through collaboration with others in the Red-Green Study Group. He is a well-known photographer and writer on natural history.

Erik Bichard is Professor of Regeneration and Sustainable Development at the University of Salford in Greater Manchester. He has spent a career in four different sectors exploring the conditions for sustainable change in organizations and in individuals. His book *Positively Responsible*, written with the psychologist Cary Cooper, tackles issues of resistance to sustainable decision-making in a business context.

Michael Brearley, psychoanalyst, is a Fellow of the Institute of Psychoanalysis in London, where he was also President. He works as a psychoanalyst in private practice. He has been a Lecturer in Philosophy at the University of Newcastle-upon-Tyne and a professional cricketer, captaining England. He has written and lectured in the areas of psychoanalysis, philosophy and leadership and is author of the book *The Art of Captaincy*.

Irma Brenman Pick, psychoanalyst, trained first at the Tavistock Clinic as a Child Psychotherapist, then at the Institute of Psychoanalysis in London as an Adult and Child Psychoanalyst. She is now a Senior Training Psychoanalyst and Supervisor of the Institute of Psychoanalysis, where she was also a past

President. She has a particular interest in the subject of difficulties in coming to terms with painful emotional experiences.

Stanley Cohen is Professor Emeritus of Sociology at the London School of Economics. He has written about states of denial, criminological theory, prisons, social control, criminal justice policy, juvenile delinquency, mass media, political crime and human rights violations. He is now working on *The Distant Other*, a collective research project about humanitarian communication.

Tom Crompton, PhD, is Change Strategist at the World Wildlife Fund UK. In recent work he has explored the importance of cultural values in underpinning public expressions of social and environmental concern. His most recent report, *Common Cause: The Case for Working with Our Cultural Values*, published in September 2010 (available at: www.valuesandframes.org), has led to extensive debate across the third sector, and its recommendations are now being incorporated into the strategies of many UK-based NGOs.

Clive Hamilton is Professor of Public Ethics at Charles Sturt University. He has held visiting academic positions at the University of Cambridge, the University of Oxford and Yale University and is the author of several best-selling books, including *Growth Fetish, The Freedom Paradox* and *Requiem for a Species: Why We Resist the Truth about Climate Change*.

Mike Hannis, PhD, is an Honorary Research Fellow in Environmental Philosophy and Politics at Keele University. His academic research centres on issues arising at the interface between ecological sustainability and personal freedom. He also works as a freelance writer and consultant and is an editor of *The Land* magazine.

Stephan Harrison, PhD, is Reader in Quaternary Science at Exeter University and a Senior Research Associate at the Oxford University Centre for the Environment. He is Director of Climate Change Risk Management. With a background in quaternary science, since 1991 he has worked on glaciers and climate change.

Bob Hinshelwood, psychoanalyst, is Professor in the Centre for Psychoanalytic Studies, University of Essex, and Fellow of The Institute of Psychoanalysis. He was previously a Consultant Psychotherapist in the British National Health Service and Clinical Director of the Cassel Hospital in London. He has written extensively on Kleinian psychoanalysis and also on social and political issues of various kinds.

Paul Hoggett is Professor of Politics and Director of the Centre for Psycho-Social Studies at the University of the West of England in Bristol. He is also a practicing psychoanalytic psychotherapist, a Member of the Severnside Institute for Psychotherapy and Associate Member of the Lincoln Centre for Psychotherapy. His most recent book is *Politics, Identity and Emotion*.

John Keene is a Training and Supervising Psychoanalyst of The Institute of Psychoanalysis in London and works as a psychoanalyst. He was formerly a member of the Senior Staff of the Tavistock Clinic, where in addition to clinical commitments he taught on its Institutional Processes programme. His interest in the planetary ecosystem combines his first academic studies in geology with later degrees in philosophy and psychology. He has an interest in the functioning of groups, organizations and political processes.

Johannes Lehtonen, MD, is a psychoanalyst with the Finnish Psychoanalytical Society and Professor Emeritus of Psychiatry at the University of Eastern Finland. He was chairman of the Finnish Psychiatric Association, 1996–1999, and Dean of the Medical Faculty of the University of Eastern Finland in Kuopio, 2004–2007. He has published on neurophysiology, psychiatry and psychoanalysis, focusing on the relationship between the mind and brain, and also on human responses to climate change.

Renee Aron Lertzman, PhD, is a senior research fellow at Portland State University. Her work is concerned with the relations of psychoanalytic research and theory with contemporary environmental crises. She is Special Editor of Environment and Sustainability for the journal *Psychoanalysis, Culture and Society* and is currently working on a book, *The Myth of Apathy*, based on her doctoral research.

Angela Mauss-Hanke, PhD, is a Training and Supervising Psychoanalyst for adults and groups with the German Psychoanalytic Association (DPV) in Munich and a child psychoanalyst. She has written many psychoanalytical papers on topics relevant to society, e.g. 'The killing of the So-called Handicapped in Germany and the Nuremberg Medics Trial 1946/47' (2000); on 9/11 ('The Low Voice of Sanity', 2004); about revenge and school shootings ('Revenge Doesn't Know Its Bounds', 2009) and on 'National Socialism and Its Impact on German Self-conceptions Today' (2011).

Rosemary Randall is a psychoanalytic psychotherapist working in private practice and a member of the Cambridge Society for Psychotherapy. She was co-founder of the 'Carbon Conversations' project, which takes a psychological approach to personal carbon reduction and is used by many organizations across the UK. She has written many papers on our relationship with climate change, and she writes a regular blog on the subject, available at www.rorandall.org

Margaret Rustin is a Child and Adult Psychotherapist and an Associate of the Institute of Psychoanalysis, London. She was Head of Child Psychotherapy at the Tavistock Clinic for many years. She has a special interest in thinking psychoanalytically about literature and has co-written, with Michael Rustin, *Narratives of Love and Loss: Studies in Modern Children's Fiction* (Verso 1987; repub. Karnac 1999), and *Mirror to Nature: Drama, Psychoanalysis and Society*, Karnac: Tavistock Series 2002.

Michael Rustin was Professor and Head of the Department of Sociology at the University of East London from 1974 to 1988 and Dean of Faculty of Social Sciences from 1991 to 2001. His current roles at UEL are primarily in research and research supervision, and as academic link between the University and the Tavistock Clinic. He has written several books, including *The Good Society and the Inner World: Psychoanalysis, Politics and Culture*.

John Steiner, MD, is a Senior Training and Supervising Psychoanalyst for the Institute of Psychoanalysis in London and works in private practice as a psychoanalyst. He is the author of several psychoanalytic papers and the editor of several books, and he has written two books. The first, *Psychic Retreats* (1993), describes how patients may withdraw to defensive internal mental organizations, which protect them from anxiety and loss. The second, *Seeing and Being Seen* (2011), describes the situation of patients emerging from a psychic retreat.

Jukka Välimäki, MD, is a Training and Supervising Psychoanalyst, former chairman of the Training Institute and past President of the Finnish Psychoanalytic Society. He has acted as the Finnish editor for the Scandinavian Psychoanalytic Review (1979–1989) and as a member of the editorial board of the Finnish Psychoanalytic Society, publishing psychoanalytic books in Finnish. He has written and lectured on psychoanalytic and psychotherapeutic technique, as well as on our responses to climate change.

Bob Ward is Policy and Communications Director at the Grantham Research Institute on Climate Change and the Environment at the London School of Economics and Political Science (chaired by Nicholas Stern, author of the influential Stern Review on the economics of climate change). Bob joined the Institute in 2008 from Risk Management Solutions, the leading provider of computer models for quantifying the risk of catastrophic events, where he was Director of Public Policy. He previously worked at the Royal Society and the UK National Academy of Science, where his responsibilities included leading the media relations team.

Sally Weintrobe, psychoanalyst, is a Fellow of The Institute of Psychoanalysis in London and chairs its Scientific Committee. She was formerly a Member of Senior Staff at the Tavistock Clinic and Hon. Senior Lecturer at University College London in the Department for Psychoanalytic Studies. She has written on entitlement attitudes, grievance and complaint, prejudice, greed, climate change denial and our relationship with nature.

Foreword

Chris Rapley CBE[1]

After 12,000 years of unusual stability, the world's climate is on the move. The magnitude of the changes and their impacts on humans have so far been modest. But the scientific evidence shows that evolving patterns of temperature and precipitation will become increasingly apparent and significant, as will slow but ineluctable sea level rise.

Climate change is not new. Over the long history of the planet, the climate has varied on many timescales driven by many factors. But this time there are two important differences. First, the driving forces result from human activities such as greenhouse gas emissions and the transformation of the Earth's land surface. We are therefore collectively responsible, as well as being capable, in principle, of taking avoiding actions. Secondly, the well-being of 7 billion humans depends materially on the stability and character of the climate system we inherited. The agricultural and civil infrastructures of the twenty-first century are not robust against climate changes. Examples abound of the social and economic disruption caused by extreme variations within the existing state of the system, such as severe droughts, floods and storms. So to provoke systematic changes is to place humanity under threat.

What would it take to avoid the problem? The answer is 'much more than has been achieved to date'. Despite twenty years of negotiations carried out under the auspices of the United Nations, and despite countless initiatives by governments, businesses, citizens' groups and individuals, the human driving forces, especially greenhouse gas emissions, continue to grow. The forces at play are rooted deep in the activities upon which our survival and comfort depend. Technical solutions offer a necessary but insufficient way forward. Fundamental attitudinal and behavioural changes are required in which we weave into our every action the need to respect and protect our environmental life-support system. To do so entails a degree of collectivism and intervention that strikes at the heart of fashionable 'laissez faire' ideologies and challenges the economics of growth, upon which, it is claimed, our prosperity relies.

The nature and scale of the challenge is daunting. Indeed, it is already too late to avoid some climatic change as the Earth's systems respond to the disturbances we have already created. However, history shows that we are capable of extraordinary feats, and on an otherwise finite planet, our ingenuity, at least, seems unbounded. We still have the chance to limit the scale of our disruption.

The key is actively to confront the problem and to give it due priority. But here lies a profound difficulty, well illustrated by Nicolò Machiavelli in *The Prince* (1515: VI) in which he comments on the propensity of vested interests to defend the existing order of things and on 'the incredulity of men, who do not readily believe in new things until they have had a long experience of them'. Denial is an all-too-human reaction to a new and uncomfortable truth, and its effect is to stymie the capacity to respond.

And so it has transpired. While the evidence has convinced many of the need to take action, others, many of them influential, have exhibited the classic symptoms of denial. Well documented are the shifting sequence of 'climate sceptic' arguments in response to the growing body of facts: 'climate isn't changing' . . . 'it is changing, but it's not us' . . . 'it is us, but it doesn't matter' . . . 'it does matter, but it's too expensive or difficult to do anything about it'.

To the climate scientist, bemused by the failure of the widely held, but flawed, 'information deficit' model, in which non-experts are empty vessels who will respond appropriately once informed of the facts, it is a revelation and relief to discover that this sequence of denial is all too familiar to those who deal with the workings of the human mind. Here lies the importance and power of this book. By providing a deeper understanding of ways in which people think and feel about climate change, the psychoanalytic perspective offers a basis for understanding, and thereby hopefully better overcoming, sources of resistance to evidence and to the need for action. An important distinction is made between negation (believing something is untrue, that is true) and disavowal (unconsciously accepting that something is true, but simultaneously finding ways systematically to deny it). This allows a more tailored approach to help individuals and groups to bring their 'psychic reality' into alignment with the real world. Combined with the practitioner's experience of what works and does not as regards supporting people to bear the painful truth about climate change, this points the way to increased effectiveness in encouraging and reinforcing pro-environmental thinking and behaviour. Equally, the insights in this book cast valuable light on the human tendency to self-delusion, when the need for action is accepted but the actions undertaken fall far short of what is actually necessary.

The breaching of disciplinary barriers and the pooling of accumulated experience to allow true inter-disciplinary discourse opens up the opportunity to gain such understanding. The resulting knowledge, in turn, provides the means to gear up the level of climate-related effort to achieve real effect.

Throughout the book, we are repeatedly reminded of two most basic facts: that we are all much less rational than we care to think, and that we are of, not above, the natural world. Without such insights, our response to the problem of climate change is likely to remain inadequate, leaving us vulnerable to an overwhelming tide of events. With them, we are better equipped to strive for a future in which humanity can flourish in harmony with the Earth's environmental systems upon which we depend.

Note

1 Chris Rapley CBE is Professor of Climate Science at University College London. He was Director of the Science Museum in London between 2007 and 2010. Prior to this he was Director of the British Antarctic Survey (BAS), and before that the Executive Director of the International Geosphere-Biosphere Programme (IGBP) at the Royal Swedish Academy of Sciences in Stockholm. This followed an extended period as Professor of Remote Sensing Science and Associate Director of University College London's Mullard Space Science Laboratory. In 2008 he was awarded the Edinburgh Science Medal 'For professional achievements judged to have made a significant contribution to the understanding and well-being of humanity'.

Reference

Machiavelli, N. (1515) *The Prince* [Italian: *Il Principe*]. Liberty Library of Constitutional Classics. Available at: www.constitution.org

Preface

Sally Weintrobe

It is a great privilege to edit this book, in my view a most valuable resource for understanding more about our engagement with climate change. The essays give a rich and multi-faceted picture, one that illuminates and also opens up areas for further enquiry. In inviting these particular authors to contribute, I was inspired by two beliefs: first, that psychoanalysis has an important contribution to make towards understanding people's engagement with climate change, and, second, that an interdisciplinary exchange is vital to further this understanding.

The book had its origins in an interdisciplinary conference on our engagement with climate change held at the Institute of Psychoanalysis in London in 2010. The conference and the book were planned from the outset as a conversation: one between a psychoanalytic perspective and those from other disciplines. Gathered together here are voices and approaches from across what might be called the human sciences: psychoanalysis, psychology, sociology, politics, social theory, philosophy, ethics, human rights, advertising, marketing, history and public policy. As with all real and significant conversations, authors from different disciplines can be seen to feel their way together and are sometimes challenged, both by points of disagreement but also by the difficulty of relating to approaches that may be very different from their own. Insularity and prejudice are further challenges with any interdisciplinary exchange – even greater when one discovers them in one's own theoretical approach – and there is nothing like discussion with other disciplines to make one more aware of these. But insularity and prejudice, both within and across disciplines, are ill-afforded luxuries in the face of the need to understand our responses to what is happening to our climate and our world, and they are mitigated through genuine conversation between colleagues from different disciplines. The reader is warmly invited to join the conversation: one that leads to new integrations.

Chapter I

Introduction

Sally Weintrobe

Climate change

It is increasingly clear that understanding human responses to climate change is just as important as – if not more important than – understanding climate change itself. We already know enough about anthropogenic (human-made) global warming to have triggered action to reduce CO_2e^1 emissions if our response was to be rational and not destructive. The question is, why is knowledge of climate reality being so resisted? In the West we, as societies, have known about anthropogenic global warming for at least 20 years, since NASA scientist James Hansen testified before the US Congress that the planet is heating because we are burning so much fossil fuel and hence emitting so much carbon dioxide (June 1988; Royal Society 2010). Stephan Harrison, in the final chapter of this book, outlines what we know about the science; he usefully divides his analysis into two sections: what we are more certain (in a scientific sense) about and what we are less certain about. Our certainties are the message that Hansen gave to Congress: that global warming is happening and is largely man-made. Our models of what this will lead to, when and with what regional variability are where most of the uncertainty lies.

In 2009 Hansen, among others, brought bad news about one part of the predictive modelling. 'The dangerous threshold of greenhouse gases is actually lower than we told you a few years ago. Sorry about that mistake. It does not always work that way. Sometimes our estimates are off in the other direction, and the problem is not as bad as we thought. Not this time. The bad news emerged clearly only in the past three years' (Hansen 2009: 139).

The almost throwaway 'sorry about that mistake' serves brilliantly to illuminate the dangerous and cavalier attitude to risk currently shown by governments in relation to climate change. From Hansen, 'sorry about that mistake' poignantly brings home what a heavy if not intolerable weight of responsibility is placed upon climate scientists in this situation.

In 2011 McKibben, chronicling all the record-breaking global weather events of 2010 (heat waves, drought, wildfires, tornados, the acceleration of the already rapid melt of the Greenland Ice Sheet and signs of melting permafrost), said that 'the earth was getting a taste of what global warming feels like in its early stages'

(2011b: 60). Friedman (2008) has referred to our sensing the climate 'weirding'. This has very different implications for people and for animals, depending on where they are geographically. In northern climes such as in Britain, its tangible impact on daily life may currently be home-grown strawberries ripening too early for Wimbledon and hosts of golden daffodils flowering too early for Easter tourists in Wordsworth country. For some farmers in Bangladesh it has meant that seawater from flooding exacerbated by global warming has rendered their arable land salt-logged and not usable for growing crops. I heard one Bangladeshi woman, paid for by an NGO to come to the United Kingdom to represent the plight of her community, describe what this meant for her family. She said they were forced to sell cheaply the land owned by her family for generations in order to survive in the short term. It is now being prepared by new commercial owners for cultivation for pasture for sheep farming, as grass for sheep can better tolerate the salty soil. A tiger ate her husband when he and other men took to the jungle to find food. She now tries to support her children through help from relatives, themselves poor, and with any small-scale domestic work she can find.

As McKibben noted, the extreme weather events we have been witnessing are occurring with a temperature increase of only slightly less than 1°C (over pre-industrial levels) and with atmospheric CO_2e concentrations of only 390 parts per million. However, there is growing recognition by climate scientists that an increase to roughly 4°C may by now be unavoidable. This led Hamilton and social psychologist Kasser (2009) to write their paper, 'Psychological Adaptation to a Four Degree World'. Some researchers say that without drastic action to move economies off dependence on fossil fuels, the temperature increase will be higher than 4°C – more than 550 parts per million – by the end of the century (Anderson and Bows 2008).

Many people who accept anthropogenic global warming continue to locate it as a problem of the future – one for our children and grandchildren – and one that is still largely avoidable and reparable. The tragedy for humans and animals, however, is that climate stability has already been damaged and that the carbon dioxide and other greenhouse gases already released by our coal and oil-hungry economies will remain in the Earth's atmosphere for thousands of years. McKibben (2011a), in his latest book, *Eaarth: Making a Life on a Tough New Planet*, adds an extra 'a' to Earth to mark the change to instability.

The book

Our engagement with this extremely difficult reality is the subject of this book. It begins with a chapter on political and historical aspects of our engagement and ends with the science of global warming. Between these two important 'bookends' are seven chapters that focus on different aspects of our engagement with climate change and with nature. Each of the seven chapters comprises a main essay followed by two discussion papers and, in some cases, a reply. Some discussions are by psychoanalysts, and others are by authors from other disciplines. The respondents were invited to discuss a given essay, but also to bring in their own ideas so as to enrich the exchange.

The main essays in the middle seven chapters are by authors who are psycho-analytically informed, four of them – Hoggett, Keene, Randall and Weintrobe – with clinical experience working with individuals and/or groups. Lertzman, a researcher on environmental attitudes, uses psychoanalytic theory to guide and inform her work, and Michael Rustin has a long track record as a sociologist bringing psychoanalytic concepts to bear on understanding social issues.

Any grouping of authors is inevitably selective and involves omissions. In this book, unfortunately, none of the contributors are psychologists, but several (see especially Bichard, chapter 6; Crompton, chapter 9) do draw from social psychology research. This includes the important body of research on 'frames and values' (Common Cause Handbook 2011; Crompton 2010; Darnton and Kirk 2011; Kasser (2008); Kasser et al. (2007)). So, psychology's voice is part of the conversation, as is the voice of deep ecology (see Alexander: chapter 8 and Weintrobe: chapter 9). The focus of the book is on people in the West, currently the biggest carbon polluters, and very little is said about how people from other cultures and economies think and feel about climate change and about nature. This is a significant lack. Bichard, in his discussion paper (chapter 6), makes the point that an assumption of a generalized dominant Western culture can itself be too simple. He charts some significant regional differences in Europe – particu-larly in Scandinavia and Germany – in relation to cultural feelings of stewardship for nature.

Each chapter stands alone, and chapters can be read in any order. However, for those readers not familiar with psychoanalytic ideas, I suggest reading chapters in the order given, as important psychoanalytic concepts are gradually introduced and also illustrated in ways that, it is hoped, will make them accessible. The chap-ters build, within the main essays and across the interdisciplinary discussions, to give a rich and multi-faceted picture of our engagement with climate change, one that illuminates and also opens up areas for further enquiry.

The strength of an interdisciplinary approach

The interdisciplinary exchange in this book offers new ways of seeing our indi-vidual and collective engagement with climate change – perspectives that emerge from the exchange and transcend insights that the various disciplines alone could provide. There are no false attempts to reduce one discipline to another or to apply the findings of one to another. Rather, the exchange opens up the possibility of taking up what might be called a 'third position' – one that, by situating psychic and social realities side by side, allows for points of creative integration to emerge. This genuine interdisciplinarity is not only achieved across essays. It occurs within the main essays as well. In Hoggett's essay (chapter 4), perverse organiza-tions at a psychic and at a social level are described, structurally similar under-lying features analysed and startling commonalities revealed. Keene's, Lertzman's,

Randall's and my chapters focus on subjective experiences of individuals as well as characterize groups of people within a culture. This approach does not seek to *apply* understanding of the individual to the group. That would be misplaced. Rather, it relies on taking a third position from which to see commonalities between ways individuals and groups of people think and feel within a particular dominant culture. Michael Rustin's essay (chapter 8) is also in this tradition.

Cohen, in his discussion (chapter 4), suggests that an account 'should make sense both in psychological/individual terms and social/collective terms'. His requirement is fulfilled in the main essays in the book. I suggest Hoggett's essay (chapter 4) achieves this in the most clearly argued way. His analysis of perversion, drawing on a psychoanalytic account of perverse internal organizations (Steiner) and on a sociological account of perverse social organizations (Long), makes sense in both accounts.

The exchange also provides corroboration across disciplines with different evidence bases. An example is Crompton's discussion of my essay on nature (chapter 9). Crompton cites findings from 'values and frames' based empirical research from social psychology that supports my psychoanalytically based argument.

Moments of integration, corroborations achieved and new perspectives opened up in this book are not simply the result of bringing different disciplines together. They rely at a deeper level on all the authors sharing certain commonalities of approach – what might be called common underlying frames of reference. I will go into three of these, as they are not explicitly stated in the chapters. First, all analyses, whether of the social or individual, construct human beings primarily in terms of their relationships, with conflict being a key part of their relationships. Conflict is seen as a key part of relationships, with conflict over who is dominant and who is in power being a particular focus. As important is the wish to understand the underlying more hidden sources of conflict and the deeper level structures and organizations that serve to maintain power in relationships. There is a common interest in studying the felt experience of people living within their conflictual relationships. This 'relationships-and-conflict' approach ranges from sociological views of conflict between groups to psychoanalytic views of internal conflict between different parts of the self, to psychological views of the impact of conflicting frames and values on behaviour.

Second, all the authors see engaging with climate change as part of a wider engagement with issues of social justice. With human beings as the object of study, to be human, whether as an individual or as part of humanity, is to struggle with issues of moral conflict involving rights, responsibilities and fairness in relation to self and others.

Third, and importantly, there is a common underlying approach to theory as well as to subject. The approach, involving the search for deeper meaning and positing underlying structures not manifest at a surface level, give due weight to human complexity.

A further commonality, I suggest, reached towards if not yet found, is a frame of reference in which 'social' has a wider meaning than 'human', and 'social justice' a wider meaning than 'human justice'. 'Social' includes other species.

In the West we still swim in the water of a prevailing and pervasive background philosophy to which we are mostly as oblivious as fish are to being in water. We believe that we are the dominant species, the species that wields the power and is entitled to exploit other species who are there solely for our benefit. But seismic shifts are beginning to occur in our ways of thinking about our relationship with other species. We are recognizing that we share with animals the capacity to feel empathy and a moral sense. The work of evolutionary biologists like de Waal (2009) shows that morality is not a human preserve but has evolutionary roots. And as we face loss of biodiversity, we are also more openly acknowledging that we share the Earth with fellow sentient living beings, beings we are pushing to the margins of existence.

Any background philosophy will have profound effects on how we think, and more so when not explicit but part of the social fabric. The background philosophical view that it is a done deal that we are entitled to hold dominion over all life forms still holds sway – Rustin in his essay (chapter 8) identifies this view as a particular *structure of feeling*. This view powerfully legitimizes the exploitative and instrumental side of *all* our relationships, not just our relationship with nature and with animals. The struggle for universal human rights was rooted in the fight to overturn the idea that some humans (such as the poor, women, children) are inherently less equal than those 'entitled' to dominate and exploit them. This instrumental entitled view may also affect how we 'use' science and technology. Hamilton (chapter 2) goes into how within this frame we turn against science when it gives us findings like anthropogenic global warming. We have no instrumental use for this kind of science. In my nature essay (chapter 9) I look at ways that mainstream scientific discourse itself can become prejudiced against certain kinds of data, in particular those that cannot be measured, so silencing important conflicts about what counts as data. Ward in his discussion (chapter 5) reflects on his need as a scientist to be more open to different ways of seeing and understanding.

Essentially the old background philosophy removes conflict from the picture: we face no moral conflicts in relationships when we claim a God-given entitlement to dominate. And, since engagement means facing our conflicts, the old philosophy lends support to a position where engagement is not really necessary.

We are sorely in need of a new background philosophy, a new Ethics, one that acknowledges conflictual moral struggle in all our relationships and one that acknowledges our true dependencies and responsibilities. We do not control an Earth there just for us, and our task now is not, in that debased and objectionable phrase, to 'save the planet', as if Earth depended on us and not the other way round. All the authors in this book (see, in particular, Alexander: chapter 8; Benton: chapter 8; Hannis, chapter 9) are rooted in a new Ethics of this kind.

A psychoanalytic perspective

Psychoanalysis is a theory about the human mind. In a psychoanalytic view we are primed as a species to relate and to search for meaning in relationships – in other words to engage – from the beginning of life.

A psychoanalytic way of understanding sees humans as inherently divided between love and hatred of reality. Reality is hated when it thwarts our wishes, which are at times irrational and dominated by unconscious phantasies[2], and also when it exposes us to too much emotional pain. We need support and containment to bear reality. Psychoanalytic ideas also extend our ordinary understanding of what it means to think in a rational way. We may 'think' something intellectually while not being emotionally connected to it and not seeing it as something to do with us personally. Our thoughts may be distorted by unconscious processes, which include defences against knowing what we feel and think as a way of protecting ourselves from facing 'too much reality'. The focus in this book is on what we 'think' and feel about climate change.

Psychoanalysis as a theory of mind has three main foci. First, the focus is on what we experience – our affects, our wishes, our anxieties, our sense of ourselves and who we are. Second are the mental processes we use to organize our experience and defend ourselves against it when it gets to feel intolerable or causes us too much anxiety. These defences include processes such as mental splitting, projection and idealization, and they are described in the chapters that follow. Third, psychoanalysis looks at the way we represent our experience of ourselves, and of our relationships with figures in the outside world, internally within the psyche.

Psychoanalysis is not only a theory of mind focusing on human beings in their subjectivity; it is also a way of seeing man that involves elements of both irony and tragedy (Strenger 1991). The ironic can be found in sanguine, debunking conclusions like Freud's when he said, 'man is far less moral than he would like to think he is but also far more moral than he realises' (Freud 1923: 52). The tragic comes through in psychoanalysis's view of man as a moral agent in search of the truth about himself and his place in the world while subject to powerful forces beyond, or only on the edge of, his awareness. Unconscious ideas and processes can have powerful effects in a psychoanalytic account.

Themes

Here I outline as signposts for the reader only some of the major themes this book covers. These themes are picked up and elaborated in different ways in most of the chapters. I also highlight some distinctions drawn and issues raised.

Three forms of denial: denialism, disavowal and negation

Climate change denial is an important topic in the book, and three forms are distinguished. These are denialism, disavowal and negation. This brings new and much needed clarity to the subject. It is important to distinguish the three as each form is radically different in cause and has different effects.

1. *Denialism* involves campaigns of misinformation about climate change, funded by commercial and ideological interests. Denialism seeks to undermine belief in climate science, and authors such as Monbiot (2006) have charted the techniques it uses. Denialism has been termed an industry and doubt is its main product (see Orestes and Conway 2010).

    Cohen (author of *States of Denial*, 2000) points out in his discussion of Hoggett's essay (chapter 4) that 'denialism is expressed in a learned, shared public language; the activities of claim makers and moral entrepreneurs are organized, planned, intentional and – sometimes less obviously – ideological'. Hamilton, in chapter 2, charts the way that: 'global warming has been made a battleground in the wider culture wars' in the United States. He points out that denialists have 'adroitly used the instruments of democratic practice to erode the authority of professional expertise'. He means scientific expertise in particular. He observes that one can now predict a person's attitude to global warming if one knows their attitude to same-sex marriage, abortion and gun control.

2. *Negation* involves saying that something that is, is not. Negation defends against feelings of anxiety and loss and is often resorted to when the first shock of a painful reality makes it too much to bear, for now, all in one go. In a psychoanalytic account this is the first stage of mourning, where a person may begin by saying 'it's not true', then angrily accept it is true, and only then start to feel grief and acceptance.

3. In *disavowal* reality is more accepted, but its significance is *minimized*. In his discussion Cohen writes: '"True denial" requires the special paradox of knowing and not-knowing *at the same time*.' His definition of 'true denial' corresponds with the psychoanalytic concept of disavowal.

    The distinction between negation and disavowal is an important one when looking at climate change denial. On the face of it, to deny reality in an outright way (negation) can seem a more serious evasion than seeing it, but with one eye only (disavowal). However, when one looks beneath the surface and studies the underlying structure of the defences in each case, disavowal is a more serious and intractable form of denial. Negation is a more transient defence and can be a first step towards accepting the painful reality of climate change. And, while negation says no to the truth, it does not distort the truth. Disavowal, by contrast, can be highly organized at an unconscious level and can become entrenched. It distorts the truth in a variety of artful ways. Disavowal can lead us further and further away from accepting the reality of climate change. This is because the more reality is systematically avoided through making it insignificant or through distortion, the more anxiety builds up unconsciously, and the greater is the need to defend with further disavowal. In the long run disavowal can lead to a spiral of minimizing reality with an underlying build-up of anxiety and this makes it dangerous.

Because disavowal involves an entrenched 'quick fix' approach to problems, it actually only stores them up for later with interest accrued. It involves a destructive attack on the rational mind and is anti-meaning. Disavowal can arise in individuals or in groups of people, and it can also characterize a culture. Hoggett describes in illuminating detail the features of a perverse culture of disavowal.

The prevailing view across the chapters is that currently denialism and disavowal are the dominant forms of climate change denial in Western societies.

Destructiveness

Many essays address how we most disavow our destructiveness. One caricature of a psychoanalytic view is of mankind as inherently destructive – a position that does not give sufficient weight to our loving and reparative wishes and behaviour. The psychoanalytic point is different, however: that what is truly destructive is disavowing our destructiveness. When the psychoanalyst Hanna Segal (1987) said (about the issue of nuclear weapons) 'silence is the real crime', she meant silence about our destructiveness. In states of disavowal of reality our destructiveness is minimized and a delusional state of inner tranquillity is maintained as our own dissenting and protesting inner voices are silenced.

Different aspects of our destructiveness are highlighted in the chapters. One aspect, raised by Keene (chapter 7), is the sadism and glee we can take in destroying things quickly that it takes so long to build and repair. Brearley, in his discussion of Keene quoting Homer on Sin and Prayer, conveys this inner situation beautifully: 'Destructiveness, sure-footed and strong, races around the world doing harm, followed haltingly by Prayer, which is lame, wrinkled, and has difficulty seeing, and goes to great lengths trying to put things right' (*The Iliad*, Book 9: lines 502ff, Brearley's own translation).

Keene also discusses disavowal of guilt and pain about our destructiveness to others and to the Earth, especially through our current levels of Western exploitation. He cites the Seattle Convention (1999) in arguing for continuing economic growth, 'chillingly describing as "zones of sacrifice" those whose environments or communities are destroyed in the process'. Keene writes, 'I would add here as long as they can remain out of sight and so out of mind'.

One theme is how disavowing destructiveness can go together with feeling part of a superior in-group and viewing the out-group with an eye that distorts it with dehumanizing prejudice. Rustin describes the way we split into groups of superior us and inferior them. I give examples of this kind of splitting in chapter 9 in relation to how we denigrate animals we then exploit and maltreat. It is easier to exploit others and treat them with violence if they are seen as denigrated and not sharing common ground and common cause with 'us'. Cohen talks of the way we create 'distant others': if we can keep our emotional distance, we can exploit people more easily. In the chapter on nature I suggest how the 'distant other' might be represented within the psyche.

Randall in her essay (chapter 5) discusses the way we turn a blind eye to where our consumer products come from and the environmental and human costs they entail. She also makes links with issues of social justice, adding that most of us prefer to keep obscure our relationships of exploitation with those who work to provide our consumer goods. We may like to think that we are ignorant of where our food, clothes and machines come from – 'gosh, I just never thought about it' – and it is true that the media makes it difficult to get information, but in a general culture of disavowal we also unconsciously choose to remain blind. If knowledge of the damage we cause were felt and owned, it would trigger guilt and shame.

In Brenman Pick's (chapter 6) evocative use of the title of Pinter's play *Not I*, it is NOT I who shoulders any of the blame for wanting to 'have it all and be it all'. Hamilton (chapter 2) notes that it is responsibility for both the problem and the solution that is disavowed. Randall's chapter is a detailed exploration of some of the difficulties in confronting the shock of realizing that it 'IS I' who shoulders some of the blame.

One of the consequences of disavowal is an increasing difficulty in thinking with any sense of proportion about issues of guilt and responsibility for our share of the damage. With disavowal we can simultaneously feel it is none of my fault while unconsciously increasingly feeling it is all my fault, thereby losing an ordinary sense of mea culpa – that it is some of my fault.

Disavowal of our destructiveness is discussed in several chapters as a failure to work through ambivalence in our conflicting self-representations. In the West we feel narcissistically entitled to consume what we want from wherever we want when we want, and we also simultaneously want to protect the environment. Facing this conflict and working it through would involve facing our destructiveness towards the environment and towards our own minds.

Anxiety

The ways in which we resort to irrationality as a means to try to cope with too much unacknowledged anxiety is one of the most important obstacles to our effective engagement with climate change. In my essay on anxiety (chapter 3) I go into two main and conflicting sets of anxieties about the meaning of climate change for us. I look at disavowal as an organized means of trying to minimize *both* sets of anxieties. I also argue that we need support to bear the anxieties that come with facing climate change.

Apathy

Apathy is the subject of Lertzman's essay (chapter 6), and the topic is also raised from different perspectives in several other chapters. Lertzman argues that rather than feel too little about environmental degradation – the common explanation for apathy – we feel too much. Being unable adequately to mourn natural landscapes we have loved and lost to pollution and environmental degradation, we remain trapped in what she calls an environmental melancholia. Here she uses Freud's ideas on melancholia, taken particularly from his paper 'On Transience' (Freud 1916). She highlights Freud's idea that we lose our pride when we allow our world to be robbed of its beauties. Freud was describing the general devastation brought about by the Great War, which

> had robbed the world of its beauties. It destroyed not only the beauty of the landscapes through which it passed, and the artworks that it encountered on its way, it also shattered our pride at the accomplishments of our civilization, our respect for so many thinkers and artists, our hopes of finally overcoming the differences among peoples and races. . . . In this way it robbed us of so much that we had loved, and showed us the fragility of much that we had considered stable.
>
> (Freud 1916: 307).

Here war is evoked by Freud as a destructive force trashing all that has meaning in its wake and being, in Hanna Segal's phrase, 'anti-mind'. Several chapters support Lertzman's analysis that melancholia is a good diagnostic description of our difficulties in mourning our lost trashed environments and a stable climate.[3]

Mauss-Hanke (chapter 3) discusses apathy as a position of claustrophobia between a fear of change and the scorching pain of getting in touch with our difficult feelings of guilt and loss, feelings that involve us in revisiting earlier painful childhood situations of trauma and loss. Keene writes: 'I believe it is the problem of how to influence policy, more than apathy or individual greed, that makes individual impulses to care for the planet seem hopeless or futile.' Keene situates as apathy our feelings of hopelessness and futility about influencing current destructive policies. This is a somewhat different view to Lertzman, who seems to see the lack of a political response as part of the apathy. For Keene, the apathy refers more to an experience of feeling a lack of political power and voice to make a difference, whereas for Lertzman the issue is of apathy experienced more as depression. Both perspectives are important. When we feel a lack of strength and a lack of pride due to underlying depression, we are also not so able to mount political resistance. The psychoanalyst Eric Brenman (1985) noted that it takes inner strength to stand up to omnipotent ways of thinking when they are powerfully in charge.

Cultural influences

Several chapters make the point that in the West we live in cultures that encourage narcissism and encourage us as consumers; attention is drawn to ways a culture may be internalized within the psyche. Randall (chapter 5) suggests that 'the needs of late capitalism are well served by personalities who are alienated from the rest of the natural world and who are dependent on material satisfactions to sustain their sense of self-worth and identity'. In my chapter on nature (chapter 9) I look at some ways that advertising and current TV programmes can promote this sense of alienation. Hinshelwood (chapter 7) argues that 'cultural icons grab us deep in our souls, at the place where we were once children', and Keene (chapter 7) points out that 'the cultural expectations that surround us are the medium in which our individual superegos swim and develop'.

Doing the work of engaging with our feelings

With all these difficulties, how do we come to face reality and engage with climate change? This question is addressed from different perspectives in the book. From a psychoanalytic standpoint, facing any painful reality is always hard emotional work that needs to be ongoing. The work involves facing our self-idealizations, mourning our illusions and bearing difficult feelings. It involves knowing as much as possible about the facts of human nature and mourning our illusions about human nature too.

The work also includes understanding the sorts of defences we use to deny reality. Examples of the defences we use are discussed in some detail in the chapters. They include splitting, projection and the way we may identify defensively with idealized figures to 'big ourselves up' when we feel small, dependent and anxious. Keene, Hinshelwood, Randall and I all look at different aspects of idealization and its effects. Another kind of idealization is thinking we will be saved by idealized leaders (Steiner makes this point in his discussion in chapter 4).

An important part of the impetus for engaging with a painful reality is the wish to repair damage. This is what is meant by the psychoanalytic concept of reparation, where reparation is the emotional work required to enable necessary change. Randall (chapter 5) looks at situations where people start to do the emotional work necessary for making life-style 'carbon repair' changes. It is noticeable that in all cases the problem is personally owned in a feeling way. Repairing involves facing destructiveness but also involves seeing the self in an entirely new and shockingly different light. Randall uses Dickens' story *Great Expectations* to illustrate the shock and pain of recognizing true environmental dependence and indebtedness. She charts how Pip was shocked to realize that whereas he thought he was dependent on Miss Havisham, it was actually to Madgwick that he owed his good fortune. Randall, in describing her work with people seeking to reduce their carbon emissions, tells of people undergoing a moment of shock, where, as she puts it, the truth 'would not go back in the box'. Probably many small moments of shock go into producing a moment of shock that breaks through defensive processes of negation and disavowal.

Several essays highlight that change can be fearsome and potentially destabilizing. This is particularly the case when reality has been disavowed and 'good' authority figures – on the side of facing the truth – are held in contempt. With no good authority recognized, there is no containing support for change.

Reparation is ongoing and involves the work of managing emotions, a view Randall puts forward (chapter 5) and I argue in my anxiety essay (chapter 3). Randall and I both underline the importance of developing a sense of proportion about personal guilt for climate change as central to reparation. Randall writes:

Those who managed best were those who had developed a clear sense of proportionality and placed some boundaries round their responsibility. For one person this meant protecting herself from the amount of news she read. For another it was creating a plan for the personal changes she would make. For several, it helped to see the political dimension and the power relationships clearly. It helped to understand neo-colonialism and globalization, to contribute to a political programme, or simply to point the finger at BP or bankers and say, 'It's not all my fault.'

Once some responsibility has been admitted, the eternal manic–depressive swing of 'pass the parcel of blame' ends (it's all your fault; no it's all my fault) and awareness of one's own part in a perverse collusion can begin.

Our dependency on the Earth

Many chapters go into our dependency on the Earth for our survival and the ways we deny this dependency. I suggest (chapter 3) that this dependency is the source of our deepest underlying anxieties about climate change. Lehtonen and Välimäki, in their discussion, argue that denial of our dependency on the Earth has come to constitute a modern neurosis. Anxieties about climate change are seen to revive feelings of dependency we had on our parents as small children and can revive traumatic experiences of being abandoned in states of utter need (see, in particular, Margaret Rustin's discussion, chapter 5). Mauss-Hanke argues that when we think of 'saving the planet', we may be projecting our dependency on the Earth onto the Earth, which is then seen as needing us. Keene describes us as treating the Earth as a 'breast-and-toilet mother', there solely to provide for our needs and to absorb our waste. Brenman Pick (chapter 6) talks of how environmental damage revives our earliest anxieties of having damaged the mother with our greed.

The issue of hope

Part of working through our feelings involves allowing ourselves to feel depressed. Steiner (chapter 4) outlines Klein's description of our experience of depression when we face our destructiveness: 'It arises because . . . attempts to protect (the good things we value) have been weak in comparison with the power of destructive forces mounted against them.'

Steiner observes that when he read Hoggett's essay, he felt depressed – a reaction that he regards as appropriate when faced with the reality that we are living in a perverse culture of denialism and disavowal of climate change. He argues for knowing as much as possible about perverse mechanisms and the perverse culture. He writes, 'The best we can do is to be alert to the likelihood that we are under the sway of a perverse argument and to be aware of our own propensity to join in the collusions.'

Facing reality involves finding the strength to face one's and others' destructiveness so as to be able to make what repairs we can. This is a situation of sadness and depression that, if worked through, can lead to greater hopefulness and renewed energy to work for change.

Some policy implications

Questions researchers ask are profoundly influenced by their underlying ways of seeing, by their theoretical models and by what counts for them as legitimate data. Much current writing on our engagement with climate change reveals a lack of interest in formulating underlying theories of any sophistication about how the mind actually works, how experience is represented within the mind and about the deeper structures that organize our experience, both at an individual and at a group level. Underling models in much current research on our engagement with climate change typically cast humankind as rational and see people's conscious attitudes as an accurate reflection of what they think (for instance, in opinion polls). The models tend to assume a unitary non-divided self. Nearly all research confines itself to looking only at behaviour that can be measured. The zeitgeist is currently that if it cannot be directly seen and measured, it is not legitimate, and we do not want to know about it.

But, measurement is far from all. Within this framework, issues of subjectivity and meaning – not measurable or losing meaning when measured – can be 'safely' ignored. Deeper structures are also not measurable.

All this has profound implications for policy about how to engage people in thinking about climate change. Engaging people means finding ways to relate to them about what climate change and degradation of the natural world actually means to them in a way that supports their anxieties and feared losses. It also means taking serious account of the organized ways we defend against reality when it feels too much to bear. All the psychoanalytic essays in this book make this point.

Currently popular are 'nudge-and-incentivize' polices to encourage us towards more pro-environmental behaviour. Based on Thaler's theory of behavioural economics and cognitive theory (see Thaler and Sunstein 2009), these policies, while recognizing us as conflicted and often irrational, are designed to spare us any difficulty in engaging emotionally with climate change. Elsewhere (Weintrobe 2011) I suggested that what they actually promote is the idea that we should rely on (and presumably vote for) ideal leaders who are magically able to bring about changes in our behaviour in ways that will spare us any difficulties. Policies such as 'nudge and incentivize' do not help us to begin to face our anxieties and our depressing realities, both necessary for engagement. Indeed, there are no 'quick fixes' for engagement that can lead to a radical, felt and lived reorientation in our relationships to ourselves, to others and to nature.

Genuine support and leadership that is mindful can make the ongoing difficult work of engagement easier. Real un-idealized leadership *supports* people in facing their feelings to make necessary difficult changes. It can do this by relating to their anxieties and their need to mourn what they have lost and by providing leadership and public space for facing our conflicts and working through our private feelings. Real leadership bases policy on a deeper understanding that while people are conflicted and do want to avoid difficulty, they do need to face reality and experience their feelings of anger and grief at what they have lost before they are able to move on.

NGOs involved in the project Common Cause[4] use an approach that is based on a conflict model of people – that of 'values and frames' – which supports people in making environmentally friendly changes in real and more lasting ways. The approach recognizes that 'transcendent values' inevitably vie with 'instrumental values'. It identifies underlying deeper frames that leads 'Common Cause' NGOs, for instance, to argue that banning advertising to children can be a climate change engagement measure; it also leads to their arguing that giving people financial inducements to save energy might in some circumstances actually be counterproductive to effective engagement with climate change, because it promotes instrumental values in an underlying way. Crompton outlines this position in his discussion of my chapter on nature (chapter 9).

This book, based on psychoanalytic and interdisciplinary exchange, breaks new ground, providing new and much needed perspectives on our engagement with climate change. The chapters that follow are a feast.

Notes

1 Carbon equivalents, a combined measure of greenhouse gases.
2 Phantasy when spelled with ph indicates elements are present that are unconscious.
3 Lertzman brings in how we can set up static nostalgic pictures of loved places and not make repairs to our real environments. However, it would seem that the situation is complex. Naess (2008), for instance, discusses how we may set up in our imagination what he calls 'places' that are our loved physical landscapes. It may be that we are in some cases able to preserve a memory of places we love, untouched and unpolluted, as a way to keep our love of environment alive in the face of the degradation.
4 Including World Wildlife Fund, Action for Children and Oxfam.

References

Anderson, K., and Bows, A. (2008) Reframing the climate change challenge in light of post-2000 emission trends. *Philosophical Transactions of the Royal Society*, The Royal Society.
Brenman, E. (1985) Cruelty and narrow-mindedness. *International Journal of Psychoanalysis*, 66: 273–281.
Cohen, S. (2000) *States of Denial: Knowing about Atrocities and Suffering*. Cambridge: Polity Press.
Common Cause Handbook (2011) Public Interest Research Centre. Available at: www.pirc.info
Crompton, T. (2010) *Common Cause: The Case for Working with Our Cultural Values*. Godalming, UK: WWF-UK.

Darnton, A., and Kirk, M. (2011) *Finding Frames: New Ways to Engage the UK Public in Global Poverty*. Available at: www.findingframes.org

De Waal, F. (2009) *The Age of Empathy: Nature's Lessons for a Kinder Society*. New York: Harmony Books.

Freud, S. (1916) On Transience. In J. Strachey (Ed.), *The Standard Edition of the Complete Psychological Works of Sigmund Freud, Vol. XIV*. London: Hogarth Press.

Freud, S. (1923) *The Ego and the Id*. In J. Strachey (Ed.), *The Standard Edition of the Complete Psychological Works of Sigmund Freud, Vol. XIX*. London: Hogarth Press.

Friedman, T. (2008) *Hot, Flat and Crowded: Why We Need a Green Revolution*. New York: Farrar, Straus and Giroux.

Hamilton, C., and Kasser, K. (2009) Psychological adaptation to the threats and stresses of a four degree world. *Four Degrees and Beyond Conference*, University of Oxford, 28–30 Sept.

Hansen, J. (2009) *Storms of My Grandchildren*. London: Bloomsbury.

Kasser, T. et al. (2007) Some costs of American corporate capitalism: A psychological explanation of value and goal conflicts. *Psychological Inquiry*, 18:1–22.

Kasser, T. (2008) Values and ecological sustainability: recent research and policy possibilities. In J.G. Speth and S. Kellert (Eds), *The coming transformation values to sustain human and natural communities*. New Haven, C.T: Yale School of Forestry and Environmental Studies.

McKibben, B. (2011a) *Eaarth: Making a Life on a Tough New Planet*. New York: St Martin's Griffin.

McKibben, B. (2011b) Resisting climate reality. *New York Review of Books*, *LVIII*, Part 6: 60–64.

Monbiot, G. (2006) *Heat*. London: Penguin Books.

Naess, A. (2008) *The Ecology of Wisdom*. Berkeley, CA: Counterpoint.

Orestes, N., and Conway, M. (2010) *Merchants of Doubt: How a Handful of Scientists Obscured the Truth on Issues from Tobacco Smoke to Global Warming*. New York: Bloomsbury Press.

Royal Society (2010) *Climate Change: A Summary of the Science*. Available at: http://royalsociety.org/climate-change-summary-of-science

Segal, H. (1987) Silence is the real crime. *International Review of Psychoanalysis*, 14: 3–12.

Strenger, C. (1991) *Between Hermeneutics and Science. An Essay on the Epistemology of Psychoanalysis*. Madison, CT: International Universities Press.

Thaler, R., and Sunstein, C. (2009) *Nudge: Improving Decisions about Health, Wealth and Happiness*. New York: Penguin Books.

Weintrobe, S. (2011) *Anxieties about Our Shared Environment: Engaging with Climate Change as Psychic Work*. Paper presented to the Annual Conference of the European Psychoanalytic Federation 2011.

Chapter 2

What history can teach us about climate change denial

Clive Hamilton

Repudiating science

Let me begin with a pregnant fact about US voters. In 1997 there was virtually no difference between Democratic and Republican voters in their views on global warming, with around half saying warming had begun. In 2008, reflecting the accumulation and dissemination of scientific evidence, the proportion of Democratic voters taking this view had risen from 52% to 76% (Maibach, Roser-Renouf and Leiserowitz 2009). But the proportion of Republican voters fell from 48% to 42% – a 4% gap had become a 34% gap. What had happened?

The opening of the gulf was due to the fact that Republican Party activists, in collaboration with fossil fuel interests and conservative think tanks, had success-fully associated acceptance of global warming science with 'liberal' views.[1] In other words, they had activated the human predisposition to adopt views that cement one's connections with cultural groups that strengthen one's definition of self (e.g. Kahan 2010). In the 1990s views on global warming were influenced mostly by attentiveness to the science; now one can make a good guess at an American's opinion on global warming by identifying their views on abortion, same-sex marriage and gun control.

That global warming has been made a battleground in the wider culture war is most apparent from the political and social views of those who reject climate science outright. In 2008 they accounted for 7% of US voters, rising to 18% if those with serious doubts are added (Maibach et al. 2009). Among those who dismiss climate science, 76% describe themselves as 'conservative' and only 3% as 'liberal' (with the rest 'moderate'). They overwhelmingly oppose redistributive policies, programs to reduce poverty and regulation of business. They prefer to watch Fox News and listen to Rush Limbaugh. Like those whose opinions they value, these climate deniers are disproportionately white, male and conservative – those who feel their cultural identity most threatened by the implications of climate change (Kahan, Braman, Gastil, Slovic and Mertz 2007).

Those on the left are as predisposed to sift evidence through ideological filters; but in the case of global warming it happens that the evidence overwhelmingly endorses the liberal beliefs that unrestrained capitalism is jeopardising future well-being, that comprehensive government intervention is needed and that the environment movement was right all along. For neo-conservatives accepting these is intolerable, and it is easier emotionally and more convenient politically to reject climate science.

The United States is a deeply polarized society. In Europe, the absence of a long-running and rancorous culture war explains the relative weakness of climate denial. Where it does prevail, it is associated with parties of the far right. It seems perfectly natural, for example, that the British National Party should adopt a denialist stance. In Italy and in some former Eastern bloc countries, where anti-communism and remnant-fascism still influence right-wing politics, denial is more potent.

The aggressive adoption of climate denial by neo-conservatism was symbolized by the parting gesture of George W. Bush at his last G8 summit in 2008. Leaving the room, he turned to the assembled leaders to say: 'Goodbye from the world's biggest polluter.'[2] It was a defiant 'joke' reflecting the way US neo-conservatives define themselves by their repudiation of the 'other' – in this case, the internationalist, environmentally-concerned, self-doubting enemies of 'the American way of life'. Conceding ground on global warming would have meant bridging two implacably opposed worldviews. Bush's words, and the fist pump that accompanied them, were read by those present as a two-fingered salute to everything the Texan opposed.

The fragility of the Enlightenment

In these circumstances, facts quail before beliefs, and there is something poignant about scientists who continue to adhere to the idea that people repudiate climate science because they suffer from inadequacy of information. In fact, denial is due to a surplus of culture rather than a deficit of information.[3] Once people have made up their minds, providing contrary evidence can actually make them more resolute (Kahan 2010) – a phenomenon we see at work with the upsurge of climate denial each time the IPCC publishes a report. For those who interpreted 'climate-gate' as confirmation of their belief that scientists are engaged in a conspiracy, the three or four reports that subsequently vindicated the scientists and the science proved only that the circle of conspirators was wider than previously suspected.

In a curious twist, climate deniers now deploy the arguments first developed by the radical social movements of the 1960s and 1970s to erode the authority of science. This was perhaps first noticed by Latour (2004) when he lamented the way climate deniers set out to explain away the evidence using a narrative about the social construction of facts. However, while constructivists developed an epistemological critique of science, climate deniers, adopting the heroic mantle of 'sceptic', claim to be protecting official epistemology from internal corrosion. The strategy required an attack on the system of peer review (Furedi 2010) and sustained attempts to 'deconstruct' the motives of climate scientists. They are always on the lookout for biases and prejudices that could lie behind the claims of climate scientists, explaining away the vast accumulation of evidence by impugning the motives of those who collect it. That was the genius of the 'climategate' scandal: the emails were hard evidence that the 'hard evidence' had been fabricated. The leaking of routine private exchanges between professional colleagues tarnished the public image of scientists as white-coated experts too preoccupied with their test tubes and retorts to be political.

Since the founding of modern science, matters of fact have been established through the common assent of those qualified to judge under rules laid down in the seventeenth century by the Royal Society. The break from the past lay in the fact that the 'potency of knowledge came from nature, not from privileged persons' (Shapin and Schaffer 1985). 'Climategate' allowed deniers to claim that climate science indeed emerged from privileged persons rather than disinterested nature. In their study of Robert Boyle's struggle to found the new scientific method of experimentation observable by suitably qualified others, Shapin and Schaffer noted that 'democratic ideals and the exigencies of professional expertise form an unstable compound' (1985: 336). Deniers have adroitly used the instruments of democratic practice to erode the authority of professional expertise, including skilful exploitation of a free media, appeal to freedom of information laws, the mobilization of a group of vociferous citizens, and the promotion of their own to public office.[4] At least in the United States and Australia, democracy has defeated science.

Innocently pursuing their research, climate scientists were unwittingly destabilizing the political and social order. They could not know that the new facts they were uncovering would threaten the existence of powerful industrialists, compel governments to choose between adhering to science and remaining in power, corrode comfortable expectations about the future, expose hidden resentment of technical and cultural elites and, internationally, shatter the post-colonial growth consensus between North and South. Their research has brought us to one of those rare historical fracture points when knowledge diverges from power, portending a long period of struggle before the two are aligned once again.

Popular forms of denial

The fragility of Enlightenment thinking appears not only in outright denial of climate science, but also in the reluctance of the public to take in the warnings of the scientists. After all, the conservative counter-movement's success in undermining climate science and slowing policy responses would not have been possible unless it had been able to exploit a weakness in the popular psyche – the desire to discount or disbelieve the warnings of scientists.

When climate scientists conclude that, even with optimistic assumption about how quickly emissions can be cut, the world is expected to warm by 4°C this century, it is too much to bear (Hamilton 2010a: ch. 1). Who can believe that within the lifetime of a child born today, the planet will be hotter than at any time for 15 million years? When scientists say we will cross tipping points leading to chaotic weather for centuries, we retreat to incredulity.

In 1930 Martin Heidegger commented on a rash of popular books that drew on broad philosophical ideas to characterize the contemporary situation and make prophecies about the future. The leading work was Oswald Spengler's *The Decline of the West*, first published in 1918. Today, books such as *The Clash of Civilizations* (Samuel Huntington, 1996), *The End of History and the Last Man* (Francis Fukuyama, 1992) and *The Collapse of Globalism* (John Ralston Saul, 2005) show that the appetite for this kind of world-historical prognosis is undiminished. Heidegger explained their popularity in this way: 'Is there anyone who does not wish to know what is coming, so that they can prepare themselves for it, so as to be less burdened, less preoccupied and affected by the present' (Heidegger 1995: 75)? Well, the answer is 'yes': there are many who would prefer not to know what is coming if the forecast is based on distressing facts rather than entertaining speculation. And that is why, to a greater or lesser extent, we are all climate deniers.

If the Earth seems to be locked on a path leading to a very different climate, a new and much less stable era lasting many centuries before natural processes eventually establish some sort of equilibrium, how do we respond psychologically to the scientific warnings? A paper by Kasser and myself (Hamilton and Kasser 2009) draws on psychological research into the various 'coping strategies' we might use to defend against or manage the unpleasant emotions associated with the dangers of a warming globe: fear, anxiety, anger, depression, guilt and helplessness.

Many members of the public engage in what might be called 'casual denial'. Less vociferous than outright denial of the science, casual denial relies on inner narratives such as 'Environmentalists always exaggerate', 'Didn't those leaked emails show it's all rubbish?' and 'I'll worry about it when the scientists make up their minds.' Anxiety can be reduced simply by restricting exposure to upsetting information or viewing it through a cloud of doubt. The desire to disbelieve is activated by conservative news outlets each time they give undue prominence to stories that create the impression that climate scientists cannot agree or that the science is politically tainted.

Most people do not deny climate science but use various techniques to blunt the emotional impact of the scientific warnings. We might 'de-problematize' the threat by making its scale seem smaller or distance ourselves from it by emphasizing the time lapse before the consequences of warming are felt. Narratives such as 'Humans have solved these sorts of problems before' and 'It won't affect me much' are effective. Alternatively, we might divert attention from anxious thoughts and unpleasant emotions by engaging in minor behaviour changes (like changing light-bulbs) that mollify feelings of helplessness or guilt.

Blame-shifting is a form of moral disengagement whereby people disavow their responsibility for the problem or the solution. Belittling out-groups can help solidify one's sense of self and ward off threats to it – a tactic in play whenever we hear someone say: 'China builds a new coal-fired power plant every week.' Or we might cultivate indifference to global warming and its implications. Apathy is typically understood as meaning the absence of feeling, but it can often reflect a suppression of feeling that serves a useful psychological function (Lertzman 2008). Who at times has not thought: 'If I don't care, I won't feel bad'?

One of the most widespread methods of avoiding the full force of the warnings is to practice wishful thinking. Cultivating 'benign fictions' can be comforting in an often unfriendly world, yet such fictions become dangerous delusions when they are clung to despite overwhelming evidence (Taylor 1989). The climate debate is rife with wishful thinking, deploying narratives such as, 'Technology – carbon capture and storage, nuclear power, biochar, geoengineering, etc. – will save us', 'We've solved these problems before and we will do it again' or simply, 'Something will come along'.

History can illuminate the present in a way contemporary analysis cannot. So let me dwell on three historical episodes that can give us a more nuanced under-standing of the nature of climate denial. The first, the campaign against Einstein's general theory of relativity, provides an uncannily complete template for the conservative attack eight decades later on climate science.

Anti-relativism in Weimar Germany

It is hard to imagine a scientific breakthrough more abstract and less politically contentious than Einstein's general theory of relativity. Yet in Weimar Germany in the 1920s it attracted fierce controversy with conservatives and ultra-Nationalists reading it as a vindication of their opponents: liberals, socialists, pacifists and Jews. They could not separate Einstein's political views – he was an internationalist and pacifist – from his scientific breakthroughs, and his extraordinary fame made him a prime target in a period of political turmoil.

The year 1920 was a turning point. A year earlier a British scientific expedition had used observations of an eclipse to provide empirical confirmation of Einstein's prediction that light could be bent by the gravitational pull of the sun. Little known to the general public beforehand, Einstein was instantly elevated to the status of the genius who eclipsed Galileo and Newton (van Dongen 2007: 213). But conservative newspapers provided an outlet for anti-relativity activists and scientists with an axe to grind, stoking nationalist and anti-Semitic sentiment among those predisposed to it (219). In a similar way today, conservative news outlets promote the views of climate deniers and publish stories designed to discredit climate scientists, all with a view to defending an established order seen to be threatened by evidence of a warming globe. As in the Weimar Republic, the effect has been to fuel suspicion of liberals and 'elites' by inviting the public to view science through political lenses.

At the height of the storm in 1920, a bemused Einstein wrote to a friend, 'This world is a strange madhouse. Currently, every coachman and every waiter is debating whether relativity theory is correct. Belief in this matter depends on political party affiliation' (Buchwald et al. 2006: 234).

The controversy was not confined to Germany. In France, for example, a citi-zen's attitude to the new theory could be guessed from the stance he or she took on the Dreyfus affair, the scandal surrounding the Jewish army officer falsely convicted of spying in 1894, whose fate divided French society. Anti-Dreyfusards were inclined to reject relativity on political grounds (Buchwald et al.: 234). In Britain, suspicions were less politically grounded, but relativity's subversion of Newton was a sensitive issue, leading Einstein to write an encomium for the great English scientist prior to a lecture tour.

Like Einstein's opponents, who denied relativity because of its association with progressive politics, conservative climate deniers follow the maxim that 'my enemy's friend is my enemy'. Scientists whose research strengthens the claims of environmentalism must be opposed. Conservative climate deniers often link their repudiation of climate science to fears that cultural values are under attack from progressives – witness the natural incorporation of climate denial into the story of elite conspiracy that drives the Tea Party, the movement of those who demand their fair share of injustice.

In Weimar Germany the threat to the cultural order apparently posed by relativity saw Einstein accused of 'scientific dadaism', after the anarchistic cultural and artistic movement then at its peak. The epithet is revealing because it reflected the anxiety among conservatives that Einstein's theory would overthrow the established Newtonian understanding of the world, a destabilization of the physical world that mirrored the subversion of the social order then under way. Relativity's apparent repudiation of absolutes was interpreted by some as yet another sign of moral and intellectual decay. There could not have been a worse time for Einstein's theory to have received such emphatic empirical validation than in the chaotic post-War years.

Although not to be overstated, the turmoil of Weimar Germany has some similarities with the political ferment that characterizes the United States today: deep-rooted resentments, the sense of a nation in decline, the fragility of liberal forces and the rise of an angry populist right. Environmental policy and science have become battlegrounds in a deep ideological divide that emerged as a backlash against the gains of the social movements of the 1960s and 1970s (Jacques, Dunlap and Freeman 2008; McCright and Dunlap 2003). As we saw, marrying science to politics was a calculated strategy of conservative activists in the 1990s (Mooney 2005), opening up a gulf between Republican and Democratic voters over their attitudes to climate science. Both anti-relativists and climate deniers justifiably feared that science would enhance the standing of their enemies and they responded by tarnishing science with politics.

Einstein's work was often accused of being un-German, and Nazi ideology would soon be drawing a distinction between Jewish and Aryan mathematics.[5] 'Jewish mathematics' served the same political function that the charge of 'left-wing science' does in the climate debate today. In the United States, the notion of left-wing science dates to the rise in the 1960s of what has been called 'environmental–social impact' science[6] which, at least implicitly, questioned the unalloyed benefits of 'technological–production' science. Thus in 1975 Jacob Needleman was writing: 'Once the hope of mankind, modern science has now become the object of such mistrust and disappointment that it will probably never again speak with its old authority'.[7] The support of denialist think tanks for geoengineering solutions to global warming can be understood as a reassertion of technological–production science over impact science.[8]

The association between 'left-wing' opinion and climate science has now been made so strongly that politically conservative scientists who accept the evidence for climate change typically withdraw from public debate, as do those conservative politicians who remain faithful to science.[9]

The motives of Einstein's opponents were various, but differences were overlooked in pursuit of the common foe, just as today among the enemies of climate science are grouped activists in free-market think tanks, politicians pandering to popular fears, conservative media outlets like *The Sunday Times* and *Fox News*, disgruntled scientists (Lahsen 2008), right-wing philanthropists including the Scaifes and Kochs and sundry opportunists such as Christopher Monckton and Bjorn Lomborg.

While Einstein's theory posed no economic threat and industrialists were absent from the constellation of anti-relativity forces, climate denial was initially organized and promoted by fossil fuel interests. In the last few years, climate denial has developed into a political and cultural movement. Beneath the Astroturf, grass grew.

Campaigning methods

While the social conditions in which anti-relativism and climate denial flourished have similarities that are suggestive, the organizational and tactical parallels between the two anti-science camps are more striking. The first requirement of a campaign is to counter the dominant science with an alternative science, one wrapped in as much credibility as possible. Between the first publication of Einstein's theory in 1905 and its explosion onto the public stage in 1920, the theory had naturally attracted intense debate and criticism within the scientific community. As we would expect with any development that overthrows established thinking, some eminent physicists rejected relativity and put forward powerful arguments that Einstein had to wrestle with. Some of his critics were eager to make their arguments in public, and the scientific debate soon spilled out of the seminar rooms and journals. The two most prominent critics were Ernst Gehrcke and Philipp Lenard.

Gehrcke was an experimental physicist who believed that the aether theory could be rescued. In 1913 he published a refutation, pointing out the absurdities and contradictions of relativity theory (Rowe 2006: 242). He challenged Einstein at various colloquia, leading Einstein to comment pungently to a friend that if Gehrcke 'had as much intelligence as self-esteem, it would be pleasant to discuss things with him' (quoted by Rowe 2006: 244). Gehrcke was the only scientist to speak at the raucous anti-Einstein meeting at the Berlin Philharmonic in 1920, described below.

Philipp Lenard was a Nobel Laureate whose experimental approach to physics was being overshadowed by the abstract theories of the mathematical physicists. Lenard's hostility to the Weimar Republic combined with professional resentments to see him link up with proto-fascists to oppose Einstein, a path that led him a decade later to become the Chief of Aryan Physics under the Nazis with the task of rooting out 'Jewish physics' from the academy.[10]

It would be incorrect and offensive to suggest that climate-denying scientists such as Frederick Seitz, Fred Singer, Patrick Michaels and Ian Plimer share Lenard's anti-Semitism or Nazi sympathies, but they do share Gehrcke's dogged resistance to the consensus view, his willingness to trade on his reputation to promote his views in public and his close association with right-wing organizations. They also mimic many of Gehrcke's claims, although not his insistence that Einstein was guilty of plagiarism (as well as fraud).

Anti-relativists became convinced that their work was being suppressed, excluded from the professional journals by the 'Einstein crowd', in the same way as some 'sceptics' believe that the 'climategate' emails vindicated their claim that their work has been buried by a self-protective in-group.[11] While opposition to relativity came from both scientists and political activists, it soon became difficult to separate the two, just as today those scientists who reject climate science are quickly drawn into the web of right-wing think tanks at the heart of climate denial. The most prominent ones now appear at the conferences of the Heartland Institute, currently the most active group.[12]

Ernst Gehrcke developed an elaborate account of 'mass hypnosis' to explain the public's gullibility in accepting a theory that was so manifestly untrue, an argument he laid out in a book published in 1924.[13] Climate deniers have also been required to explain why most members of the public accept climate science and the need for abatement policies, and to this end denier Fred Singer has channelled Gehrcke's theory with his argument that climate science is a form of 'collective environmental hysteria'.[14]

The foremost political agitator against Einstein was a proto-Nazi and anti-Semite named Paul Weyland. An engineer by training, Weyland was a minor demagogue who declared that he and his political associates would 'strive to free German science from Jews' (Goenner 1993: 120f). Towards this aim, Weyland founded the Working Society of German Scientists for the Preservation of Pure Science. Its first act, in August 1920, was to recruit Gehrcke to address a rowdy public meeting at the Berlin Philharmonic. Einstein joined the audience to hear his theory denounced and his character slandered. In the lobby, swastika lapel pins and anti-Semitic literature were on sale (van Dongen 2007: 217).

The Working Society of German Scientists for the Preservation of Pure Science was a front group set up by Weyland to create the impression that there was a credible body of scientists who resisted the 'Einstein craze'. For a time Einstein himself was deceived by the strategy, before realizing the true nature of the Society. Today, several pseudo-scientific organizations are active against climate science. An example is The Association of American Physicians and Surgeons (Oreskes and

Conway 2010: 245), a body also responsible for organizing rallies of the 'Doctors' Tea Party'. The Advancement of Sound Science Coalition was an early front group initially established by tobacco interests, which, in the 1990s, shifted into climate denial. More recently, Fred Singer has formed the Nongovernmental International Panel on Climate Change. 'As impressive as this title sounds', noted *Der Spiegel*, 'the NIPCC is nothing but a collection of like-minded scientists Singer has gathered around himself'.[15] The widespread use of the term 'sound science' by climate deniers, to contrast with the 'junk science' to be found in professional journals and IPCC reports, is similar to the anti-relativists' invocation of 'pure science', although the contrast with 'Jewish science' had racial overtones that are absent today.

In a forerunner of the petitions of recent years listing the names of scientists who reject the science of climate change, in 1931 a group that included two winners of the Nobel Prize for Physics published a pamphlet titled *One Hundred Authors Against Einstein*. It would be fair to assume that only a handful of the 100 understood relativity theory. When called to respond, Einstein asked why 100 scientists were needed to refute relativity: 'If I were wrong, one would have been enough'. Coincidentally, *One Hundred Authors Against Einstein* was published in Leipzig, birthplace of the anti-climate science tract known as the Leipzig Declaration. Organized by long-time 'sceptic' Fred Singer and initially signed by 80 scientists, many signatories turned out to be wholly unqualified or unaware that their names had been used. Of course, one research paper in a scientific journal would have carried more weight than the 80 signatures.

In the United States today several anti-climate science activists mirror the role performed by Paul Weyland,[16] adopting a demagogic, ruthless and aggressive campaigning style. They have a cynical view of scientific facts, deliberately target climate scientists to silence them and cultivate links with a network of conservative groups.

Throughout the 1920s and early 1930s, Einstein had genuine fears for his safety. After his face became widely recognized, he was called a 'dirty Jew' on the street by ultra-Nationalist activists and often received threats in the mail. In 1922 he cancelled a scheduled lecture to a scientific meeting after news emerged of protests planned by his enemies (van Dongen 2010: 79). The political climate in the United States today is a long way from that of Weimar Germany, but climate scientists have been the target of a campaign of abuse and threats both by cyberbullies and politicians (Fischer 2010). Republican Senator James Inhofe has called for climate scientists to face criminal charges; conservative media outlets, led by the Murdoch-owned Fox News and *The Times* in London, have set out to discredit climate scientists; and prominent right-wing commentators have provoked their readers to acts of intimidation.

When activist Marc Morano said recently that climate scientists 'deserve to be publicly flogged',[17] there was an eerie resonance with the headline above a photograph of Albert Einstein in a Nazi magazine that read 'Not Yet Hanged' (Jerome and Taylor 2005). That was in 1933, the year Einstein left Germany for good, soon to take up an appointment at Princeton University. There he was safe from the Nazis, although his presence in America immediately aroused the suspicion of FBI Director J. Edgar Hoover. His general theory of relativity was never dented by the political attacks – nor could it be. Only progress in science, in the form of quantum theory, caused physicists to reassess. The same will be true of climate science, although the delay in responding to the threat due to systematic denigration of the science will first have dire consequences.

Churchill's struggle against wishful thinking

My second example also comes from the inter-war period, but this time from across the English Channel. In the same year that Einstein fled Europe, Winston Churchill began warning of the belligerent intentions of Hitler's Germany and the threat it posed to world peace. In many speeches through the 1930s he devoted himself to alerting Britons to the dangerous currents running through Europe, returning over and over again to the martial nature of the Nazi regime, the rapid re-arming of Germany and Britain's lack of preparedness for hostilities. In 1936, with Germany re-arming on a massive scale, Hitler's troops marched into the Rhineland. Churchill told the House of Commons that the previous five years had been disastrous for the security of Britain. 'We have seen the most depressing and alarming changes in the outlook of mankind which have ever taken place in so short a period' (Churchill 1938: 297).

It is tempting to exploit hindsight – as if we, too, would have shared Churchill's foresight – so it should be acknowledged that in the early 1930s the arguments against rapid rearmament were persuasive, even compelling. Yet as the 1930s progressed and the signs of danger multiplied, pacifist sentiment among the British public, still traumatized by the memory of the Great War, provided a white noise of wishful thinking that muffled the warnings. Behind the unwillingness to re-arm and resist aggression lay the gulf between the future Britons hoped for – one of peace – and the future the evidence indicated was approaching – war in Europe, just as today behind the unwillingness to cut emissions lies the gulf between the future we hope for – continued stability and prosperity – and the future the evidence tells us is approaching – one of danger and sacrifice.

Throughout the 1930s, Churchill's aim was, in the words of his biographer, 'to prick the bloated bladder of soggy hopes' for enduring peace (Jenkins 2001: 482). But the bladder had a tough skin, far too tough to be penetrated by mere facts, even the 'great new fact' of German re-armament, which, said Churchill, 'throws almost all other issues into the background' (Churchill 1938: 171). The warnings of Churchill and a handful of others were met with derision. In terms akin to those now used to ridicule individuals warning of climate disaster – 'fear-mongers', 'doom-sayers', 'alarmists' – he was repeatedly accused of exaggerating the danger, of irresponsibility, of using 'the language of blind and causeless panic' and of behaving like 'a Malay running amok' (Churchill 1938: 152–3).

Among the public, his warnings fell on ears deaf to any messages but reassuring ones. In 1938 the British public cheered Chamberlain wildly when he returned from Munich waving his scrap of paper. So earnestly did the British public wish for peace that they were prepared to suspend their grasp of reality in return for a comforting delusion. To bounce the public from its torpor, in 1934 Churchill delivered a speech to the Commons in which he described in some detail the apocalyptic effects that bombing raids would have on London. He was trying to conjure up in the minds of the unwilling an image of the devastation that could become the reality were incendiary bombs to rain down on the capital. The details were provided to him, he said, 'by persons who are acquainted with the science' (Churchill 1938: 173).

Like the Murdoch press today, in the 1930s conservative newspapers, led by *The Times*, accused Churchill of alarmism. Their fear of communism caused them to overlook the threat of fascism. Churchill was no friend of dictators of any stripe, but, unlike the newspaper editors, he was unwilling to play down the Nazi menace because of its antagonism to communism, just as today the loathing of some conservatives for all things championed by environmentalists causes them to give credence to critics of climate science.

Late in 1938, Churchill's trenchant criticism of Chamberlain's Munich agreement – 'a total and unmitigated defeat' (Churchill 1941: 42) – earned him the fury of Conservative party members. Anti-Churchill forces in the party rallied, and as late as March 1939, a year before he was to become war-time Prime Minister, it seemed likely that Churchill would be ousted as a Conservative MP by Government loyalists (Jenkins 2001: 531).[18] Devotion to party, combined with the peace-dreams of the public, blinded Britain to the looming peril and brought it to the edge of the precipice. In the post-war years Britons preferred to remember the Churchill who embodied their bulldog spirit rather than the Churchill they had ignored and ridiculed.

Camus' *The Plague*

My third illustration is historical allegory rather than history. Albert Camus' 1947 novel *The Plague* (*La Peste*) is typically read as a representation of how the French responded to German occupation. Bubonic plague breaks out in Oran, a town of some 200,000 people in Algeria. It is cut off from the rest of the world for months on end as thousands succumb to horrible deaths.

Bernard Rieux, the doctor and protagonist, is the first to recognize that the mass die-off of rats and the strange symptoms of his patients had signalled the arrival of plague. It took others much longer to accept the facts before them. The citizens of Oran, wrote Camus, 'did not believe in pestilence'. They told themselves 'that it is unreal, that it is a bad dream that will end'. Camus forgave human frailty.

> [T]hey merely forgot to be modest and thought that everything was still possible for them, which implied that pestilence was impossible. They

continued with business, with making arrangements for travel and holding opinions. Why should they have thought about the plague, which negates the future, negates journeys and debate? They considered themselves free and no one will ever be free as long as there is plague, pestilence and famine.

(Camus 2002: 30)

The town's mayor, too, was reluctant to acknowledge the truth officially because doing so would have required him to take stern measures, an institutional sclerosis all too familiar today.

In a comment that applies with great force to the contemporary climate debate, Camus observed that in denying the facts 'we continue to give priority to our personal feelings' (63). As the story unfolds, Camus sees into the strategies used by the townspeople to deny or avoid the meaning of the plague. First they tell themselves the deaths are due to something else. Then they tell each other the epidemic will be short-lived, and life will soon return to normal. Later, they cling to superstitions and prophecies, unearthing old texts that seem to promise deliverance or protection. They begin to drink more wine because a rumour has circulated that wine kills the plague bacillus. Then, when drunk, they offer optimistic opinions into the night air.

Eventually, the daily count of Oran's dead overwhelms all forms of resistance to the truth. The emotional force of the realization explains why it is resisted for so long. 'At that moment', wrote Camus, 'the collapse of their morale, their will power and their patience was so abrupt that they felt they would never be able to climb back out of their hole' (57).

At one point a Dionysian spirit arrives to wipe away the gloom. 'At the beginning, when they thought it was a sickness like any other, religion had its place' wrote Camus. 'But when they saw that it was serious, they remembered pleasure. So in the dusty, blazing dusk all the anguish imprinted on their faces during the day resolves itself into a sort of crazed excitement, an uneasy freedom that enflames the whole population' (93).

There are lessons in *The Plague* for the stances we might adopt in the face of the truth about global warming. After months of the deadly epidemic, everyone confined in Oran fears that it will never end. There is Jean Tarrou, a mysterious visitor trapped in the quarantine town, who has kept a chronicle of events in which the people of Oran were viewed from a distance, as through the wrong end of a telescope. Wrote Camus, 'Yes, there was an element of abstraction and unreality in misfortune. But when an abstraction starts to kill you, you have to get to work on it' (69).

As a means of abstracting from suffering, Tarrou's telescope is akin to the approach of some scientists, like James Lovelock, who take up a position somewhere in space from which they dispassionately analyse the possible end of humanity in an abstract kind of way. After Father Paneloux, Oran's Jesuit priest, sermonizes on sin and faith, Rieux observes: 'Paneloux is a scholar. He has not seen enough people die and that is why he speaks in the name of eternal truths' (97).

In 1945 Hannah Arendt described as 'metaphysical opportunists' those who took flight from the reality of wickedness by engaging in abstract arguments about good and evil (Arendt 1994: 134–135).[19] It is a powerful temptation to escape in these ways, either by a retreat to cosmological thinking or going in the opposite direction, an inward journey to a place of reconciliation and faith.

Dr Rieux works tirelessly against overwhelming odds. He knows that any victories against the plague will be short-lived. 'But that is not a reason to give up the struggle', he tells his friend; '. . . one must fight, in one way or another, and not go down on one's knees' (Camus 2002: 98 and 102), an attitude sometimes read as a metaphor used by Camus for the stance of the French Resistance against German occupation.

Camus argued that the only way to maintain one's integrity in such a situation is to adopt what he called an 'active fatalism', in which 'one should start to move forward, in the dark, feeling one's way and trying to do good'. The novelist was acutely aware of the importance of hope – 'how hard it must be to live only with what one knows and what one remembers, and deprived of what one hopes' (176 and 225). Some will argue that, in facing the facts of warming, we must not succumb to apathy but re-imagine a different future and begin to hope that it can be the best possible in the new conditions.[20] It is a stance akin to the 'Christian hope' expressed by St Francis when he said: 'Even if I knew the world would end tomorrow, I would still plant this tree.'

Dr Rieux's active fatalism, a refusal to capitulate to hopeless odds, is similar to the distinction, drawn by Nietzsche and elaborated by Heidegger, between the pessimism of strength and the pessimism of weakness (Heidegger 1991: 54–5).

Pessimism as strength faces up to the facts as they present themselves, accepts the danger fully and engages in sober analysis of what is. It is the pessimism of Dr Rieux – in contrast to others who became absorbed in despondency, adopted a submissive stance and capitulated to the situation through a weary knowingness, taking refuge in ineluctable fate. These two correspond to what Nietzsche called active and passive nihilism, and it is fair to assume that as the full truth of climate science dawns and wishful thinking is rendered untenable – just as the piles of bodies in Oran could no longer go unheeded – then people will divide into these two camps: the pessimists of strength and the pessimists of weakness.

Humans and nature

The success of climate denialism in its various guises reveals how shallow are the roots of the Enlightenment. When superstition was swept away by science and reason, our penchant for self-deception merely lost its cover. In the most vital test of our capacity to protect the future through the deployment of rationality and well-informed foresight, the 'rational animal' is manifestly failing. We see now that the forces unleashed by science and the commitment to a rational social order had entered into a contingent alliance only. The 'autocratic subject'[21] could extract knowledge from nature but could also choose to ignore that knowledge if it unsettled the mind. It was a double-edged subjectivity that had the self-certainty to both liberate objective science and reject the facts it uncovered when convenient. The climate crisis is upon us because we are intoxicated by our subjectivity.

Those now afraid for the future are naturally aghast at the ability of climate denial to erode confidence in science and weaken political resolve. Yet it is not so much the fanaticism of the small minority of active deniers that concerns us, but the vulnerability of the majority to their influence. The soggy hopes of the pre-war British public, the wishful thinking of the citizens of Oran, the fears of economic and cultural decay that haunted Weimer Germany – these are the danger. The desire to disbelieve deepens as the scale of the threat grows, until a point is reached when the facts can be resisted no longer.

Yet the resistance to global warming goes beyond a psychological frailty. Developments in climate science have revealed a natural world so influenced by human activity that the epistemological division between nature and society can no longer be maintained. When global warming triggers feedback effects, such as melting permafrost and declining albedo from ice-melt, will we be seeing nature at work or human intervention? The mingling of the natural and the human has philosophical as well as practical significance, because the 'object' has been contaminated by the 'subject'.

Climate denial can be understood as a last-ditch attempt to re-impose the Enlightenment's allocation of humans and Nature to two distinct realms, as if the purification of climate science could render Nature once again natural, as if taking politics out of science can take humans out of Nature. The irony is that it was Enlightenment science itself, in the rules laid down by the Royal Society, that objectified the natural world, putting it on the rack, in Bacon's grisly metaphor, in order to extract its secrets. We came to believe we could keep Nature at arms' length but have now discovered, through the exertions of climate science, something pre-moderns took for granted: that Nature is always too close for comfort.

Notes

1 The story has been well told by Jacques, Dunlap and Freeman (2008); McCright and Dunlap (2010); and Oreskes and Conway (2010).
2 Available at: www.independent.co.uk/news/world/politics/bush-to-g8-goodbye-from-the-worlds-biggest-polluter-863911.html
3 The evidence contradicting the information deficit model is overwhelming, so that those who continue to cleave to it, ipso facto, demonstrate its falsity. Faith in the power of information prevails over the power of information.
4 Some have also used illegal practices, including hacking into computers and engaging in various 'black ops' (available at: www.clivehamilton.net.au/cms/media/documents/articles/abc_denialism_series_complete.pdf).
5 According to one conception, which had wide currency at the time, even among 'pro-Semites', Jews were 'innately inclined towards algorithmic, analytic, or abstract thinking, whereas Aryans tend to think intuitively and synthetically'. David Rowe, 'Jewish Mathematics' at Gottingen in the Era of Felix Klein, *Isis*, 77 (3), Sept. 1986: 424.

6 McCright and Dunlap (2010), 'Anti-reflexivity: The American Conservative Movement's Success in Undermining Climate Science and Policy'.
7 Adding: 'The crisis of ecology, the threat of atomic war, and the disruption of the patterns of human life by advanced technology have all eroded what was once a general trust in the *goodness* of science.' Jacob Needleman, *A Sense of the Cosmos: The Encounter of Modern Science and Ancient Truth*, Doubleday & Company, New York, 1975, p. 1.
8 Clive Hamilton, 'An evil atmosphere', *New Scientist*, 17 July 2010. For a longer version see 'The powerful coalition that wants to engineer the world's climate', *The Guardian* (online), 13 Sept. 2010.
9 In the United States calls are being made to ban the teaching of climate science in schools, or at least to 'balance' it with the views of climate deniers (available at: www.prwatch.org/node/9097).
10 Curiously, the English translation of Lenard's book on great men of science (1933), which excluded Einstein, was still widely used in schools and universities in Britain in the 1950s.
11 Claiming censorship, in 1921 some Einstein opponents established their own body to dispense prestige, the 'Academy of Nations', an international association that awarded honours to anti-relativist scientists and promoted 'free' science (van Dongen 2010).
12 So, for example, 'respectable' scientists such as Fred Singer, Richard Lindzen, Craig Idso, Willie Soon, Ian Plimer, William Kininmonth, Garth Paltridge and Bob Carter speak at Headland Institute conferences shoulder-to-shoulder with political extremists such as Christopher Monckton, Andrei Illarionov and Marc Morano (available at: www.heartland.org/events/2010Chicago/program.html).
13 Hubert Goenner, 'The reaction to relativity theory, I: The anti-Einstein campaign in Germany in 1920', *Science in Context*, 6 (1): 107–133, 1993: 120.
14 Quoted by Oreskes and Conway (2010), *Merchants of Doubt*, p. 133.
15 Meyer, C. (2010) The travelling salesmen of climate skepticism, *Spiegel Online*, 8 Oct. Available at: www.spiegel.de/international/world/0,1518,721846,00.html
16 For reasons that are obscure, Weyland emigrated to the United States in the 1930s (Goenner 1993: 123).
17 Available at: www.climatesciencewatch.org/index.php/csw/details/denialist-morano-rejoicing/
18 On the outbreak of war, the leader of the anti-Churchill forces in the Epping division, Colonel Sir Colin Thornton-Kemsley, wrote a humble apology to the man whose refusal to be silenced almost led to the end of his parliamentary career.
19 Also quoted by Tony Judt in his introduction to *The Plague*.
20 See the last chapter of Hamilton (2010b), *Requiem for a Species*.
21 The term is from Max Horkheimer and Theodor Adorno, *Dialectic of Enlightenment*, Allen Lane, London, 1973: xvi.

References

Arendt, H. (1994) *Essays in Understanding: 1930–1945*, ed. J. Kohn. New York: Harcourt Brace and Co.
Buchwald, D. et al. (2006) *The Collected Papers of Albert Einstein, Vol. 10*. Princeton: Princeton University Press: 428–429.
Camus, A. (1947, 2002) *The Plague*. London: Penguin.
Churchill, W. (1938) *Arms and the Covenant: Speeches by the Right Hon. Winston Churchill*. London: George C. Harrap and Co.

Churchill, W. (1941) *Into Battle: Speeches by the Right Hon. Winston Churchill*. London: Cassell and Co.

Fischer, D. (2010) Cyber bullying intensifies as climate data questioned. *Scientific American*, 1 Mar. Available at: http://climateprogress.org/2010/03/02/the-rise-of-anti-science-cyber-bullying/

Fukuyama, F. (1992) *The End of History and the Last Man*. New York: Free Press.

Furedi, F. (2010) Science's peer system needs a review. *The Weekend Australian*, 20–21 Feb.

Goenner, H. (1993) The reaction to relativity theory I: The anti-Einstein campaign in Germany in 1920. *Science in Context*, 6 (1): 107–133.

Hamilton, C. (2010a) An evil atmosphere. *New Scientist*, 17 July.

Hamilton, C. (2010b) *Requiem for a Species*. London: Earthscan.

Hamilton, C., and Kasser, K. (2009) Psychological adaptation to the threats and stresses of a four degree world. In *Four Degrees and Beyond* conference, University of Oxford, 28–30 Sept. 2009. Available at: www.clivehamilton.net.au/cms/media/documents/articles/oxford_four_degrees_paper_final.pdf

Heidegger, M. (1991) *Nietzsche, Vol. IV: Nihilism*, ed. D. Krell. New York: Harper Collins.

Heidegger, M. (1995) *Fundamental Concepts of Metaphysics: World, Finitude, Solitude*. Bloomington and Indianapolis, IN: Indiana University Press.

Horkheimer, M., and Adorno, T. (1973) *Dialectic of Enlightenment*. London: Allen Lane.

Huntington, S. (1996) *The Clash of Civilizations and the Remaking of World Order*. New York: Simon & Schuster.

Jacques, P., Dunlap, R. E., and Freeman, M. (2008) The organization of denial: Conservative think tanks and environmental skepticism. *Environmental Politics*, 17 (3)

Jenkins, R. (2001) *Churchill: A Biography*. New York: Farrar, Straus and Giroux.

Jerome, F., and Taylor, R. (2005) Einstein on race and racism. *Logos* 4 (3, Summer). Available at: www.logosjournal.com/issue_4.3/jerome_taylor.htm

Kahan, D. (2010) Fixing the communications failure. *Nature*, 463 (21 Jan.): 296–297.

Kahan, D. M., Braman, D., Gastil, J., Slovic, P. and Mertz, C. K. (2007) Culture and identity-protective cognition: Explaining the white male effect in risk perception. *Journal of Empirical Legal Studies*, 4 (3): 465–505.

Lahsen, M. (2008) Experience of modernity in the greenhouse: A cultural analysis of a physicist 'trio' supporting the backlash against global warming. *Global Environmental Change*, 18: 204–219.

Latour, B. (2004) Why has critique run out of steam? From matters of fact to matters of concern. *Critical Inquiry*, 30 (2, Winter): 225–248.

Lenard, P. (1933) *Great Men of Science*. London: G. Bell and Sons.

Lertzman, R. (2008). The myth of apathy. *The Ecologist*, 19 June.

Maibach, E., Roser-Renouf, C., and Leiserowitz, A. (2009) *Global Warming's 'Six Americas' 2009: An audience segmentation*. New Haven, CT: Yale Project on Climate Change and George Mason University Center for Climate Change Communication.

McCright, R., and Dunlap, R. (2003) Defeating Kyoto: The Conservative Movement's impact on US climate change policy. *Social Problems*, 50 (3): 348–373.

McCright, A., and Dunlap, R. (2010) Anti-reflexivity: The American Conservative Movement's success in undermining climate science and policy. *Theory, Culture & Society*, 27 (2–3): 100–133.

Meyer, C. (2010) The travelling salesmen of climate skepticism. *Spiegel Online*, 8 Oct. 2010. Available at: www.spiegel.de/international/world/0,1518,721846,00.html

Mooney, C. (2005) *The Republican War on Science*. New York: Basic Books.

Needleman, J. (1975) *A Sense of the Cosmos: The Encounter of Modern Science and Ancient Truth*. New York: Doubleday and Company.

Oreskes, N., and Conway, E. (2010) *Merchants of Doubt*. New York: Bloomsbury Press.

Rowe, D. (1986) 'Jewish Mathematics' at Gottingen in the era of Felix Klein. *Isis*, 77 (3, Sept.): 424.

Rowe, D. (2006) Einstein's allies and enemies: Debating relativity in Germany, 1916–1920. In V. Hendricks et al. (Eds.), *Interactions: Mathematics, Physics and Philosophy, 1860–1930*. Dordrecht: Springer.

Saul, J. R. (2005). *The Collapse of Globalism and the Reinvention of the World*. Toronto: Viking Canada.

Shapin, S., and Schaffer, S. (1985) *Leviathan and the Air-Pump: Hobbes, Boyle, and the Experimental Life*. Princeton, NJ: Princeton University Press.

Spengler, O. (1918) *The Decline of the West*. London: Allen & Unwin.

Taylor, S. (1989) *Positive Illusions: Creative Self-deception and the Healthy Mind*. New York: Basic Books.

van Dongen, J. (2007) Reactionaries and Einstein's fame: 'German Scientists for the Preservation of Pure Science, Relativity, and the Bad Nauheim Meeting'. *Physics in Perspective*, 9: 212–230.

van Dongen, J. (2010) 'On Einstein's opponents, and other crackpots', *Studies in History and Philosophy of Modern Physics*, 41: 78–80.

Chapter 3

The difficult problem of anxiety in thinking about climate change

Sally Weintrobe

Many environmentalists and policymakers stress the importance of not making people feel anxious when telling them about climate change. However, anthropogenic global warming is anxiety-provoking. Being able to bear anxiety is a vital part of being able to face reality, as we know that when anxiety becomes too much to bear, our thinking can become irrational and start to lack proportion. This chapter is on anxiety. I first explore the subject of anxiety and then look at what might be our central anxieties about climate change. It is important that we identify these and also that we seek to know as much as we can about the effects of our anxieties about climate change on our capacity to think and act. I conclude by looking at some implications for policy about how to engage people about climate change.

Anxiety

We can feel anxious for many different underlying reasons. Here I concentrate on anxieties about survival, tracing two main forms. I then look at some common defences we use to reduce anxiety. One of these is denial. I go into the subject of denial in some detail.

The psychoanalytic model that underpins my understanding of anxiety is that we are inherently in conflict between different parts of ourselves, that much of the conflict goes on at an unconscious level and that the biggest conflict we face in life is between the concerned part of us that loves reality and the more narcissistic, vain part of us that hates reality when it thwarts our wishes or deflates our view of ourselves.

The narcissistic part that hates reality feels ideal and special and is prone to omnipotent thinking. It uses magical 'quick fixes' to try to restore its sense of being ideal when reality brings disillusionment. It expects admiration – indeed adoration – for its 'quick fixes'.

The part that loves reality recognizes its right size and where it fits within the scheme of things, tolerates limits, tolerates having very ambivalent feelings about reality, tolerates being far from perfect, is motivated by loving concern, finds reality challenging and finds it is struggling with reality that ultimately provides meaning and self-worth. It aims to try to put right damage caused by the narcissistic part in real ways. It is able to mourn an idealized world.

Melanie Klein (1940), following Freud's (1917) pioneering work on the subject, recognized that anxiety is at the very centre of our work to face reality. She argued that the narcissistic and the reality-based parts of the self both face anxiety. The narcissistic part is anxious it will not survive if reality is accepted. The realistic part is anxious that the narcissistic part has caused damage and may imperil its survival.

Klein saw that the work of gradually accepting reality involves facing both these kinds of anxiety. They both involve anxieties about survival. Her point was that when faced with reality, especially when it can bring most hated and unwanted changes, we inevitably veer back and forth between protecting ourselves from these two very different kinds of anxiety. She also, crucially, pointed out that for the part of the self that loves reality to be more powerful than the part of the self that hates reality, we need emotional support to bear anxiety and also to bear difficult feelings like guilt, shame and loss.

An everyday example of these two different kinds of anxiety at work is a conversation a friend reported to me between herself and Katie, her three-year-old granddaughter. The background was that Katie was facing major changes at home with the arrival of a new baby. 'Grandma', Katie said, 'I've decided to marry Daddy and we are going to have lots and lots of babies.' 'I see', my friend said, 'but what about Mummy and new Baby Gemma?' 'Oh, that's alright. They are only dwarfs.' Part of the touching charm and poignancy of this ordinary story from family life is the unabashed way little Katie states out loud her wishful phantasy solution to current problems. I suggest her omnipotent phantasy – we can almost see her whooshing her magic wand – is a way for her to reduce her anxiety at the shocking new realization that she must share Mummy with New Baby and also with Daddy. Her foremost anxiety here would seem to be survival anxiety. Will the part of herself that has believed up until now that she is the adored and special centre of the family survive? Her magic solution serves to reduce anxiety about the survival of this part of herself. She is a big lady, in charge and having magicked up a powerful creative couple, herself and Daddy. Her feelings of being small, marginalized and not so in control of her fate are projected onto Mummy and New Baby, now morphed into discarded dwarfs. However, this 'quick-fix solution', designed to reduce anxiety, brings other anxieties. Has she damaged her mother's love by allowing her hatred of the new reality at home to triumph in this way? Can a diminished and hated dwarf mother provide her with the love and care she still badly needs? Her anxieties may be that not only is phantasy Mummy now minimized and useless but also that real Mummy might be cross with her.

Paranoid-schizoid anxiety and depressive anxiety

Klein identified characteristic defences used by the narcissistic part of the self to defend itself against anxiety. They include mental splitting, idealization and projection. In our example, we might say that little Katie splits Mummy into, on the one hand, a powerful idealized figure – the lady partner of Daddy who can make lots of babies with him – and, on the other hand, a depleted, ridiculed dwarf figure. She steps into Mummy's big-lady shoes and identifies with her in her imagination, and she flings little dwarf Mummy away. This omnipotent action protects the part of herself that likes to feel specially adored and powerful from experiencing her own littleness, feared insignificance and lack of power. All these unwanted feelings are projected onto dwarfed Mummy and Baby. Splitting is characterized by idealization and by black-and-white, all-or-nothing kinds of thinking. Katie is unconsciously pushed by anxiety to split in the way she does.

Klein called the anxieties experienced and defences used by the narcissistic part of the self 'paranoid-schizoid'. Calling Katie's frame of mind paranoid recognizes that her anxiety is about the survival of the narcissistic part of her. Will it survive all these changes in the family? Calling it schizoid refers to the way she uses mental splitting to reduce her anxiety about this.

Klein characterized as depressive the anxiety experienced by the part of the self that loves reality. Depressive anxiety is not meant to convey that this part is depressed in a clinical sense but, rather, that it is burdened with sadness, guilt and shame and with anxiety that the narcissistic part has caused damage. Here, there is less idealization and splitting and more love, concern and realism. Katie's depressive anxiety might be whether her loving relationship with her mother will survive the way she is rubbishing her.

Klein's point is that reality can bring most hated, unwanted and anxiety-provoking changes, and when faced with reality, we inevitably veer between protecting ourselves from different kinds of survival anxiety – those felt by the part of the self that hates reality and those felt by the part of the self that loves it. Our love of the other helps us to face depressive anxieties about their state, and our love gives us strength to withstand our more paranoid anxieties. In particular, love gives us the strength to face damage we have caused, to others and to ourselves, and leads to our wish to repair it as best we can.

Klein also pointed out that having these competing anxieties is entirely normal, and that working them through begins in early childhood and is ongoing throughout life. A further crucial point she made is that for the self that loves reality to be more powerful than the self that hates it, we need emotional support. Katie is supported by the adults in her life who love her and gently steer her towards reality by respecting her and empathizing with her and by intuitively understanding what probably lies beneath the surface of her defences.

It might be thought that a small child voicing an irrational phantasy that she is special and has magic powers is far removed from the subject of adult anxiety. However, as adults we think like Katie far more often than we care to realize. Katie essentially deals with her anxieties about impending change not by facing them but by trying to minimize them through 'quick-fix' magical and irrational thinking. There are a myriad ways in which as adults we do the same. Perhaps our biggest difference from Katie is that we have learned better to conceal our irrationality, most of all from ourselves.

Common defences against anxiety

Anxiety is most often a vital signal that alerts us to real threats and dangers to survival. It is when these anxieties become too much to bear that we can tend to apply irrational 'quick fixes' to try to reduce them. I will now look at three common 'quick fixes' that can also tend to be applied together.

Feeling magically big and powerful

Little Katie felt big and powerful. When we see people behaving in ways we identify as muscle flexing, as feeling a bit god-like and as being out of touch with real worries and real concern, it is important to bear in mind that they may be defending themselves against feeling acutely anxious, a feeling that may be too difficult to bear. This is important when looking at social groups as well as individuals behaving like this. We are familiar with the many analyses of current Western societies as narcissistic (Lasch 1978). We are less familiar with looking at the extent to which feelings of 'I/we are King of the Castle' may be a defence against fearing being in the position of the Dirty Rascal, the dwarfed social outcast.

Projection

Another way to deal with too much anxiety is to project it onto or into another or others. For instance, little Katie projected her anxieties about feeling powerless, side-lined and potentially unloved onto Mummy and Baby. We all use projection of this kind, and it is a prevalent mechanism used by our social groups.

Denial

Denial is a commonly used defence. It tries to get rid of reality altogether by maintaining that it is not there. We only deny things we have already seen, even if only dimly or out of the corner of one eye. The denial is aimed at protecting us from the anxiety and from the pain of impending loss and change that would follow if we did accept reality in a felt and owned way.

When anxiety gets too much to bear, we may resort, broadly speaking, to two different sorts of denial: negation and disavowal. It is crucial to distinguish the two, as negation is more likely to be a stage on the way to mourning illusions and accepting reality. Disavowal can involve the more stuck terrain of delusion. And, with disavowal, unreality and irrationality are not only more likely to prevail but may, indeed, escalate.

Denial as negation

Negation, the assertion that something that is, is not, can be our first response to reality when it faces us with shocking losses and changes. Negation is the first stage of mourning, that process that usually proceeds from negation to anger and only then to grief and acceptance of the loss. Negation helps us process the initial shock of loss when it is too much to bear. 'Too much' is really 'too much all in one go'.

In order to mourn what we have lost, we vitally need to feel the presence of supportive figures who will not judge us too harshly, who are warm in their feelings for us and who can forgive us and accept our human frailty. These figures are not just the actual people in our lives – parents, teachers and leaders – but are also, importantly, figures who are part of the world of relationships that we represent in our internal worlds and carry within us, mostly in unconscious forms. The degree of support from these internalized figures affects how much we are able to mourn and face reality.

So, for example, when we initially deny our loss – say, the death of a loved one – through negation, it helps if we feel the support of people who understand that we cannot bear the whole truth, just for now. Then, when in the grip of the anger phase of mourning, it helps if we feel in the presence of figures who can support and forgive us as well as be reality-oriented. Without an inner climate of forgiveness in which we have real and not ideal expectations of others and ourselves, we may become stuck in a climate of hatred, bitter recrimination and relentlessness, easily feeling harshly judged, being harshly judging and not moving towards accepting the reality of the loss; we may feel caught in the ruinous expectation that our only salvation will be to have our ideal world back again, a world in which no loss has occurred. It also helps to grieve if we feel the support of those who appreciate how painful grief feels.

Loss is far harder to face without support, empathy and forgiveness. But if we are able to work through our grief, with support, to the point of being able to think rationally, we have survived in heart and mind. Thinking is not just having an intellectual and rational understanding of a reality that causes us pain and anxiety: it is that reality felt and owned by the self; not an activity, but a process involving mourning and facing the anxieties that come with inner change.

The prospect of any significant change is itself often shocking. With change comes the unknown and anxiety about the survival of different parts of ourselves. We inevitably face myriad changes and endure myriad losses in life. We lose the past, we lose our idealizations and we lose our self-views. We can also lose our hopes for the future. Many of the different kinds of losses we face in life can feel like deaths and are, indeed, deaths in so far as death is the irrevocable. With death there is no return to how it was before.

Change can also involve accepting back and reintegrating parts of ourselves that we may have split off and disowned. Defences mounted to protect against too much anxiety need to give way if reality is to penetrate, and negation can protect against a sense of impending disintegration. For instance, feeling big and powerful may give way to feeling helpless and perhaps humiliated, and the anxieties that have been split off and minimized can return to flood and overwhelm.

Negation is hopefully worked through with strengthened inner resolve and outer support, so that reality is eventually faced and loss is mourned. But we can also resort to a different sort of denial, one that can lead us not towards accepting reality but increasingly away from it. This is disavowal.

Denial as disavowal

Disavowal involves radical splitting and a range of strategies that ensure that reality can be seen and not seen *at one and the same time*. Disavowal is often called turning a blind eye, but this description does not go far enough in distinguishing disavowal from negation. There are two key differences. First, with disavowal our more wish-fulfilling narcissistic part may have come under the sway of a more entrenched arrogant attitude that can exert a powerful hold on the psyche. Second, disavowal may be part of a more organized and enduring defensive structure, whereas negation is typically a more transitory defence against anxiety.

Psychoanalytic researchers such as Rosenfeld (1971), O'Shaugnessy (1981) and Steiner (1987) have discussed more stuck mental states the aim of which is to create a psychic retreat from reality where both paranoid-schizoid *and* depressive anxieties can be *systematically* avoided. These states, which can be resistant to influence and change, have been called pathological organizations. Here a delusion of being special – indeed, god-like – is clung to and not gradually mourned and given up. Bion in a series of papers (1957, 1958, 1959) linked this god-like attitude with an underlying arrogance that Rosenfeld (1971) later called destructive narcissism, to emphasize its destructive effects and to distinguish it from less pathological and more transitory forms of inflated self-worth. I will use Bion's term 'arrogance' in this context rather than narcissism in order to keep clear the difference from 'normal' narcissism.[1]

Brenman (1985) discussed the way that arrogance is accompanied by single-minded exploitative greed, and I (Weintrobe 2004) have discussed the way it is accompanied by a sense of narcissistic entitlement to exploit the other, with the 'justification' of being ideal, superior and special. With arrogance, a destructively narcissistic part of the psyche has gained the upper hand in a power struggle with the part that feels wedded to reality. A sense of narcissistic entitlement to be immune to emotional difficulties has triumphed over a lively entitlement to a relationship with reality.

Steiner (1993) linked the pathological organization with the experience of being in a psychic retreat from reality, with the aim of being spared anxiety and pain. Rosenfeld (1971) had originally put forward a powerful analysis of the way that pathological organizations are maintained within the psyche by phantasies of powerful internal mafia-like gangs that enforce compliance and treat the reality seeking part of the self with violence if it does not toe the line.

Disavowal is part of a pathological organization. With disavowal, anxiety may be systematically gotten rid of, sometimes in a flash, through a range of 'quick fixes'. A central quick fix is minimizing or obliterating any sense that facing reality entails facing any loss. Reality may be seen to be there, but the loss that it signals has no or little significance in this state. Disavowal aims to block mourning at the stage before sadness, grieving and reconciliation, and in this sense may be seen as a form of arrested, failed mourning, or melancholia, as Freud (1917) described it.

When we think of a hateful destructive attack, we imagine something active and violent. It is more difficult to see that disavowal – which, after all, apparently 'deals with' anxiety and apparently keeps all negative effects to a minimum – can conceal great hidden violence while being quite split off from its effects.

Triumph is an important part of disavowal. The arrogant omnipotent part of the self feels very clever for being able to 'solve' painful problems so instantly. The delusion that nothing is lost because loss itself has no meaning is perhaps the ultimate triumph. Disavowal is also artful. It can cleverly bend, reverse and warp the truth, and fraudulent thinking flourishes in this state of mind.

The kind of disintegration of the sense of self that is experienced when disavowal *is* acknowledged and reality accepted is far more severe than with negation. It may involve struggling to reintegrate back into the self crippling anxieties and burdens of guilt and shame – crippling because they have been allowed to build up through being consistently and systematically split off so as to stay in a psychic retreat.

The problem with disavowal is, not least, that it involves a severe attack on thinking.

While negation denies the truth, it does not distort its shape so much, whereas disavowal can result in confusion and an inability to think with a sense of proportion. The splitting that occurs with disavowal also leads to a breakdown of proportionality in thinking. Anxiety is minimized, guilt and shame – emotions that also cause us great anxiety – are minimized, and all this is achieved through omnipotent thinking. But human nature does not work this way. When a problem is minimized and ridiculed, the sane part of the mind – which is always there, even if eclipsed and made small – becomes increasingly anxious. The arrogant part of the mind also becomes increasingly anxious, but for different reasons. Having psychically damaged – through triumph and contempt – any internal figures who might be containing and might put a stop to the irrationality, it fears possible retaliation. Also, it is increasingly mentally vulnerable, as it has damaged any internal figures who might contain and calm anxiety and help to re-establish a sense of proportion.

Disavowal is a poor means of lowering anxiety in the longer term. Because disavowal does nothing to address the real causes of anxiety, it can lead to an escalation of underlying anxiety that can feel increasingly unmanageable. The more disavowal is allowed to proceed unchecked by reality, the more anxiety it breeds and the greater the danger that the anxiety will be defended against by further defensive arrogance and further disavowal. Disavowal leads to a vicious spiral, and this makes it dangerous.

What might cause disavowal to set in? Clinical experience suggests that the following conditions apply: the reality has become too obvious to be ignored, there is anxiety that damage is too great to be repaired, it is felt that there is not enough help, support and containment to bear the anxiety and suffering that insight brings and there is anxiety that parts of the self will not survive change that now feels catastrophic and too much to face.

Cultures of denial

Individuals use denial, but denial can also become embedded within cultures, and powerful groups and lobbies play an important part in fostering cultures of disavowal. People internalize their social groups and make them part of their inner worlds. What they may internalize is the idea of a powerful, arrogant group that threatens exclusion and punishment if one breaks ranks. It is harder for any individual to fight for sanity and truth when intimidated not only by actual external powerful groups but also when such groups become internalized within the inner world and gain strength and force there. Rosenfeld's (1971) analysis about the way in which phantasies of mafia groups can hold sway within the internal mental organization to support arrogance has profound implications for understanding the way in which powerful external social groups operating in mafia-like ways can be internalized within the psyche and there have major effects on mental functioning, both at an individual and at a group level.

Again, anxiety is a key issue. The sane self suffers survival anxiety if it speaks out, and survival anxiety if it remains silent. But the sane self can also feel puny in the face of a needed social group that threatens it with rejection, social exclusion, or worse.

How a culture of disavowal props up irrationality in our social world

We are profoundly influenced socially as to what is to be deemed rational and irrational. It is truly startling to think about how much in society is flagrantly irrational and how much we avoid really wanting to know this. If those in power tell us irrational things aimed at reducing our anxiety, we may go along with this and find it seductive. However, it only leads to the build-up of underlying depressive anxiety, including that we may have damaged our capacity to think clearly. An extreme example is the way that, at the height of the Cold War in Britain leaders advised people to shut their windows and climb under a table in the event of a nuclear attack. Imagining ourselves under a table may have served to minimize the horror of the threat to survival, but only if people gave up awareness of just how irrational leaders were being in giving this advice and they would be in following it.

In the example above it is easy to see the irrationality. However, Western culture actively seduces and threatens us into using 'quick-fix' irrational ways of reducing anxiety in many ways that are not so blatant and visible. One example is advertising. A disturbing fact is that in Western societies a significant proportion of women, especially young women, suffer from underlying depression and feelings of worthlessness.[2] They do not feel wanted or desirable. A well-known advert for L'Oréal hair and skin products involves glamorous 'A-list' celebrity women coyly saying that they use L'Oréal '. . . because I'm worth it'. I suggest L'Oréal appeals not just to women's ordinary vanity – their normal narcissism – but to their underlying more arrogant wish to be part of an in-crowd of superior women, valued by society and loveable; it also promotes and sells the phantasy that we can rid ourselves of unpleasant feelings like depression, envy and fear of social exclusion through a very simple act: that of buying a small, inexpensive plastic tub of cosmetic cream. This is magical thinking and irrational, but because it is endemic in our culture, it is not generally fully recognized as such. My point is not about one specific advertisement but advertising in general and also a culture that sanctions and appeals to the part of us that feels especially entitled in an arrogant way to deploy omnipotent fixes to life's painful problems. We are actively encouraged to use disavowal and to live within an organized psychic retreat from the anxieties that reality brings.

But, irrational 'quick fixes' for anxiety only increase underlying anxiety and also lead to loss of underlying genuine self-worth. The part of the self that struggles to face reality, that feels entitled in a lively way to a relationship with reality 'because I *am* worth it', can be dwarfed and denigrated by society and also by the narcissistic part of ourselves that feels entitled to be spared psychic difficulty.

Anxieties about climate change

I now turn, finally, to our anxieties about climate change. What is it specifically about climate change that makes us so anxious? Välimäki and Lehtonen (2009) have suggested that modern man is suffering from what they call an environmental neurosis, rooted in deep-seated annihilation anxiety resulting from our denial of our real dependence on nature and based on the illusion of our own autonomy. They also make the cogent point that much of our illusory sense of autonomy is based on our use of science, but that our use of science (not science itself) has led to imbalance and damage.[3] I think Välimäki and Lehtonen have grasped the nub of the matter. I now explore some specific survival anxieties about climate change, highlighting the radically different sorts of anxieties suffered by the reality-based and the narcissistic parts of the self and focusing on the increasingly prevalent denial of climate change through disavowal.

Starting with our depressive anxieties, they can all cause traumatic levels of 'too much' anxiety. They include first, that we need a healthy biosphere to stay alive, and the biosphere is already showing signs consistent with predictions of effects of climate change. Second, we face the loss of a predictable future and, potentially, the loss of any future. Third, leadership is not acting sufficiently to protect us; deep down we know this, and it is traumatic to feel so uncared for. Fourth, we are realistically anxious about the destructiveness of the arrogant side of our own nature, which is destructive to ourselves and to the outside world; in particular we rightly fear circumstances when the destructiveness has become split off and disavowed and where its real effects are minimized.

Alongside this, I suggest that the narcissistic part of the self dreads giving up our sense of entitlement to have whatever we want and entitlement to apply our magical 'quick fixes' to the problems of reality.

Survival anxieties

The depressive anxieties of the reality-based part of the self about climate change

1. We face the loss of the Earth as the dependable bedrock that enables and supports our very life, the life of other fellow species and future life for all. Specifically, we face the effects of a climate tipped into instability. The terrible anxieties we face about this are akin to the small child's anxieties of losing the mother he or she utterly depends on. This cogent point is made by several authors in this volume. Margaret Rustin, commenting on the class-room artwork of primary-school children about the effects of climate change, argues that little children may be more in touch with their fears about the state of Mother Earth than are adults because they are more aware of just how dependent they are on their mothers and parents for their very survival. We truly hate fully to register the depth of our dependence on nature and our attachment to nature. We much prefer to see ourselves as the exploiting King of the Castle with the Earth as the exploited and controlled Dirty Rascal. But without a bountiful and flourishing Earth we are lost and deeply anxious. Deep down I suggest most people know this, at least unconsciously. This is the annihilation anxiety that Välimäki and Lehtonen (2009) have suggested we are now having to find ways to live with.

   As psychoanalysts, we know that children's anxieties, conscious and unconscious, about losing the mother are exacerbated by fears that greedy demands on her have damaged her. When we are small, as well as loving the mother, we can tend to see and treat her in a split way as an ideal 'breast-and-toilet' mother, there endlessly to supply our needs and demands and to absorb our waste (Keene, chapter 7, this volume). Climate damage can also revive our earlier childhood fears of damage. This may feel traumatic, and the accompanying anxiety may feel unbearable (Brenman Pick, chapter 6, this volume).

2. When we register that the climate is out of kilter, and are faced with what Friedman (2008, quoted in Morris 2010, p. 600) called 'climate weirding', at stake is not only anxiety about our physical survival, but the survival of our very sense of self. It is deeply anxiety-making to have our belief in a reliable

future and our sense of regularity and continuity as a species threatened at such a basic level. Undermined is our hope that we are generative – that our children will have children who will have children into the future – and rooted within long time.

3. We depend on our leaders in the current situation, and this introduces further anxiety. We know that currently in the United Kingdom, for instance, while they are setting very ambitious targets, they are not pushing through measures to reduce carbon emissions within a viable timescale. Because of this, we know that our leaders are not looking after us. We see them, too, pulled in by and in the power of commercial lobbyists and pressure groups with interests destructive to the Earth and all its human and non-human inhabitants. The message – and I suggest we do hear it – is that we are not cared for at the level of our very survival. To feel this uncared for is deeply traumatic and can also lead to unbearable anxiety, born of a feeling of help-lessness and aloneness in the face of survival threats. This, I suggest, was the fundamental legacy of the 'Hopenhagen' summit in 2009. At Copenhagen, for the first time, world leadership came together and publicly accepted that climate change is real and man-made. This provided an iconic image of truth backed by power. But the abiding iconic image of Copenhagen is a later one – that of truth bending the knee to greater, more hidden sources of power in the wings.[4]

The anxieties of the narcissistic part of the self about climate change

If we do contemplate making changes to reduce CO_2e emissions, we, leaders and followers, can start to experience survival anxieties of a more paranoid-schizoid kind. Our identities and status are intimately bound up with our lifestyles. In current consumerist societies we are actively encouraged to express our sense of identity through our material possessions, and losing these can therefore mean losing our sense of identity. We know we need a radical shift in our expectations of what we can take from nature, a shift towards a type of thinking that is based on real observation, on real arithmetic, and not on our idealized expectations. I think in these circumstances what we dread giving up is not so much particular material possessions or particular ways of life, but our way of seeing ourselves as special, and as entitled, not only to our possessions but to our 'quick fixes' to the problems of reality. This underlying attitude, just one side of human nature, is strongly ingrained in current Western societies. As I suggested via the L'Oréal advert, advertisers play to this attitude and foster it to sell us things, and society rewards those who embody it. We know that in giving up an unsustainable consumer lifestyle, we are threatening the identity of this part of ourselves, one we are mostly not aware of but will fight tooth and nail to protect.

A culture of disavowal of climate change

Currently there are signs that we are in the grip of disavowal when it comes to climate change, with all its effects of distortion of the truth. This was argued in a paper of mine (Weintrobe 2010) and is the subject of the next chapter in this book. Chapter 4, by Paul Hoggett, is in my view a major contribution to the subject. In it Hoggett links a detailed psychoanalytic account of perversion with a thorough-going analysis of what makes for a perverse culture. He discusses perverse modes of thinking about climate change – specifically, the lies and distortions involved for society collectively to turn a blind eye to global warming.

In this paper I have focused specifically on anxiety. Within a perverse culture we find 'quick-fix' ways to reconcile irreconcilable sets of anxieties about the implications of climate change. We are so bemired by this culture – one that breeds confusion and a lack of proportionality in thinking – that it can become very difficult to discuss with any objectivity not only issues of global warming but also economic issues, such as the necessity or not for growth in the economy. In a climate of disavowal, there is the greatest possible need for support and containment of anxieties so they can, albeit with difficulty, be jointly faced. There is also the least real support available because so much reliance is placed on the 'quick fixes' of evasion, fraud and splitting by leadership.

If we look at predisposing factors to disavowal, we see that they fit current realities about climate change very well. I will repeat them:

- The reality has become too obvious to be simply denied with negation.
- There is anxiety that the damage is already too great to repair.
- There is felt to be not enough support and help to bear the anxiety and suffering that knowledge of reality brings.

As climate change progresses and its effects become ever more visible, unless greater support for facing reality is given and unless group identification with a stance of arrogant entitlement is challenged to a greater extent, we can expect disavowal to be the prevalent defence against the 'too-much-ness' of the reality. Inaction on climate change does not only lead to soaring levels of CO_2e emissions. It may lead to spiralling disavowal.

Some implications for policy

What are the implications for how policymakers engage people about climate change?

1. Feeling big and powerful

When we look at economic models that insist on growth, regardless of whether or not it is environmentally sustainable, it is important to distinguish between purely economic factors and underlying unconscious emotional factors, such as the need to feel big and powerful, which can then also become a spiraling defence against anxiety. For instance, the state of mind of traders – some of them feeling like self-confessed 'sexy masters of the universe' – has been analysed in terms of underlying emotions and not just economics (see Tuckett 2011). And, history shows that expansionist utopian narcissistic states of mind that buck reality always lead to ruin in the end.

Also, when we advocate policies about climate change measures aimed at minimizing emotional difficulties for people, we should beware lest our unrecognized agenda is to put ourselves forward as ideal leaders magically able to spare people pain. In this case, our anxiety might be about our own survival as ordinary un-ideal but real leaders. Actually, people need ordinary real un-idealized leaders to help them to face and engage with very difficult realities about climate change. When we pretend we have idealized solutions that enable people apparently not to have to face any difficulties at all, we support disavowal and can unwittingly cause people's anxieties to rise, not diminish.

2. Projection

It is vital to come to understand our own anxieties about climate change as best we can before seeking to engage with others about it. If we do not, we are in danger of projecting our anxieties onto the people we want to engage, 'passing them on', as it were. This makes it more difficult for people to think in a rational way. Unwitting projection of this kind may have been a part of some of the early, 'catastrophizing', stridently doom-laden communications about climate change.

3. Disavowal

It is very important that we understand as much as possible about how disavowal works in our culture in order to work collectively to resist it.

Concluding comments

Lertzman (2008; see also chapter 6, this volume) has argued that what can appear as public apathy about environmental issues is the result of people caring too much, not too little. I agree, and in this chapter I have focused on defences against anxiety as contributing to what can appear as public apathy.

We are poorly equipped because of our very nature as human beings to bear the truth that global warming is mostly caused by human activity. This is because the truth makes us so anxious. The truth about damage to climate stability also makes us feel guilty and ashamed, and whether or not it is rational to have these feelings, having them is also part of human nature.

One main reason we find guilt and shame such difficult emotions to bear is that they cause us considerable anxiety. If we defend ourselves with disavowal, this can lead us rapidly to lose a sense of proportion. Indeed, proportional thinking is the first casualty of the environmental crisis we are in. We are trying, unsuccessfully, to manage contrary internal positions within our psyches where we are both overwhelmed by anxiety and not anxious at all; where we simultaneously feel no guilt and it is the other person/nation/corporation who is to blame and, on the other hand, where we feel monstrously guilty and to be blamed; and where we are shameless and easily flooded with shame at one and the same time.

In truth, in current Western cultures we all bear some small individual responsibility for climate change and environmental degradation, and we are also, realistically, largely not individually responsible. While we can be incapacitated by anxiety when thinking about climate change, we are, in a realistic sense, not nearly anxious enough, given the current news that warming is proceeding faster than had been estimated.

Anxiety is, I suggest, the biggest psychic barrier to facing the reality of anthropogenic global warming. In this chapter I have looked at some of the main ways we defend against our different sorts of anxieties about climate change. My main conclusions are threefold. Avoiding the subject of anxiety does not make people's anxieties about climate change go away. The defences used to minimize anxieties drive them underground, where they are not worked through and can escalate. People need genuine emotional support to bear their anxieties, and this is particularly the case when the defences used to minimize them involve disavowal. It is important for people to bear their anxieties, because when they do not, their thinking deteriorates, and irrationality, lack of proportionality, hatred and narcissism are more likely to prevail.

Notes

1 This is Kohut's (1966) distinction. He differentiated between normal and pathological narcissism.
2 Amelia Hill, 'Mental health of women in crisis', *Guardian Newspaper*, 11 Jan. 2011. See also World Health Organization (WHO 2011) report on depression: 'Depression is the 4th leading contributor to the global burden of disease (DALYs) in 2000. By the year 2020, depression is projected to reach 2nd place of the ranking of DALYs calculated for all ages, both sexes. Today, depression is already the 2nd cause of DALYs in the age category 15–44 years for both sexes combined.'
3 Hamilton (2011) has cogently argued that the narrative of the enlightenment backs up our illusion that we are in charge of Nature and control the future, with the help of what he calls 'technological–production science'. This is an important point. In Western societies we swim in the medium of enlightenment philosophy like fishes oblivious to being in water.
4 Lest anyone think I am simply accusing governments, the relation between leaders and led is a complex collusive dance. I do, however, think that this is a dance heavily led by one side.

References

Bion, W. R. (1957) Differentiation of the psychotic from the non-psychotic personalities. *International Journal of Psychoanalysis*, 38: 266–275.

Bion, W. R. (1958) On arrogance. *International Journal of Psychoanalysis*, 39: 144–146.

Bion, W. R. (1959) Attacks on linking. *International Journal of Psychoanalysis*, 40: 308–315.

Brenman, E. (1985) Cruelty and narrowmindedness. *International Journal of Psychoanalysis*, 66: 273–281.

Freud, S. (1917) Mourning and melancholia. In J. Strachey (Ed.), *The Standard Edition of the Complete Psychological Works of Sigmund Freud, Vol. VIII* (pp. 237–258). London: Hogarth Press.

Friedman, T. (2008) *Why we Need a Green Revolution*. New York: Farrar, Straus and Giroux.

Hamilton, C. (2011) *Denial, evasion and disintegration in the face of climate change*. Keynote paper given at the 'Changing Climates: Integrating Psychological Perspectives' Conference held in London, 2 July 2011.

Hill, A. (2011) Mental health of women in crisis. *The Guardian*, 11 Jan.

Klein, M. (1940) Mourning and its relation to manic-depressive states. *International Journal of Psychoanalysis*, 21: 125–153.

Kohut, H. (1966) Forms and transformations of narcissism. *Journal of the American Psychoanalytical Association*, 14: 243–272.

Lasch, C. (1978) *The Culture of Narcissism: American Life in an Age of Diminishing Expectations*. New York: Norton.

Lertzman, R. (2008) The myth of apathy. *The Ecologist*, 19 (6): 16–17.

Morris, I. (2010) *Why the West Rules – For Now*. London: Profile Books.

Rosenfeld, H. (1971) A clinical approach to the psychoanalytic theory of the life and death instincts: An investigation into the aggressive aspects of narcissism. *International Journal of Psychoanalysis*, 52: 169–178.

Steiner, J. (1987) The interplay between pathological organizations and the paranoid-schizoid and depressive positions. *International Journal of Psychoanalysis*, 68: 69–80.

Steiner, J. (1993) *Psychic Retreats*. London: Routledge.

Tuckett, D. (2011) *Minding the Markets: An Emotional Finance View of Financial Instability*. London: Palgrave MacMillan.

O'Shaughnessy, E. (1981) A clinical study of a defensive organization. *International Journal of Psychoanalysis*, 62: 359–369.

Välimäki, J., and Lehtonen, J. (2009) Ilmastonmuutoksen torjuntaan tarvitaan johtajuutta. [Leadership is required for counteracting climate change] (in Finnish). *Kanava*, 37 (6): 341–344.

Weintrobe, S. (2004) Links between grievance, complaint and different forms of entitlement. *International Journal of Psychoanalysis*, 85: 83–96.

Weintrobe, S. (2010) On links between runaway consumer greed and climate change denial: A psychoanalytic perspective. *Bulletin Annual of the British Psychoanalytical Society*, 1: 63–75. London: Institute of Psychoanalysis.

WHO (2011) *Report on Depression*. World Health Organization. Available at: www.who.int/mental_health/management/depression/definition/en/

Discussion
The difficult problem of anxiety in thinking about climate change

Johannes Lehtonen and Jukka Välimäki

The environmental neurosis of modern man: the illusion of autonomy and the real dependence denied

The human mind is often regarded as man's evolutionary crown, and the mind of modern man as competent and powerful, whereas because of its elusive and affect-laden character it represents man's 'weak point'. This is both remarkable and poorly recognized. It is particularly clear in relation to climate change, where the mind inhibits recognition of the warning signals, as Sally Weintrobe aptly describes in this chapter. Here, the mind specifically is the anxious mind, and its functions are maladaptive.

Decisions we take or withhold are made on the stage of the mind. The topical question of how to cope with the Gordian-knot-like complex of the interdependence of multiple climate-related factors is also dealt with, solved or left unsolved, on the stage of the mind. In the simple, but poignant words of an experienced Finnish industrial leader Tauno Matomäki several years ago, the problem of controlling climate change depends on what resides between our ears.

The psychological factors involved in our adaptation to the consequences of climate change are numerous. Together they form a complex that has many different roots in the sphere of our minds, such as our affects, basic sense of security of life, social orientation, economic adaptation, individual wishes and fears and, last but not least, our psychological make-up – the structure of the mind that has developed from infancy and adolescence to its adult forms. In addition, our social ideals and the capacity to feel shame and guilt about the exploitation and destruction of nature are also involved in our responses to signs of climate change.

Together, these factors have created a psychological condition that merits being called an environmental neurosis of modern man. We badly need the resources of nature that we cannot live without, and simultaneously we do not want to acknowledge these needs since their recognition ensures that we can no longer expect our lives to be safe or our self-centred demands guaranteed to be fulfilled in the future.

In this discussion, we consider two points to be of particular importance in the complex psychology of facing climate change.

The first is the tacit assumption of the autonomy of man in relation to the physical, chemical and biological conditions of life on our planet. We like to forget that the dominant position of mankind in nature is, in reality, based on the availability of living and inorganic natural resources. The real condition of man with respect to nature is not autonomous. On the contrary, our welfare is based on an uncompromised dependence on food, water, energy and a biologically feasible atmosphere, all of which make the idea of man's independence an illusion.

Because of our profound dependence on nature, climate change shakes the security of the human sense of being at a very basic level. This is already true at the present uncertain stage of knowledge of its consequences. The current effects of climate change and its imminent future effects pose and evoke a threat to the continuity of our present way of life, one in which we in Western societies are accustomed to technological efficiency, affluence and comfort. It is thus perhaps understandable that attempts to prevent the experience of deep anxieties about the future development of living conditions on our planet will inevitably be mobilized by any information that tells us of the dangers of the increase of carbon dioxide and the other greenhouse gases in the atmosphere.

Trust in the ultimate independence of human intelligence over nature is nurtured by scientific discoveries and technological inventions that are expected to continue endlessly. We believe that we are able to solve all the riddles posed by nature for the benefit of our well-being and prosperity. The fact that environmental problems are largely caused by the application of these very discoveries has been a severe blow to the illusion of the sovereignty of technology. Science has guaranteed us development and prosperity. Now, it has revealed its hidden face: the dangers of its uncontrolled use and our inclination to exploit nature beyond its tolerance. In the same vein, the unwelcome reality of the dependence of man on nature instead of the illusion of full autonomy in relation to nature is becoming more conscious, and this awareness is followed by increasing anxiety and a sense of helplessness.

Our second point is the unfathomable quality of the anxiety that tends to be mobilized when basic conditions of life are threatened. The human personality with its conscious and unconscious functions is a result of long development, with major roots in infancy and adolescence. The sense of human security is embedded in deep psychological layers that stem from vital, absolute dependence of the infant on her or his caretaker and from the basic trust that has developed when care has been adequate (Winnicott 1965). Using the basic Kleinian concepts of paranoid-schizoid and depressive anxiety (Klein 1975), Weintrobe's discussion of these deep issues is truly illuminating. Emphasizing the psychological survival aspects inherent in both concepts, she demonstrates how in the midst of anxieties about climate change these two positions are activated and aim for psychological survival by using different strategies, the former in a maladaptive and the latter in an adaptive way. Also, her thorough analysis of the concept of disavowal deserves special mention.

It follows from the structure of the mind that the developmentally early and functionally most primitive mental manoeuvres are mobilized when a massive anxiety, covered or open, is actualized. Due to its non-verbal and all-encompassing nature, the dependence of man on nature as a supplier of vital means for life is very difficult to acknowledge consciously. From this point of view, man's relationship to nature and its resources bears an important analogy to the original absolute dependence of a baby in her/his union with the caretaker in the beginning of the life-cycle (Lehtonen 1994; Lehtonen et al. 2006). We suggest our inability to recognize the influence of the limitations in the man–environment relationship and the tendency to succumb to denial and disavowal of the real threats may derive from these primitive psychological sources. *Modern man is like a baby-adult in her or his relationship to the basic survival issues that arise from the present conflict between natural resources, their usage and the modern vision of successful life.*

Nonetheless, anxiety that hardly has words for its expression needs to be recognized, shared and to become accepted as a valid aspect of the problem and to be taken into account in questions of how to deal with climate change. Otherwise, the weak part of our mind cannot be changed, nor can its implicit tendency to denial when problems without a clear shape arise. The effects of denial and disavowal as depicted by Weintrobe are seen all over in the debate on the nature and dangerousness of climate change. Arguments that it is not yet actual but will only happen sometime in the future and that the evidence is not fully confirmed, or that the United States and China first have to decide on action, or a little warming is not bad, and so on, are all responses revealing partial acknowledgement and simultaneous denial that only end in non-commitment and non-verification of the global signs of the changes. At bottom, the problem continues to be by-passed.

The point is not in looking to cure our psychological make-up when problems exceeding our coping capacity are encountered. The anxieties mobilized by climate change cannot be blown away or rendered neutral by any psychological measures. The real climate problems that are part of the present environmental neurosis cannot be resolved or removed by any means. On the contrary, they have become a part of our living conditions. Climate change and its consequences constitute limiting factors in our physical and biological as well psychological existence. The imbalance in the ratio between population growth and available safe energy, as well as the imbalance between energy demands and oil resources, are facts that together will make a critical oil-price factor around the year 2015, according to recent forecasts (Sackinger 2011).

Under these unwelcome conditions, it is important to pay attention to the effects of primitive psychological measures, denial as negation and disavowal first and foremost, that are activated by the threats, and to show ways to cope with the threats without seeking security from reality-distorting denial. Understanding the deep, anxiety-evoking psychological impact of the threats activated by climate change can provide an opportunity to find alternative, better adaptive modes of coping with the psychological malaise that is increasingly being felt. As long as the primitive psychological mechanisms continue their blurring effects on our relationship with the environment, we will be invalidated and incapable of thinking in a mature and productive way about the challenges imposed upon us by man-made climate change, and of seeking constructive means to handle them, whatever that may imply.

The point made by Weintrobe, that primitive anxiety leads to loss of proportionate, sensible thinking and may lead to an attack on further development of the human capacity to think, is, in our opinion, extremely important. Thus, the question is not to diminish the anxiety, but to make it tolerable so that constructive thinking can proceed.

We would like to end with a reminder that what has been analysed and suggested above as pertaining to our psychological maladaptation to climate change creates a mental scene that exceeds the adaptive powers of any individual. Coping with issues of the magnitude of climate change is not possible at an individual level. Facing the uncertainties posed by current threats is only possible by joint effort in a social community, and for that purpose real, not idealized, leadership is required, as Weintrobe points out (see also Välimäki and Lehtonen 2009 on the role of leadership). As quoted by Harold Bloom (1997: xxxvi), this principle had already been elegantly expressed by Francis Bacon: 'Certain it is, though a great secret in nature, that the minds of men in company are more open to affections and impressions than when alone.'

Highlighting the psychological, largely unconscious, aspects of human responses to coping with climate change can be of aid in this effort and can increase social trust in the human community, enabling it to face and respond creatively to the unwelcome signs of the changes that are already visible.

References

Bloom, H. (1997) *The Anxiety of Influence* (2nd ed.) Oxford: Oxford University Press.

Klein, M. (1975) *Love, Guilt and Reparation & Other Works 1921–1945*. London: Hogarth Press and The Institute of Psycho-Analysis.

Lehtonen, J. (1994) On the psychology of oil-dependence. *Mind and Human Interaction*, 5: 3–5.

Lehtonen, J., Partanen, J., Purhonen, M., Valkonen-Korhonen, M., Könönen, M., Saarikoski, S., and Launiala, K. (2006) Nascent body ego: Metapsychological and neurophysiological aspects. *International Journal of Psychoanalysis*, 87: 1335–1353.

Sackinger, W. (2011) *Prospects of World Energy Economy until 2050*. Paper presented at a Senior Expert Advisers' meeting, Katajanokan Casino, Helsinki, 21 Jan.

Välimäki, J., and Lehtonen, J. (2009) Ilmastonmuutoksen torjuntaan tarvitaan johtajuutta. [Leadership is required for the counteracting climate change, in Finnish]. *Kanava*, 37 (6): 341–344.

Winnicott, D. W. W. (1965) From dependence towards independence in the development of the individual. In *The Maturational Processes and the Facilitating Environment*. London: Hogarth Press.

Discussion

The difficult problem of anxiety in thinking about climate change

Angela Mauss-Hanke

In her excellent chapter Sally Weintrobe describes one of the basic conflicts of human beings in our attitudes to climate change: that between our realistic part, concerned not only about ourselves but also about those we feel related to, and our narcissistic part, concerned about nothing but ourselves and the fulfilment of our egocentric wishes. In the example of little Katie, Weintrobe shows us vividly the basic anxieties that can arise within us when we have to face unwanted, frightening changes in our lives: the fear of the narcissistic part that it will not survive if it accepts the reality of those changes and adapts itself towards them in a reasonable way, and the anxiety of the realistic part that what and whom we depend upon in life might have been damaged by our narcissistic rage and will therefore cut benevolent connection with us.

We are familiar with the idea that there is no other time in life in which we are more dependent on these benevolent relationships than during early childhood. Babies who have nobody to feed and caress them die. But when we empathize with a baby, we assume that in the earliest stages of life there is no conscious conception of what relationships are, what is 'me' and 'you'; the other is perhaps felt as an extension of the self. A newborn baby sees its surroundings and other people as a part of itself. In a way it expects the other to have just one assignment: to serve the baby's needs and to comfort it. Little children do not yet have any consideration about the needs of others. Mummy is being woken up and her breast has to be full of milk whenever I am hungry and regardless of whether Mummy is totally worn out. In early childhood hunger is felt like an existential threat. In order for me to survive, Mummy cannot have needs herself – she must be there to serve my needs. And whenever those needs are not fulfilled sufficiently, little children can become immensely angry and terribly frightened at the same time: angry because Mummy does not function the way I expect, and frightened because Mummy might turn away or becomes angry herself because she has been hurt by the attacks of the angry child.

I will transpose this situation between baby and mother into the situation between us and 'Mother Earth'. Weintrobe describes three ways to defend ourselves against such existential anxieties in combination with ongoing climate change. The first is feeling 'magically big and powerful' – that is, going on to insist on economic growth and the needlessness of changing (i.e. adapting) our thinking and behaviour to real circumstances. The second is projecting our anxieties into others, and I wonder whether the most powerful and at the same time most destructive way of doing this might be to project our anxieties onto our environment by insisting on economic growth and the needlessness of changing anything. Because, by doing this, we would seem to turn the situation upside down by forcing this very environment on which we existentially depend into the role of the one (the baby) who is desperately dependent on us in order to survive.

The third way of defending ourselves is denying the damage being done to the climate. Denial takes centre stage in Weintrobe's examination of possible ways that we have to cope with our anxieties. She distinguishes two main forms of denial: denial as negation – that is, a sort of denial that can be 'worked through' with good enough 'outer support' and growing inner strength – and denial as disavowal. In disavowal Weintrobe sees a 'more organized and enduring defensive structure' based on 'radical splitting': reality is noticed, and at the same time it is ignored. When this defensive structure is dominated by the side of the ego that denies reality, the arrogant tendency that Weintrobe describes is at work and a feeling of triumph spreads out because narcissistic greedy wishes have won over the cognition of reality. But it is, paradoxically, this very triumph that may cause even deeper anxieties as the healthy realistic part, though being ignored, still silently knows that something is rotten in the inner state. When we look around at the political and economic decisions being made worldwide with respect to ongoing anthropogenic climate change, we can observe this domination of disavowal on many occasions and many levels.

Climate change is something that splits our inner and outer world into normal and at the same time deeply threatening circumstances. It is a change that does not necessarily affect all our daily lives, and at the same time it threatens mankind at the most basic level. 'We need a healthy Earth and biosphere to stay alive', Weintrobe says. But we know we have already damaged 'Mother Earth' in a way that is irreversible by having used up within a century or so most treasures of the soil – treasures that were formed over millions of years. Nevertheless we still fly from A to B, though we could easily take the train – and when we read the newspaper while sitting in the plane and see pictures of arid landscapes and starving children, we are shocked.

Weintrobe describes several 'realistic survival anxieties' about climate change: the anxiety about loss of the Earth, the anxiety about loss of the future and generativity, the anxiety about not being protected by our political leaders and anxiety about our destructiveness. But she also points out that 'climate change can revive our early childhood fears of damage'. I think it is worth while to take a closer look at the threatening circulus vitiosus she describes here about our early childhood fears – namely, that the revival of frightening feelings can cause emotional apathy, and growing emotional apathy can cause an intensification of early childhood anxieties. This apathy as a mental state marks a cul-de-sac that, on a psychic level, resides in an abysmal inner no-man's-land, as it were, in which the split between the illusionary feeling of living in a healthy and 'good-enough' environment on the one hand and the knowledge that this environment is being threatened even more if we go on to pretend that we are able to stick to this illusion is to the fore. In this apathetic state neither emotional cognition nor development seems possible because any progression is anticipated as realization of climate change that must and can be avoided, whereas in reality it is already a matter of fact. It is a claustrophobic position, with little room for backward or forward movement.

I suggest that we need to distinguish between two forms of anxiety at play in this psychodynamic state. First, the anxiety of entering a terra incognita – that is, the fear of the unknown which requires letting go of the familiar without knowing the new; and, second, a *terra cremata* that involves the fear of re-entering psychic territories that had once been experienced as something most threatening and were therefore 'burned down' (from the Latin *cremare* – to burn) – that is, they were psychically destroyed.

What does this mean with respect to climate change? I suggest that terra incognita is being faced with our task to develop totally new approaches concerning the use of natural resources. The *terra cremata* is the inner 'land' of an existential vulnerability and dependence – a terribly frightening and traumatic experience we all went through as babies (though, of course, at very different levels, frequencies and intensities) and which we overcame by developing our autonomy in order never ever again to be so vulnerable and dependent!

In this way of conceptualizing the situation we face, the encapsulating of trauma, involving splitting, creates a psychic 'void' that is strenuously defended and in which the delusion is maintained that there is no damage, At the same time, the emotions and thought processes that were involved in the traumatic event as well as the psychic surroundings undergo an active, albeit unconscious, change *themselves*.

Weintrobe speaks about 'attacks on thinking' – that is, in order to hold on to an illusionary standpoint, we can not only think something untrue though we know better, but we might furthermore attack and therefore damage our thinking capability itself. Any development that is anticipated and at the same time vehemently resisted, like ongoing climate change, involves a psychic movement in which an inner *terra cremata* must be reinvigorated in order to reach a *terra incognita*. It involves a retreat to a primitive developmental state in order to work through a situation in which the new and the damaged are intertwined. In this primitive state, mature (realistic) means of communication and functions may be destroyed and replaced by immature (illusionary, narcissistic) ones. When the immature gains the upper hand in a mature stage, it loses its meaningful place in the structure of the whole and thus puts that very psychic structure at risk. The paradoxical result is the outbreak of dreaded and unbearable catastrophic anxiety.

I think it is this anxiety that Weintrobe describes when she speaks about 'unbearable anxiety' as 'the biggest psychic barrier to facing the reality of anthropogenic global warming', and I totally agree with her conclusion: 'Perhaps one step towards engagement is to recognize the difficulty.' As psychoanalysts, we should engage ourselves first of all by providing our knowledge about psycho-dynamic processes, as Weintrobe does, by showing some of the main obstacles that hinder us from engaging more intensely in activities against climate change. Let us as a last step in this discussion of Weintrobe's very helpful and clarifying thoughts remind ourselves of what we have learned about childhood develop-ment: namely, that when facing any existential threats like that of climate change, we regress to early childhood states. But, as no regression is endless and absolute, we can at the same time remind ourselves how we learned to let go of the illusion that our mother is nothing but a wish-fulfiller. We can remind ourselves how we even learned to understand that our mother has her own needs and must be treated with respect, especially after we have treated her badly, and even more so when she becomes seriously weak. And we can become aware of Mother Earth being so many generations older than all of us without being replaceable in the way we can be.

Chapter 4

Climate change in a perverse culture

Paul Hoggett

A fragile consensus

In the wake of Copenhagen there is accumulating evidence that the public consensus around climate change is very fragile. For example, in the United Kingdom a BBC survey revealed that between November 2009 and January 2010 there had been an 8% rise in the proportion of adults not believing in global warming (Guardian 8 Feb. 2010). Two weeks later, an Ipsos Mori survey indicated that the proportion of adults who believed climate change is 'definitely' a reality had dropped from 44% to 31% over the previous year (Ipsos Mori 2010). Whether the swing in public attitudes was influenced by the failure of Copenhagen, by the media furore surrounding accusations of malpractice by researchers at the Climatic Research Unit of the University of East Anglia (UEA) and criticisms of the Intergovernmental Panel on Climate Change (IPCC) or by the unusually cold winter in the United Kingdom and United States is open to question. What cannot be doubted, however, is the fickleness of public opinion on this issue. Even before the attacks on the IPCC, in the late autumn of 2009 the UK Department of Energy and Climate Change published research indicating that over 50% of UK citizens did not believe that climate change would affect them, and only 18% believed that it will have an impact during their children's' lifetime (DECC 2009). Meanwhile in the United States the Pew Research Centre released findings from their latest survey of public opinion, which indicated that over the previous year the percentage of US citizens believing that there was no solid evidence of global warming had increased from 21% to 33% (Pew Research Centre 2009).

In contrast to this weakening of public belief in anthropogenic climate change, many of the contributors to the IPCC's Fourth Assessment Report (AR4) now believe that the original aim of Kyoto, to limit temperature rises to 2°C (capping emissions at 450 parts per million), is already unrealizable and that the best that can be hoped for is to limit rises to 4°C. The problem is that despite the overwhelming scientific evidence there appears to be widespread public denial that we are facing a crisis.

Two kinds of fatal disconnections seem to be at work here. First, there appears to be a gap between scientific knowledge and public opinion, something I explore further on in this chapter under the heading of 'perverse thinking'. Second, there is a gap between opinion and behaviour; thus, even those who express concern about climate change may do little about it. A good review of research findings from social science is provided by Kollmuss and Agyeman (2002). Individuals may have formed opinions that are favourable to taking action, and yet action may still not occur because: (a) there may objectively be little they can do (e.g. no public recycling schemes, no sympathetic political party to vote for); (b) they have little belief in their own ability to effect changes in their circumstances (a low internal locus of control) and there are no wider networks of like-minded people to act in concert with; (c) the framework of government policies, taxes and subsidies either fails to incentivize pro-environmental behaviour (e.g. the absence of feed-in tariffs to encourage the use of domestic renewables) or provides a disin-centive to such behaviour (e.g. public transport is too expensive to use); (d) people perceive that there is little they can do to make a difference because they believe either that it is too late or that the key changes need to be made by others (e.g. one's own or other governments), an attitude illustrated by the following contribution to an online debate:

> How much of the overall world CO_2 emissions will be reduced if the UK stopped producing CO_2 altogether? Answer less than 1.6%, and if it stopped all forms of emissions from cars it would be a drop of less that 0.01%. In other words, no effect whatsoever.
>
> (Times online, 12 Oct. 2009)

Much of this research is eminently useful and offers practical indications about how climate change communications can be made more effective. However, there are problems with the research, not least the way in which the notion of a 'gap' (between knowledge, opinion and action) oversimplifies what may be much more complex relations (Lertzman 2010). Indeed, much of this research is not based upon a particularly complex understanding of the human mind and necessarily operates with rather simplified models of human behaviour. It tends to assume a unitary and rational self, not one that is torn, ambivalent and in two minds (or several minds, for that matter); nor one whose sense of self, other, environ-ment and so on is governed by powerful narratives, meanings and imaginings; nor one besieged by potentially overwhelming emotions such as fear, despair, anxiety, guilt, love or hope.

A second problem is the tendency to separate the psychological from the social. Much of the research and many of the models are primarily psychological in focus, and yet it is possible that some of the essential clues to understanding the fatal disconnections I mentioned earlier may only come from an analysis that integrates psychological with socio-political perspectives. The danger of a psychologizing analysis is that it can collude unwittingly with policymakers who may be tempted to locate the problem in the individual rather than in the culture in which the individual is situated. As Hamilton indicated in his reflections on

Monbiot's book *Heat*, 'it is quite consistent for a person who does not opt to buy green electricity to vote for a party that promises to compel us all to buy it. Insisting on a collective response to a collective problem is far more politically practical and environmentally responsible than a politics of guilt' (Hamilton 2007: 101).

In this chapter I argue for the value of examining some of the socio-political underpinnings of climate change denial. In particular I suggest that there is a perverse dimension to the culture of advanced Western societies, one particularly pronounced in neo-liberal societies such as the United States and the United Kingdom, and it is this dimension that provides part of the cultural support for climate change denial.

The perverse structure

Three decades of neo-liberal economic and social policies finally came to a singular crisis with the financial crash, which began in September 2008. In an interesting analysis of the crash, Lent (2008) argued that it was the destruction of civility that lay at its heart. He construed civility as the capacity and willingness to think beyond self to other and to accept restraint upon one's own desires in order to protect the well-being of others. He noted that even conservative thinkers such as David Willets and John Gray believed that civility has been systematically undermined by the avid free-market economics of neo-liberalism. He suggested that the resulting crisis of civility found expression on the streets (rising crime and anti-social behaviour), in the workplace (increased stress levels, bullying), in rising levels of childhood unhappiness and, crucially, in economic life itself.

One of the first writers to explore the re-emergence of anti-social behaviour in corporate life in a critical and analytic way was Long in her book *The Perverse Organization and its Deadly Sins* (Long 2008). Long's book is particularly valuable because it provides a psycho-social analysis of the practices of organizations such as Enron and Long Term Capital Management (LTCM) whose anti-social practices can now be understood not as one-off aberrations but as precursors for the way in which the whole financial services sector operated in London and New York. Long argued that the malpractices at Enron and LTCM must be seen not in terms of the deviant behaviour of powerful executives but as an organized structure, something she calls *the perverse structure*. Long outlined five dimensions of this structure:

1   It involves the pursuit of individual pleasure at the expense of others (excessive bonuses, share options, the use of tax havens, etc.).
2   It occurs in a situation where reality (i.e. the reality that the wealth being generated by the firm is largely fictitious and illusory) is simultaneously accepted and denied.
3   The deviant practices require the collusion of others (auditors, accountants, tax lawyers) as accomplices.

4   It flourishes where instrumental relations dominate (i.e. where the 'other' has no intrinsic worth or value but is seen purely as a means to an end).
5   Once such practices take hold they become normalized, and perversion begets perversion.

Long is well aware of the psychoanalytic literature on perversion, but what is particularly interesting about her analysis is the way in which she pushed us to think of perversion as an organized phenomenon.

Loss and the perverse response

Within the psychoanalytic world, denial has been linked to perversion since Freud. Freud develops his ideas on denial in his papers on 'Negation' (Freud 1925) and 'Fetishism' (Freud 1927). Faced with an unpalatable reality, Freud suggested that we may resort to one of two mechanisms – outright rejection, where we simply do not see what is in front of us, and disavowal, where one part of the mind sees while another discounts what is seen (this is Long's second dimension).

While classical psychoanalysis specifically locates perversion in terms of sexuality (fetishism being one form of sexual perversion), more recently there has been considerable interest in perversion as a corruption of thinking, as a state of mind that can characterize an individual or group. In a way perhaps particularly pertinent to climate change denial, Steiner (1993) sees perversion as a way of not coming to terms with loss. For Steiner, if we are to truly come to terms with the fundamental aspects of the human condition – our dependency on others, our mortality, the necessary constraints upon our desires – then we must face up to loss.[1] But in the perverse state of mind such realities are denied. Steiner (1993: 89) goes so far as to suggest that sexual perversion may be a special instance of a more general perverse attitude. In this more general sense perversion involves a turning away from what is true and right or, more strongly, an obstinate or stubborn persistence in what is untrue and unreasonable (here the resonance with climate change denial seems particularly strong). In this sense perversion also has connotations of deviance, of leading oneself or another astray. At this time Steiner was developing a very interesting theory concerning the existence of what he called a 'pathological organization' in the mind and hence his belief that one part of the mind could be 'perverted, led astray, or corrupted by an agency working against what is true or right' (Steiner 1993: 89). Crudely put, we could say that whereas Freud suggests (through his idea of the superego) that there is a policeman inside our head, Steiner adds that there may also be a 'pimp' inside our head (a fixer who seduces us with his promises and propaganda and tells us that we should be able to have what we want). This focuses our attention on the 'relational' character of perversion in which the role of collusion is paramount. From this perspective there is not only a collusion going on internally and in the outside world but there is also a collusion going on between internal and external forces.

Returning to the theme of loss, the perverse aim is to protect us from having to face reality rather than helping us to confront it (Steiner 1993: 93). It arises at the point where outright and sustained rejection of reality (the psychotic response) becomes increasingly untenable. To use an analogy, the well-known phenomenon of 'mid-life crisis' emerges at that point where it becomes increasingly unrealistic to deny the intimations of one's own mortality. Our earlier child-like rejection becomes increasingly anomalous as our parents die, our hair recedes and our flesh droops. Whereas in outright rejection, reality and belief are kept completely split apart and there is a retreat from truth to omnipotence (Steiner 1993: 129), the perverse attempt to deal with reality occurs when some kind of integration between belief and reality has begun. Steiner, reflecting on Freud's discussion of fetishism (Freud 1927), reminds us that the perverse response is 'artful', and I think this helpfully prompts us to consider a state of mind and set of practices that thrive on ambiguity, illusion, evasiveness, trickery, collusion and guile. This is the territory of half-truth, of distortion, of compliance with the letter while defeating the intention or spirit of the law. Returning to Long, this is the territory of Enron, Barclays Offshore Funds, Jersey Finance, and so on.

Once more, I believe this is very pertinent to climate change. While, particularly in the United States, there remain a large number of 'outright deniers', they are no longer the majority. Despite the recent criticisms of climate science, the sheer weight of scientific evidence is forcing intimations of reality upon us all; it is at this point that the perverse response comes into its own. The majority of us in the West 'know' the facts, but we turn away from what we know. The value of Long's work is that she provides us with a map or framework with which to explore the different dimensions of this perverse structure.

Perverse pleasure

Greed has increasingly become good, not bad. We should have what we want, and we should have it now. The expansion of consumer credit, a particular phenomenon of the neo-liberal regimes in the United Kingdom and the United States, reinforced this illusion. As psychoanalytically informed commentators such as Mishan (1996) have argued, here was the cultivation of that omnipotent, greedy, child-like part of the subject. An instrumental orientation to nature was no longer just a characteristic of science and industry but increasingly of a greedy citizenry. This lay at the heart of Lasch's lament about the decline of some kind of authority that could set a limit to desire, a lament that continued throughout several of the books he wrote from the mid-1970s onwards (Lasch 1978, 1984).

Long argued that the perverse state of mind involves the pursuit of one's individual pleasure at the expense of others. This connects to the element of cruelty in perversion, the callous indifference to the fate of the other upon whom one's own pleasure depends. There seems to be an arrogant element of entitlement here (Weintrobe 2010), one perhaps widely shared by Western consumers in their unwillingness to face the costs to others of their lifestyles, but exemplified by the greed of the corporate executives in the investment banks and hedge funds. This is a parasitic form of capital that, like the private equity company, feeds off the wealth created by more productive forms of capital such as manufacture and personal services. But while these parasitic relations are exemplified by finance capitalism, they also characterize relations between the developed and developing world, a perspective particularly associated with the 'underdevelopment theory' of Frank (2001) and the theory of 'unequal exchange' of Amin (1977). Climate change threatens greatly to amplify this dynamic. Current estimates suggest that warming is proceeding quicker on the African subcontinent than elsewhere, with dire estimates concerning desertification, the collapse of food production and famine. The *Human Impact Report: Climate Change, the Anatomy of a Silent Crisis* produced by the Global Humanitarian Forum in 2009 and chaired by Kofi Anan estimates that 300,000 people a year are already dying as a direct result of climate change.[2]

In a further twist to the theme of perverse pleasure, Davar (2004) suggested that the perverse state of mind is one in which the subject confuses his individual pleasure with the other's good. In the sexual perversions this is illustrated by the propaganda of the paedophile, where he (and occasionally she) convinces himself that his victim was a willing partner to the relationship. This reminded me of the reflections of Waddell and Williams (1991) on the perverse state of mind in which they note the way in which attacks on truth often assume the form of internal propaganda which distorts and inverts reality in a way reminiscent of Orwell's *Newspeak* – War is Peace, Freedom is Slavery – and Shakespeare's Macbeth – 'Fair is foul and foul is fair'. With this in mind, I was reminded of one of the core rationales of neo-liberalism, namely 'trickle-down theory', which argues that tax cuts for the rich and other forms of regressive redistribution will benefit the common citizen as the activities of these wealth creators will trickle down to benefit us all (selfishness is beneficence).

Perverse thinking

One problem facing citizens in the developed world is that we are cursed by our knowledgeability. Information saturates the world in which we live, and as a consequence we cannot but help know about things we would rather not know about: things such as global inequality and poverty, or massacres and pogroms, some of which, as in Bosnia, occur on our very doorstep. In his compelling book *States of Denial*, Stan Cohen (2001) argues forcefully that in post-Holocaust society organized denial has become a crucial mechanism for sustaining citizen apathy in the face of violence, injustice and disaster. We 'know' and yet we seem ill-equipped to bear the pain of what we know. In the perverse state of mind reality is not rejected outright but is simultaneously acknowledged and disavowed. Rather than imagining a single mechanism at work here, it is more useful to consider the existence of a range of perverse stances.

Scepticism

At what point does scepticism become perverse? In the early phases of any scientific inquiry, such as that which investigated the links between smoking and cancer, scepticism plays a constructive role in the development of a robust body of evidence. But once such a body of evidence has been established, then the stance of the sceptic increasingly becomes an obstinate or stubborn persistence in what is untrue or unreasonable – that is, it becomes increasingly perverse.

Doubt is central to scepticism, yet doubt is a complex and slippery thing. Steiner gave the example of the troubled individual who has gained some insight into his condition and yet does not change. Steiner noted that 'chance seems to play an important role in this process, as it forms the vital flaw through which truth can be attacked. Everything may point to the initial truthful observation but it has not been proved beyond doubt; there is still a chance that it may be wrong' (Steiner 1985: 168).

The capacity for doubt has been seen by some as one of the most important *virtues* of a contemporary society (Beck 1997). But many climate change sceptics use the enlightenment virtue of doubt as their defence, and the reliance of climate change science on estimates regarding future trends provides such sceptics with the flaw through which truth can be attacked. Sceptics argue that estimates are estimates, not proof. Absolute truth is demanded, and in its absence the truth-value of accumulated evidence and theory is annihilated. This is exactly the same process that occurs in creationist attacks on evolutionism and provides the former with the rationale for asserting that evolutionism is an 'opinion' with no greater claim to truth than religion. This is a perverse misrepresentation of the process of science. Philosophers of science (Lakatos and Musgrave 1970) have demonstrated that all scientific communities are faced with anomalies – that is, with evidence that does not fit with the emerging scientific consensus. In other words, no scientific truth can ever achieve absolute verifiability. But ideologists use this as the basis for questioning the entire truth-value of a scientific outlook.

Within the perverse logic of the ideologist, those outside the consensus are the real bearers of truth; in contrast, the 'consensus' is construed as an exclusive group of insiders, a conspiracy against free-thinkers, a 'highly politicized scientific circle', according to the Republican populist Sarah Palin. As Hulme noted, in areas like climate science, where the attempt is made to understand the behaviour of large complex systems that cannot be replicated in the lab, consensus-building is the only way forward. He added,

> reaching consensus about climate change, recognizing that these statements emerge from processes of deliberation and discussion rather than from pure observation, experimentation and falsification, can therefore be an uncomfortable thing for scientists and public alike. Scientists need to be prepared to argue about their 'considered opinions', to embrace consensus but without closing down argument or suggesting that matters are settled. And the public

need to recognize that sometimes consensus is the best that science has to offer about a topic.

(Hulme 2010)

Of course there are also plenty of corrupt agencies willing to spread doubt as a way of supporting vested interests. Monbiot's valuable examination of the 'denial industry' in his book *Heat* reveals some of the tactics used by the tobacco industry when faced with the campaign against smoking. As one leaked tobacco industry memo put it: 'Doubt is our product since it is the best means of competing with the "body of fact" that exists in the mind of the general public' (Monbiot 2006: 34).

Turning a blind eye

A second perverse strategy draws upon the human desire 'not to know'. Climate change science covers an enormous range of disciplines and seeks to monitor changes across innumerable ecosystems. The ordinary citizen, who is not a full-time student able to study these issues in depth, encounters evidence in little bits. We hear about things – things that make us anxious and deter us from finding out more. Primo Levi, writing about his experience of the 'Holocaust deniers' who lived in Germany and German-occupied territories at the time of the transportations to the concentration camps, argued 'at that time among the German silent majority, the common technique was to try to know as little as possible, and therefore not to ask questions' (Levi 1986: 222). Speaking of Dr Muller, the officer in charge of the chemical lab at the IG-Farben works, which were within sight of the chimneys of the Buna crematorium at Auschwitz, Levi called him 'a typically grey human specimen . . . one of the not so few one-eyed men in the Kingdom of the Blind' (Levi 1986). Interestingly enough, Steiner also used the phrase 'turning a blind eye' as a key device to understand the way in which perverse denial operates, including denial of the possibility of nuclear or ecological catastrophes (Steiner 1985). Taking the phrase from Vellacott's reinterpretation of the Oedipal myth, 'turning a blind eye' is a method whereby a truthful experience is drained of its emotional significance, leaving it simply as a 'useless fact'. We 'know' – and yet what we know no longer disturbs us, the meaningfulness of the thought has been drained away, denuded by the corrupt agency inside our head. For the American social theorist Mestrovic (1997), this has become part of a wider cultural phenomenon, the phenomenon of disposable emotion. Mestrovic, shocked by the absence of Western reaction to the slaughter occurring in Bosnia in the early 1990s, argued that emotions are no longer designed to disturb us: they are throw-away or post-emotions, part of a throw-away society.

Internal propaganda

Perversity involves an *artful* engagement with the truth and propaganda and is essential to this process. But this is internal propaganda, the distortions, rationalizations and little half-truths we tell ourselves. Hamilton and Kasser (2009) have catalogued many of these. Besides selective inattention, the scale of the threat or its imminence can be reduced (Homburg, Stolberg, and Wagner 2007), the degree of scientific dissent can be overemphasized, the technological resourcefulness of humanity can be overestimated ('they'll come up with something before things get too bad') or the resilience of nature can be exaggerated. Or, if some of the emotional disturbance does break through, then the individual can engage in token actions like carbon offsetting to mollify feelings of helplessness and guilt (Stoll-Kleeman, O'Riordan, and Jaeger 2001). They can also escape feelings of anxiety by resorting to pleasure seeking ('make hay while the sun shines'), escape feelings of guilt by resorting to 'blame shifting' ('it's the fault of Americans/Chinese/Indians etc.') or can escape any feeling by 'emotional numbing'. The danger is that as such artful attempts to avoid facing the truth break down, denial can become increasingly tinged with despair and a sense of imminent catastrophe, leading to either a cynical, resigned, survivalist or redemptive stance (Hoggett 2011).

Perverse thinking in a virtual world

For social theorists such as Lyotard (1984) and Baudrillard (1994), one of the defining characteristics of the last decades of the twentieth century was the ascendancy of the image. As images became more powerful and pervaded more and more areas of life, they began to insinuate themselves upon us as somehow more real, more comforting, more vivid and more alive than the 'real thing' (which increasingly got put into inverted commas). Concepts such as Disneyfication (Zukin 1996) and McDonaldization (Ritzer 1993) were flourishing long before the rapid development of Internet-based 'virtual worlds' such as Second Life. The boundary between image and reality, between signifier and signified, was becoming increasingly blurred. Within many areas of postmodern social theory the validity of such distinctions as real/unreal and true/false was itself subject to sustained challenge, a process that encouraged the development of relativism, as any stable criteria on which to make judgements and distinctions (including ethical ones) were subject to attack. But it was not only our orientation to our world that took on an *as if* quality, but also our orientation to ourselves and our own actions. It became increasingly difficult for us to tell when we were simulating and when we were not – a predicament captured by Hochschild in her concept of 'deep acting' (Hochschild 1983).

A virtual economy

There is an ongoing argument about the legitimacy of distinguishing between the 'real' economy on the one hand and the 'virtual' economy on the other. First, some authors such as Zizek (2009) regard the distinction as misleading, whereas others see the distinction as a useful way of understanding the distinctive characteristic of neo-liberalism. What cannot be doubted is that financial transactions can now occur in 'real time' on a global scale, making it possible for traders to 'bet' against movements in prices on a continuous basis (and, because of the instantaneousness and unmediated nature of communication in global financial markets, this provides the precondition for amplified crowd dynamics such as hysteria, panic and contagion).

Second, economic activity in this sector has become increasingly 'disembedded' (Carrier and Miller 1997) – that is, abstracted from social relations. This is a process that also enhances the tendency of economists, politicians and ordinary citizens to reify the market, to view the market as a thing in itself, a phantasmagoria existing beyond human interference (as Margaret Thatcher used to say: 'you can't buck the markets') that has no connection to the human activities and relations – including relations of power – that are its real foundation.

Third, the new technologies have provided the conditions of possibility for a range of new forms of finance capital (new products and services such as Collateralized Debt Obligations) whose abstracted nature has become so exaggerated that those who work with these new products and those who manage those who work with them have found themselves increasingly at the limits of their comprehension of the very things that they have created (Seivers 2010). One consequence was that, as the crunch approached, banks and other financial institutions were unable initially to identify the 'extent of their exposure to the credit crisis' (Poynter 2009: 3). As Seivers put it, 'many if not most role holders in the financial industry were unable to calculate the risk of their transactions, much less to understand the instruments and products they were dealing with' (Seivers 2010: 132). Long mentioned that, even at Enron, it was difficult to know precisely whether it was the senior executives' arrogant certitude and hubris, their ruthless self-interest *or* their capacity for self-deception that drove the corporation to destruction (Long 2008: 36–37).

As the real economy became increasingly eclipsed by the virtual one, it became more difficult for actors in the financial sector to know what was real and what was false. An illusional space opened up, riddled with ambiguity, in which transgression was invited precisely because the boundaries between truth and lie, propriety and corruption, rule bending and rule breaking, and so forth, had become fatally blurred. It is this kind of space in which perverse practices flourish. This is the soil on which self-deception, or internal propaganda, can thrive.

Virtual governance

Neo-liberalism has had a significant impact on the conduct of government itself through public sector reform programmes, often referred to as the New Public Management, which have attempted to apply private-sector principles and methods to the operation of the public services. Using another Orwellian mantra, 'private is good, public is bad', neo-liberalism propounded the progressive deregulation of markets (facilitating the practices of Enron and all), while at the same time it prescribed the very opposite (i.e. less trust, more regulation and the phobic avoidance of risk) for the public sphere. As a result, a 'targets-and-indicators' culture emerged through which government sought to control the public sphere by attempting to specify, measure and monitor all aspects of the performance of public agencies and of those who worked in them. The attempt to control such complex systems was, of course, futile and only made system failure more likely, with each failure (whether in the sphere of public order, counterterrorism, the protection of children at risk or educational attainment) leading to the reassertion of more controls. Slowly a body of research and scholarship began to accumulate documenting what are often (interestingly) referred to as the 'perverse effects' of government target systems (Bevan and Hood 2006; Coulson 2009). These include the selective reporting and manipulation of information, the 'crowding' of performances to meet the required targets, 'gaming' and so on.

More importantly from the point of view of my argument here, the new systems contributed to the creation of a virtual reality, an 'auditable surface' (Cummins 2001), which then became confused with the reality that it represented. This auditable surface of signifiers (targets, output and outcome indicators and returns, inter-organizational comparators, activity plans and reports, risk assessments and reviews, etc.) acted as a proxy or stand-in for what was actually going on – a phenomenon Miller (2005) referred to as 'virtualism'. The problem was that governments began to believe that this virtual reality was actually the real thing. A good illustration of the problems this leads to is education policy under Labour governments in the United Kingdom. A ground-breaking recent independent review of primary education undertaken over several years by Cambridge University (Alexander et al. 2009) reveals that: (a) British children are subject to more perform-ance testing than children in any other European country; (b) while their test results have shown significant improvements over time (i.e. it looks *as if* things are getting better), their actual attainment levels compared to children in other OECD coun-tries have stagnated or declined in the same period (discussed in Hoggett 2010).

A virtual politics of climate change?

The danger is that virtual governance may already be infecting the politics of climate change. First, there is the problem of carbon markets. There is an uncanny resemblance between carbon trading and derivative trading schemes, 'with EU carbon permits being traded like securitized debt or derivatives, carbon trading looks potentially like the next sub-prime market' (Prins 2009). As Tickell (2008) indicated, carbon credits under the Kyoto Protocol offered the appearance of a strategy for mitigating climate change while actually providing all sorts of methods of dissimulation (e.g. receiving credits for renewable projects such as hydroelectric schemes, which were already under construction and were therefore not 'new' initiatives at all).

But there is a much greater danger than the creation of quasi-market mecha-nisms, which, rather than driving policy, lead to policy failure. The language of

Kyoto and Copenhagen is the language of targets, and the danger is that it is precisely this language (refined to an extensive degree by successive Labour governments in the United Kingdom) that will appeal to governments who need to look *as if* they are doing something while safe in the knowledge that they will not be in power when it becomes clear that the targets are not being met. As Monbiot said: 'the thought that worries me most is this. . . . We will wish our governments to pretend to act. . . . My fear is that the political parties in the rich nations have already recognized this. They know that we want tough targets, but that we also want those targets to be missed (Monbiot 2006: 41–42).

Much of the evidence available suggests that Kyoto achieved very little. According to Prins and Rayner: 'Kyoto protocol is a symbolically important expression of governments' concern about climate change. But as an instrument for achieving emissions reductions, it has failed. It has produced no demonstrable reductions in emissions or even in anticipated emissions growth (Prins and Rayner 2007: 973).

The UK Climate Change Act of 2008 provides a legally binding target of at least an 80% cut in greenhouse gas emissions by 2050, to be achieved through action in the United Kingdom and abroad, together with a reduction in emissions of at least 34% by 2020 (both these targets are against a 1990 baseline). The Act established an independent Committee on Climate Change whose first annual report (available at: www.theccc.org.uk/reports/progress-reports) in October 2009 made it clear that the apparent good progress on emissions reduction in the United Kingdom to date was a 'false impression' created by the recession and, before that, by the closure of much of manufacturing industry. But the anachronism of a 'world-class' piece of legislation in (a) one of the most deregulated market economies in the world, where (b) the use of renewable energy is lower than in virtually all comparable EU nations (after Malta and Luxembourg), should give us pause for thought.

The joint Oxford University/London School of Economics report *How to Get Climate Policy Back on Course* (Prins et al. 2009) is scathing in its assessment of the Act. Speaking of the targets that have been set, the authors argue:

> It requires Britain, by law, to achieve by 2016 a carbon efficiency of its economy equivalent to that of the world-leading major economy, France. That would require, for example, building and putting into operation 30 nuclear power stations in 7 years. Thereafter, assuming a GDP growth of 2% p.a., a year-on-year annual rate of decarbonization of 5.3% is required to reach the Act's target; whereas there is no record of any economy having achieved greater than 2.0%, and then only for short spells. In sum, this Act requires the UK to achieve the impossible.
>
> (Prins et al. 2009: 9)

Pielke Jr, who writes on public policy and science, concludes that it appears that the world-leading British Climate Act has failed even before it comes into effect and that it will either have to be revisited by Parliament or will simply be ignored by policymakers (Pielke, 2009).

Conclusion

Denial can be seen as a 'solution' to the predicament of what Sloterdijk (1984) called 'the unhappy consciousness' of the socially knowledgeable but materially comfortable citizen of advanced Western-type democracies – an intelligent citizen, but one who must perform his work in spite of this unhappy consciousness. In this chapter I have attempted to situate the psychology of climate change denial in its cultural context. I have construed it as a form of perverse thinking and action, one that has been greatly facilitated by the spread of virtualism in economic and social life. I have speculated that such perversity may have infected the practice of politics itself, leading to a kind of virtual or 'as if' politics in which enormous energy is put into the specification of objectives, targets and indicators and the corresponding demonstration that one's performance is moving towards such targets. The attempt by the British and other governments to set themselves targets for achieving emissions reductions and the attempts to reach international agreement around climate change, first embodied in the Kyoto Protocol and more recently in the failed Copenhagen Summit, in some ways bear an uncanny resemblance to such perverse forms of politics, as though government actors themselves no longer know whether they are simulating or not.

In the post-Copenhagen world the efficacy of politics is in doubt. But perhaps the demise of the top-down regulatory approach to climate change epitomized by Kyoto and Copenhagen is no bad thing. After all, many argue that Kyoto did little more than symbolize political agreement that international action was necessary without being able to achieve it. Regulation is no substitute for direct state intervention through a mix of pricing, taxing, investment support, ownership and control and legal sanctions. The state at national, regional and global level could have a huge role to play in fostering bottom-up developments pioneered by small and large firms, empowered local governments, NGOs, communities and households. But this requires the return of a confident and authoritative state, one with real potency and one not in awe to the phantasm of 'the markets'.

Notes

1 Both Mishan (1996) and Randall (2009) have written specifically about the challenge of facing up to loss in the context of our relations to nature.
2 Available at: www.ghf-geneva.org/Portals/0/pdfs/2009forumreport.pdf

References

Alexander, R., Armstrong, M., Flutter, J., Hargreaves, L., Harlen, W., Harrison, D., et al. (2009) *Children, Their World, Their Education: Final Report and Recommendations of the Cambridge Primary Review*. London: Routledge.

Amin, S. (1977) *Imperialism and Unequal Development*. New York: Monthly Review Press.

Baudrillard, J. (1994) *Simulacra and Simulation*. Ann Arbor, MI: University of Michigan Press.

Beck, U. (1997) *The Reinvention of Politics: Rethinking Modernity in the Global Social Order*. Cambridge: Polity Press.

Bevan, G., and Hood, C. (2006) What's measured is what matters: Targets and gaming in the English public health care system. *Public Administration*, 84 (3): 517–538.

Carrier, J., and Miller, D. (Eds.) (1997) *Virtualism: A New Political Economy*. Oxford: Oxford University Press.

Cohen, S. (2001) *States of Denial*. Cambridge, UK: Polity Press.

Coulson, A. (2009) Targets and terror: Government by performance indicators *Local Government Studies*, 35 (2): 271–282.

Cummins, A. (2001) 'The road to hell is paved with good intentions': Quality assurance as a social defence against anxiety. *Organisational & Social Dynamics*, 2 (1): 99–119.

Davar, E. (2004) The perils of conviction: Addiction, terror, and leadership. *Psychodynamic Practice*, 10 (4): 439–458.

DECC (2009) Department of Energy and Climate Change, 9 Oct. Available at: www.egov-monitor.com/node/29412/print

Frank, A G. (2001) The development of underdevelopment. In: S. Corbridge (Ed.), *Development: Critical Concepts in the Social Sciences*. London: Routledge.

Freud, S. (1925) On negation. In J. Strachey (Ed.), *The Standard Edition of the Complete Psychological Works of Sigmund Freud, Vol. XIX* (pp. 235–239). London: Hogarth Press.

Freud, S. (1927) Fetishism. In J. Strachey (Ed.), *The Standard Edition of the Complete Psychological Works of Sigmund Freud, Vol. XXI* (pp. 149–157). London: Hogarth Press.

Hamilton, C. (2007) Building on Kyoto. *New Left Review*, 45 (May–June): 91–103.

Hamilton, C., and Kasser, T. (2009) *Psychological adaption to the threats and stress of a four degree world*. Paper presented at the 'Four Degrees and Beyond' Conference, Oxford, 28–30 Sept.

Hochschild, A. (1983) *The Managed Heart: The Commercialization of Human Feeling*. Berkeley, CA: University of California Press.

Hoggett, P. (2010) Government and the perverse social defence. *British Journal of Psychotherapy*, 26 (2): 202–212.

Hoggett, P. (2011) Climate change and the apocalyptic imagination. *Psychoanalysis, Culture & Society*, 16 (3): 261–275.

Homburg, A., Stolberg, A., and Wagner, U. (2007) Coping with global environmental problems: Development and first validation of scales. *Environment and Behavior*, 39 (6): 754–778.

Hulme, M. (2010) *The IPCC, Consensus and Science*. 19 Feb. Available at: www.mike-hulme.org

IPCC (2007) *Intergovernmental Panel on Climate Change: Fifth Assessment Report*. Available at: www.ipcc.ch

Ipsos Mori (2010) *Climate Change Omnibus: Great Britain*. London, 24 Feb.

Kollmuss, A., and Agyeman, J. (2002) Mind the gap: Why do people act environmentally and what are the barriers to pro-environmental behavior? *Environmental Education Research*, 8 (3): 239–260.

Lakatos, I., and Musgrave, A. (Eds.) (1970) *Criticism and the Growth of Knowledge.* Cambridge, UK: Cambridge University Press.

Lasch, C. (1978) *The Culture of Narcissism: American Life in an Age of Diminishing Expectations.* New York: Norton.

Lasch, C. (1984) *The Minimal Self: Psychic Survival in Troubled Times.* New York: Norton.

Lent, A. (2008) A crisis of civility. *Renewal*, Sept.

Lertzman, R. (2010) *The Myth of Apathy: Psychosocial Dimensions of Environmental Degradation.* Unpublished PhD Thesis: University of Cardiff.

Levi, P. (1986) *The Periodic Table.* London: Abacus.

Long, S. (2008) *The Perverse Organization and the Seven Deadly Sins.* London: Karnac.

Lyotard, J.-F. (1984) *The Postmodern Condition: A Report on Knowledge.* Manchester: Manchester University Press.

Mestrovic, S. (1997) *Postemotional Society.* London: Sage.

Miller, D. (2005) What is best 'value'? Bureaucracy, virtualism and local governance. In: P. Du Gay (Ed.), *The Values of Bureaucracy.* Oxford: Oxford University Press.

Mishan, J. (1996) Psychoanalysis and environmentalism: First thoughts. *Psychoanalytic Psychotherapy*, 10 (1): 59–70.

Monbiot, G. (2006) *Heat: How to Stop the Planet Burning.* London: Allen Lane.

Pew Research Centre (2009) *Fewer Americans See Solid Evidence of Global Warming.* 22 Oct., people-press.org/report/556/global-warming

Poynter, G. (2009) *The Crunch and the Crisis: The Unravelling of Lifestyle Capitalism.* London: Soundings.

Pielke, R. A., Jr (2009) The British Climate Change Act: A critical evaluation and proposed alternative approach. *Environmental Research Letters*, 18 June. doi: 10.1088/1748–9326/4/2/024010

Prins, G. (2009) *Earthquakes Happen: Recent Developments in Climate Policy.* LSE Mackinder Programme for the Study of Long Wave Events. Available at: www.lse.ac.uk/collections/mackinderProgramme/

Prins, G., and Rayner, G. (2007) Time to ditch Kyoto. *Nature*, 449: 973–975.

Prins, G., Cook., M., Green, C., Hulme, M., Korhola, A., Korhola, E. R., et al. (2009) *How to Get Climate Policy Back on Course.* Institute for Science, Innovation and Policy (University of Oxford) and the LSE Mackinder Programme, 6 July. Available at: www.lse.ac.uk/collections/mackinderProgramme/

Randall, R. (2009) Loss and climate change: The danger of parallel narratives, *Ecopsychology* (Sept.): 118–129.

Ritzer, G. (1993) *The McDonaldization of Society.* Thousand Oaks, CA: Sage Publications.

Seivers, B. (2010) Beneath the financial crisis. In: H. Brunning and M. Perini (Eds.), *Psychoanalytic Perspectives on a Turbulent World* (pp. 117–137). London: Karnac.

Sloterdijk, P. (1984) Cynicism – the twilight of false consciousness. *New German Critique*, 33, 190–206.

Steiner, J. (1985) Turning a blind eye: Psychotic states and the cover up for Oedipus. *International Review of Psychoanalysis*, 12 (2): 161–172.

Steiner, J. (1993) *Psychic Retreats.* London: Routledge.

Stoll-Kleeman, S., O'Riordan, T., and Jaeger, C. (2001) The psychology of denial concerning climate mitigation measures: Evidence from Swiss focus groups. *Global Environmental Change*, 11: 107–117.

Tickell, O. (2008) *Kyoto 2.* London: Zed Books.

Waddell, M., and Williams, G. (1991) Reflections on perverse states of mind. *Free Associations*, 22: 203–213.

Weintrobe, S. (2010) On links between runaway consumer greed and climate change denial: A psychoanalytic perspective. *Bulletin Annual of the British Psychoanalytical Society*, 1: 63–75. London: Institute of Psychoanalysis.

Zizek, S. (2009) *First as Tragedy, Then as Farce*. London: Verso.

Zukin, S. (1996) *The Cultures of Cities*. Oxford: Blackwell.

Discussion
Climate change in a perverse culture

Stanley Cohen

The elementary forms of denial

There is very little that I disagree with in this stimulating chapter by Paul Hoggett. I would merely like to think a bit further about the central role given to the concept of denial and locate the term 'climate change denial' on a wider conceptual grid. I believe that there is near-universal agreement that something like denial plays a central role in assessing the prospects of the climate change movement. 'The problem,' says Hoggett, 'is that despite the overwhelming scientific evidence, there appears to be widespread denial that we are facing a crisis.' There would also be agreement with the opening words of Weintrobe's (2010) paper: 'Why are so many people denying climate change?' This is not a problem of marginal dissidence or maladjustment but is 'widespread' and shared by 'many people'.

Denial as personal defence and social critique

Denial is invariably invoked as a 'gap' or 'disconnect' problem. Hoggett, however, is quite right that there are two very different disconnections at work: one is the gap between scientific knowledge and public belief, the other is the gap between belief (opinion, attitude) and action. In neither case am I concerned with first-order questions about the substance of the claims and counter-claims about climate change but, rather, with the reasons for the existence of climate change denial as a causal link as well as an object of study in itself.

Denial is not a specific concrete social phenomenon. But there are some common threads running through all those diverse cases categorized as 'denial'. We might be tempted by a nihilist version of social constructionism: denial is whatever is called denial. But there is surely some consensus about the lowest common denominator of all states of denial: something like 'the refusal to accept unpleasant realities'. I have traced (Cohen 2001) the original genealogy in psychoanalysis (denial as an unconscious defence mechanism) and its different versions in existential philosophy (self-deception and bad faith) and cognitive psychology (cognitive error). For my pragmatic purposes here, it is enough to use a composite definition: an unwillingness to accept the reality of uncomfortable, painful facts (and/or unconsciously) the repression of such facts. In the Catch 22 version: if the presented reality is too terrible to be true, then it cannot be true; if it were true, things would be too terrible.

There are two lowest common denominators that give a distinctive meaning to the concept of denial. First, strictly speaking, the concept 'should' only be used when the difference between knowing and not-knowing is not what it seems to be. Labelling a state or process as 'denial' implies that something special is going on, something that cannot be explained as genuine inadvertent ignorance or straight-forward chosen lying, but indicates a state of knowing and not-knowing at the same time. You are aware of a fact, yet you fail to acknowledge: (a) its very exist-ence, whether anything at all happened (this is what I have called *literal denial*) or (b) its conventional interpretation – for example, its scientific or legal meaning (*interpretive denial*) or (c) its emotional, moral and political implications (*implicatory denial*).

At first glance this typology applies smoothly enough for climate change denial. First, there is *literal denial*: the records show that nothing like climate change or global warming has happened: this is myth, invented by the left-liberal media, there is no evidence one way or the other. (This, the strongest and most primitive form of denial, is especially present in the climate change case.) Second, there is *interpretive denial*: yes, there might have been some changes, but these could be random fluctuations, they were not anthropogenic (caused by humans), nor can they be attributed to social change, nor are they reversible. Finally, *implicatory denial*: this is a technical, not a moral problem; anyway, why should I feel or do anything about this? Alternatively (but sometimes simultaneously): why should the government do anything?

'True denial' requires the special paradox of knowing and not-knowing *at the same time*. Some of the dialectics of knowing and not knowing were infamously captured by the then US Secretary of State for Defence, Donald Rumsfeld, at a press conference about the Iraq War:

> Reports that say that something hasn't happened are always interesting to me, because, as we know, there are known knowns; there are things that we know that we know. We also know there are known unknowns. That is to say that we now know we don't know. But there are also unknown unknowns. There are things that we don't know we don't know.
>
> (Rumsfeld, 6 June 2002)

He ignored, of course, 'things that we know but say that we don't know'. But even this does not capture the paradoxes of 'knowing' nor the emotional (as opposed to purely cognitive) dimension of the threat: fear about knowing what might be revealed if you look too closely.

The second requirement for a working conception of denial is that it should make sense both in psychological/individual and social/collective terms. Such formulations as 'a culture of denial' or 'British society was in denial about racism', or 'the regime was in denial about its violent past' require not only the special denial paradox, but one or another version of the following links between the personal and the social: (a) the link is *causal* in the sense that the psychic forces determine the social pattern and cultural expressions of denial; (b) the *causal* sequence is reversed: political power and cultural scripts determine the expressions of personal denial; (c) the link is *symbiotic* in the sense that the personal and the political always appear together, the one reinforcing the other; (d) the link is purely *symbolic* – that is, a psychological model (for example, the psychoanalytical reading of denial as a defence mechanism) is projected onto the whole society. Hoggett rightly warns us against the tempting first link: invoking psychological models to explain the social. He offers us instead an ambitious version of link number (c): 'an analysis that integrates psychological with socio-political perspectives'.

This is perhaps too ambitious. Furthermore, the psychic nuances of being in denial might be literally self-contained – that is, contained within the inner world of the self, even the unconscious – and not connected to any cultural, organized or political phenomena. On the other hand the genesis and momentum of the 'denial industry' identified by Monbiot (2009) and others can be understood in political economic terms without much reference to the arcane refinements of Freudian theory.

In the typology that has evolved over the last decade, the specific term 'in denial', is reserved for those personal psychic states that exhibit the denial paradox. These states are private and unique to each person. Other states are public and shared by whole cultures and institutions. This is the vast territory increasingly referred to as cultures of denial (for example, in the police, army, hospitals, civil service, government.) These are the spaces in which Hogget's 'perverse culture' belongs – with its distortions, virtualism and collusion – the illusions that result when self-deception is faced only by moral ambiguity. Criticism of opponents for being 'in denial' has become a fixed part of political rhetoric. The term is used to bestow a spurious strength and psychological depth to certain positions and people. Consider these examples from British and Canadian newspapers in 2009[1]:

> Why the Pakistani security services did not prevent a fatal terrorist attack on the Sri Lankan cricket team: '. . . most of the Pakistani elite are in denial. . . . Pakistan's denial is a bigger problem than analysts usually acknowledge.'
>
> Reporting a UN study on people trafficking: 'Many of the world's governments are in denial about the extent and seriousness of human trafficking.'
>
> The Washington based Policy Institute stated that the UK Government was: 'Stuck in a state of denial on the scale of its illegal immigrant problem.'
>
> 'The Colombian government is painting a positive picture of the human rights situation in Colombia . . . the authorities are in absolute denial, even refusing to admit there's an armed conflict in their country.'

Doing denial

Over the last decade, the major focus of theory and research in the sociology of denial has become the nature of public reactions to knowing about the suffering of distant others. This focus comes from many different interests: the reconstruction of environmental problems into social problems; the status of scientific knowledge about the environment; the 'spectatorship of suffering' (Chouliaraki 2006) and the 'politics of pity'.

The ideology of the 1960s gave rise to many of the concerns and conflicts reflected in the climate change debate. The concerns of the original environmental ('ecological') movement (pollution, energy policy, climate change) do not obviously belong to the categories of either human rights or humanitarianism. There are disagreements within the green movement about whether to pursue such conceptual and political alliances. There are two extreme positions: (a) environmentalism is a meta or mega problem itself – in its religious version, there has been a violent disruption of the natural harmony between humankind and nature; (b) in the secular version, climate change is the greatest man-made threat to the future of the planet. Only concerted and massive political action can 'save the planet'. In a third and more banal view of social problems theory, denial is a stupid, ignorant, Luddite view. The basic scientific consensus agrees with the entire paradigm of climate change. As Monbiot notes, even if you were to exclude every bit of evidence that could possibly be disputed, the evidence for man-made global warming would still be unequivocal.

An increasing proportion of the public, though, do not accept the consensus. Somewhere close to 20% of US voters have 'serious doubts' about climate change. The scientific response is not much more than repeating the bad news: that the public do not realize how bad things are, and when they do understand, they do not do anything. This response may, in turn, leave people feeling even more helpless and threatened, thus reinforcing existing inclinations to remain 'in denial'.

This passive denial merges into the more active (even pro-active) responses that Seu (2010) classified as ways of 'doing denial'. The number and type of verbal accounts for socially problematic behaviour – whether by perpetrators, victims or bystanders – is finite. The repertoire of climate change denial is remarkably close to the accounts that Seu showed are used in response to actual Amnesty International appeals: for example, 'shoot the messenger' – the moral gaze is shifted to the defects of the agencies that collect, interpret and disseminate the information. Questions are asked about their competence, integrity and trustworthiness; their historical record, degree of expertise and sources of funding; their likelihood of delivering on the promise to 'do something now'.

Denialism

Human resistance, however, to knowing (and still greater to 'facing up to') harsh, ugly and unacknowledged realities is profound and ingenious. There seem to be no lengths to which people will not go, no measures, however desperate, they will not devise or improvise to hide partly known realities from self and other. We are talking not about a psychotic refusal to accept visual or verbal evidence, but about a willed and knowing refusal to see the logic and implications of an obvious conclusion, or else an ideological screen that makes people unable to see the world in any other way than they always have.[2] Reactions, however, that appear to be immediate, automatic, even natural, are the products of socialization, education and indoctrination.

These projects constitute denialism, yet another variant of generic denial. In a sense denialism is the polar opposite of 'in denial'. Instead of a personal and private state that might last a lifetime, denialism is expressed in a learned, shared public language; the activities of claim makers and moral entrepreneurs are organized, planned, intentional and – sometimes less obviously – ideological.

The climate change denial industry meets the pure case: institutions and people that are dedicated to advance the denialist programme – corporations and NGOs, research institutions and public relations firms, foundations and the mass media. This work may be ideologically quite open – or in the special sense that commitment to an unregulated free market (and its associated perversities) is ideological. So too is the extreme anti-science strain pervading the US right wing.[3]

Hamilton, in chapter 2 in this volume, shows in fascinating detail how global warming has become a battleground in the wider cultural wars. Denialism correlates with shifts to the right on issues such as gun control, social redistributive policies, creationism and abortion. The opening of the gulf between the new conservatives and the moderate centre was due to the fact that Republican activists, in collaboration with fossil fuel interests and conservative think tanks, 'had successfully associated acceptance of global warming science with "liberal" views' (Hamilton, chapter 2, this volume). Limbaugh knows the enemy: 'The four corners: government, academia, science and media. These institutions are now corrupt and exist by virtue of deceit . . . science has become a home for displaced socialists and communists.'

Scepticism defended

Faced with daily repeat doses of political nonsense, bizarre conspiracy theories and sheer venom, it is easy to understand the refusal of mainstream environmentalists to give – in the name of parity and fairness – 'equal time' to denialism. Whether in a court-room or a research journal, the right to reply leads only to repeating slogans like 'GREEN IS THE NEW RED' – or theories like 'When communism didn't work out, environmentalism became the anti-capitalist vehicle of choice, drawing cash and adulation from business, Hollywood, media and social elites' (Horner 2007: 3).

Two final comments on the anti-denial criticism. First, it seems to me misleading to conceive of climate change denialism as analogous to Holocaust denialism. Some activists have called for Nuremberg-like trials to establish legal responsibility for climate disasters. The comparison is wrong not because some metaphysical reason makes the Holocaust special, but because of a simple non-comparability: The one refers to a well-documented set of events that happened in recorded history; the other is a scientific prediction of what is likely to happen in the future.

Second, we must note that the sad tales, told to win sympathy, support, moral and financial resources for combating denial take for granted the quite extraordinary way the environmental movement has ascended the political agenda. The climate change message – however diluted, compromised and caricatured – has got through to the major social institutions: to the educational system, the mass media, some sections of big business, even to governments. To be sure, action is not congruent with knowledge – but this would also be true for racism, sexism and world poverty.

The soft and cuddly components of the environmentalist movement have become accepted parts of middle-class life style: living green, using recycled toilet paper, batch cooking, insulating pipes, unplugging the printer, not boiling a full kettle for one cup of tea, cosmetics that are 'organic, fair-traded, chemical-free and non-toxic'. The Sunday Supplements and special features in the *Observer, Guardian* and *Telegraph* provide regular guides to living a carbon-friendly life-style.[4]

Everyday life has been successfully penetrated by the anti-denialist message. But the more this knowledge piles up, the more perplexing (and pressing) becomes the question posed in my opening paragraph: how do we explain widespread denial despite the overwhelming evidence?

To be discussed further

Let us start with the social composition of the 'we' who are so worried about the gaps, disconnections and paradoxes for which denial is a strategic solution. The environmental movement has always been elite-driven. The scientists, professionals, economists, politicians plus the more enlightened middle class and some radical post-1960s activists were responsible for the translation of scientific problems into social problems. They were moral entrepreneurs who drew on the classic repertoire of moral panics to create new rules – for example, new laws (including criminal law), regulations and government policy to prevent or ameliorate dangers such as global warming. In the public arena, this project was immediately opposed – whether rationally by interest groups from big business and government or irrationally from anti-science and pseudo-science. Soon enough, evidence became claims; claims generated counter-claims; some counter-claims became fully-fledged denials – literal, interpretive and implicatory.

I believe that we need a flowing, fluid narrative like this, rather than the static image of 'gaps', to study both the internal discourse and how (or whether) this reaches the everyday concerns of ordinary people. Thomas (2006) places these subjects together:

In the macho world of politics and ecological debate, it is all too easy to get sucked into a war of words and clever arguments. . . . For the past eight years or so, most people's response to climate change has been played out on this mental plane, ultimately making the major challenges we face seem distant and abstract . . . stressing the large scale of global warming and then telling people they can solve it through small actions such as changing a light bulb, brings about a disconnection that underlines the urgency of the message and encourages people to think that individual action is meaningless.

(Thomas 2006)

Furthermore, the notion of a 'gap' between knowledge and action – useful as it is for rhetorical and pedagogic purposes – makes little psychological sense. There are no phrenological compartments in the brain, neither spatial nor strictly sequential – that is, there are no separate boxes marked '*What I Know* (about climate change); *What I feel about it* and *What am I going to do about* it'. In cognitive terms, a single perception will contain all three. Nor is there a fixed biographical sequence in which you go through demarcated stages of thought and emotion and only then proceed to a separate stage of either action or avoidance, indifference or evasion.

The cognitive sciences now work with more complex and integrated models: the initial perceptual schema, for example, has already 'decided' on modes of action or avoidance. Concepts like 'cognitive morality', 'moral minds' and the 'empathic civilization' do not undermine denial theory, but they do make it more complicated. And this is before we even consider the sociological differences – history, culture, class, gender – that might explain the many variations of denial.

Notes

1 I am grateful to Paul de Canio for this and other searches of media texts.
2 For a summary of the social psychology of self-deception – why we justify foolish beliefs and hurtful acts – see Tavris and Aronson (2007).
3 For a brief summary, see 'Science Scorned' *Nature*, 476 (9 Sept. 2010): 133.
4 The examples in this paragraph come from Everyday energy: The essential guide to reducing your carbon footprint: 52 eco dilemmas solved. A year's worth of green living. *The Guardian* and *Observer*, over 2010.

References

Chouliaraki, L. (2006) *The Spectorship of Suffering*. London: Sage Publications.
Cohen, S. (2001) *States of Denial: Knowing About Atrocities and Suffering*. Cambridge, UK: Polity Press.
Horner, C. C. (2007) *The Politically Incorrect Guide to Global Warning and Environmentalism*. Washington DC: Regnery Publishing.
Monbiot, G. (2009) The climate denial industry is out to dupe the public. And it's working. *The Guardian*, 8 Dec.

Rumsfeld, D. (2002) Press Conference at NATO Headquarters, Brussels, Belgium, June 6, 2002. Available at: www.youtube.com/watch?v=jtkUO8NpI84

Seu, I. B. (2010) Shoot the messenger: Dynamics of positioning and denial in response to human rights appeals. *Journal of Human Rights Practice*, 3 (2): 139–161.

Tavris, C., and Aronson, E. (2007) *Mistakes Were Made (but not by me). Why we Justify Foolish Beliefs, Bad Decisions, and Hurtful Acts*. New York: Harvest Books.

Thomas, P. (2006) How to beat denial – a 12 step plan. *The Ecologist*, 1 Dec. Available on: www.theecologist.org/search.php?q=how+to+beat+denial+a+12+step+plan&offset=0&submit=Go

Weintrobe, S. (2010) On links between runaway consumer greed and climate change denial: A psychoanalytic perspective. *Bulletin Annual of the British Psychoanalytical Society*, 1: 63–75. London: Institute of Psychoanalysis.

Discussion
Climate change in a perverse culture

John Steiner

Paul Hoggett's excellent account of the perverse culture leaves very little for me to add. He has described the essential points that arise from Freud's (1927) discussion of fetishism and extended the psychoanalytical findings to the larger social sphere in a convincing manner. The overall effect was, however, at least initially, to leave me depressed. What does the ubiquity of the perverse culture say about the outlook for the planet and about human nature in general? I believe that this depression is appropriate and that it is better to face it while we can, knowing that sooner or later we will slip into the familiar evasions that we all rely on. I think this means that we have to accept that our views of human nature have been simplistic and, perhaps because of this, that attempts to prevent climate change have largely failed.

The feeling of depression is not due to an absence of goodness or decency, or of natural and cultural richness and creativity; rather, it arises because the good things we value are precisely those most under threat. Moreover, the attempts made to protect them have been weak in comparison with the power of the destructive forces mounted against them. This is the situation that Melanie Klein considered to be at the heart of our experience of depression – namely when we come to appreciate and value our good objects and at the same time are unable to protect them from destructive attacks.

That ordinary methods of thinking have failed is increasingly being accepted. Of course it is right to continue to do everything we can to bring about climate change reduction and to use every argument that we can muster in order to create a more rational world, but I think it is clear that it has not worked. George Monbiot himself admitted defeat in his wish to 'teach the world how to stop the planet burning'. Recently he wrote,

> Climate change enlightenment was fun while it lasted, but it is now dead. To compensate for our weakness we indulged in a fantasy of benign paternalistic power acting . . . in the wider interests of humankind. We allowed ourselves to believe that, with a little prompting and protest, somewhere, in a distant institutional sphere, compromised but decent people would take care of us. They won't. They weren't ever going to do so.
>
> (Monbiot 2010)

Monbiot asked, 'What do we do now?' but admitted that he does not know. 'All I know', he said, 'is that we must stop dreaming about an institutional response that will never materialize and start facing a political reality we've sought to avoid'.

In this chapter Hoggett points out how simplistic are our views of human nature. And, we have to recognize that this is true also of the views held by psychoanalysts who, like everyone else, can only appreciate a limited amount of reality and are subject to the same perverse culture. Even though we are aware of unconscious mechanisms and destructive forces operating in the setting of the consulting room, many psychoanalysts, and I include myself, regularly expect people to behave rationally and decently in the world at large, and can become outraged when they do not. The most signal failure in our understanding of human nature in general is surely our failure to understand and to confront the inevitability and universality of destructive forces.

In my approach to this theme I am going to raise the issue of the universality of a destructive drive, and connect it with the death instinct. It is central to our understanding of perverse mechanisms, which depend on the capacity to accept and to deny something at the same time. Freud (1927) first applied it to the problem of recognizing the difference between the sexes, but as Hoggett affirms it has a wider application, indicating a more general 'turning away from what is true and good'. How many types of perversion are there? In addition to the sexual perversions, I have argued that a perverse denial of the reality of death is the most pervasive and perhaps the most disabling. It leads to an unconscious belief in our immortality and accounts for many of the failures to rein in our phantasies of omnipotence.

The perverse attitude seems particularly designed to defend us from the unwelcome perception of difference. Freud began by describing the case of a boy who becomes aware of the fact that women do not have a penis. The boy finds this unacceptable because of a primitive belief that the penis was originally there and must have been lost by castration, in which case his own penis could be lost in the same way. Today we are more likely to see the problem in terms of the difficulty of the recognition of differences between the sexes and as an instance of reluctance to recognize difference in general. Any difference has the potential to give rise to envy and leads to defensive attempts to deny its existence.

The intolerance of difference between the generations and between the sexes gives rise to varieties of sexual perversion, and the intolerance of ageing, illness and death is also dealt with by perverse means. In a classic paper Money-Kyrle (1971) described these issues as the 'facts of life'. Most significant of all is his third fact of life, which concerns the reality of the passage of time. It is this latter fact that forces us to recognize 'that all good things come to an end', including life itself, and brings us up against the reality of ageing, infirmity, and death. The huge difference is that between being alive and being dead.

It is the fact of our own mortality that is most difficult for us to bear and elicits the most powerful defences and denials, among which perverse mechanisms are prominent. We are constantly reassured through fantasies of an afterlife, and this may well be one of the reasons for the shift towards beliefs that concretize immortality such as creationism and other types of fundamentalism.

The awareness of difference is so provocative because it gives rise to envy and mobilizes destructive attacks fuelled by the death instinct. Indeed, Freud (1920) believed that all conflicts, at their deepest level, involve a struggle between the life and death instincts. The life instinct creates structure and meaning, and the death instinct attempts to destroy meaning to create an amorphous uniformity in which no structure is discernible. It is really more accurate to consider the death instinct as an anti-life instinct, which is most vividly expressed through destructive attacks on goodness, truth and creativity.

Envy is commonly split off, projected, and attributed to others, and what is more, the projection is often preceded by a shift towards concrete thinking. This is why an intolerance of difference may provoke a shift towards fundamentalism in which the opposing factions come so closely to resemble each other. Each idealizes itself and sees the other as the embodiment of evil. If we can become aware of this propensity to project, our capacity to examine our own motives may allow for a different kind of dialogue. The point that arises from these considerations is that destructive attacks against things we value are always going to be there. They will not go away and be replaced by a rational and cooperative attitude. Our understanding of these processes is gradually deepening, but we do have to be realistic and not believe in simplistic solutions. I believe this applies to psychoanalysts and climate change reformers as much as to the fundamentalists who seem to present such an intransigent obstacle to change.

It may be that considerations of this kind can deepen our understanding of perverse mechanisms and hence of the perverse culture. In my view, Paul Hoggett, George Monbiot and others are moving towards a spirit of realism in which a more complex and less naïve model of human nature is being used. I consider this to be an important advance even though it does not answer questions like what to do now. Maybe these cannot be answered at any deep level and perhaps the best we can do is to become alert to the likelihood that we are under the sway of a perverse argument and to be aware of our own propensity to join in the collusions.

References

Freud, S. (1920) *Beyond the Pleasure Principle*. In J. Strachey (Ed.), *The Standard Edition of the Complete Psychological Works of Sigmund Freud, Vol. XVIII* (pp. 1–64). London: Hogarth Press.

Freud, S. (1927) Fetishism. In J. Strachey (Ed.), *The Standard Edition of the Complete Psychological Works of Sigmund Freud, Vol. XXI* (pp. 149–157). London: Hogarth Press.

Klein, M. (1940) Mourning and its relation to manic-depressive states. *International Journal of Psychoanalysis*, 21, 125–153. Reprinted in *The Writings of Melanie Klein, Vol. 1* (pp. 344–369). London: Hogarth Press.

Monbiot, G. (2010) Climate change enlightenment was fun while it lasted. But now it's dead. *The Guardian*, Monday, 20 Sept. Available at: www.guardian.co.uk/commentis-free/2010/sep/20/climate-change-negotiations-failure

Money-Kyrle, R. (1971) The aim of psycho-analysis. *International Journal of Psychoanalysis*, 52: 103–106. Reprinted in *The Collected Papers of Roger Money-Kyrle* (pp. 442–449). Perthshire: Clunie Press, 1978.

Reply
Climate change in a perverse culture

Paul Hoggett

It is a great pleasure to engage with two thinkers whose work I have continually drawn upon over many years. Perhaps, almost inevitably, each develops my own thinking in different ways – John Steiner deepening the psychoanalytic dimension and Stan Cohen the sociological. For more than twenty years now I have tried to think and write in a way that brings together these two perspectives without reducing one to the other. Cohen wonders whether this is too ambitious. I think if the aim was to bring about a comprehensive integration of these perspectives, then I agree that this would be unrealistically ambitious. But I actually do not believe that such an integration between 'personal' and 'political' perspectives is possible. Some of what is 'personal' will always remain just that, part of a human nature that is the product of thousands of years of civilization, and some of what is 'political', such as the organized climate change denial lobby in the United States, is, as Cohen notes, perfectly explainable in terms of political economy (the pursuit of economic self-interest by Exxon Mobil, etc.). But even though these two perspectives cannot be integrated, this does not mean that they do not overlap, enrich and inform each other in places. In this chapter I have tried to bring these perspectives together through the idea of a 'perverse culture' – a concept that combines the psychoanalytic notion of the perverse with the sociological notion of an organized culture.

Regarding the cultural dimension, Cohen very usefully develops some distinctions between denialism, anti-denialism and the rhetorical political device of accusing another of being 'in denial'. Of course, as Cohen's example of the Pakistani security forces reveals, the use of this rhetoric does not mean that a culture of denial is not present in the security forces, and it made me think just how widespread denial may be as a characteristic of institutional cultures (which, of course, brings us back to Susan Long's work on Enron, etc.). The question is, does this qualify as a sociological phenomenon? In other words, is there something distinctive about the world in which we live now that makes denial a more pervasive aspect of institutional life than, say, a century ago? I believe so, and in my essay I try to itemize some of the factors that make this a uniquely contemporary phenomenon by drawing attention to the strength of the 'virtual', or what we might call the 'as if', in postmodern societies. In doing so I am trying to make the point that I see denial as a cultural phenomenon, as organized self-deception, that *we all* participate in. I definitely do not want to pathologize a small minority of 'deniers' if to do so is to imply that there is a larger group of non-deniers who are facing up to reality. Rather, by emphasizing the cultural dimension of denial, I seek to draw attention to the 'unhappy consciousness' or bad faith, which is, I believe, the lot of all of us who live in late-modern Western societies. But Cohen is also correct in highlighting how the 'denialists' have become a real and powerful movement, far larger than the 'denial lobby' that Monbiot analysed (Monbiot 2006), and here, as Cohen notes, the work of Clive Hamilton tracing the links between the denialists and the fundamentalist Republican right is very thought-provoking (Hamilton, chapter 2, this volume).

Thinking of the perverse, John Steiner suggests that perhaps what we really cannot face up to, and therefore seek to deny, is the reality of human destructiveness – 'the inevitability and universality of destructive forces', as he puts it. He insists strongly, and in a way that made me think, that the climate change movement has suffered from having a simplified view of human behaviour, perhaps one that was itself based upon a denial of an unpalatable reality. But in facing this reality we must beware of using this depressive stance as a form of quietist resignation, for we must not forget that Melanie Klein also linked the depressive position to the capacity for hope (Klein 1957), and hope is essential to human agency. There are some former environmental activists such as Paul Kingsnorth who now face climate change without hope – indeed make a virtue of this stance by insisting that this 'is concerned with being honest about reality' (Kingsnorth and Hine 2010: 4). But I do not think this is honesty; rather, their ecocentrism conceals a bitter disenchantment with (and at times a discernible contempt towards) humankind – theirs is a pessimism of both the intellect and the will. In contrast, I much prefer the 'dark optimism' of writers and activists such as Shaun Chamberlin (2011) when he says:

> Dark Optimism is, in part, a way of seeing life which is not afraid of seeking the truth – even when that truth is unpalatable or feels overwhelming. By exploring the unknown we can see it for what it is, rather than what we might fear it to be. Where there is darkness present we face it with an indomitable belief in the potential of humankind.
>
> (Chamberlin 2011)

Once we lose our hope in each other, then there is no hope for nature. Sure, living systems on earth will survive, just as they have done for the last four billion years. But there is no consolation to be had from looking at things through the lens of geological time. Many scientists say now that even if we manage to get carbon dioxide emissions under control in the next two decades, it is highly likely that global temperatures will rise by 4°C by 2080. The implications are horrendous, but if we lose hope and fail to struggle for a better future, then in all likelihood the temperature rise could be 6° C or worse. We owe it to this beautiful and complex planet to fight our desecration of it rather than resign ourselves to a long descent into darkness.

References

Chamberlin, S. (2011). Available at: www.darkoptimism.org
Kingsnorth, P., and Hine, D. (2010) Introduction. *Dark Mountain*, Issue 1.
Klein, M. (1957) *Envy and Gratitude,* in *The Writings of Melanie Klein, Vol. III, Envy and Gratitude and Other Works 1946–1963*. London: Hogarth Press.
Monbiot, G. (2006) *Heat: How to Stop the Planet Burning*. London: Allen Lane.

Chapter 5

Great expectations

The psychodynamics of ecological debt

Rosemary Randall

Introduction

The idea that people do not know themselves well, hide uncomfortable truths from themselves and are frequently mistaken in their estimations of themselves and of others is central both to psychoanalysis and to literature.

In this chapter I explore this capacity for self-deception in relation to a scale of ecological debt that, although it dwarfs any debt that bankers have run up in the financial world, provokes only a limited political or personal response. A number of writers have used a psychoanalytic perspective to explore the phenomenon of climate change denial and the reasons why so little attention is paid to environmental problems (see, for example, Lertzman 2008, Mishan 1996, Randall 2005, Rust 2008). I am also interested in the other side of the picture: what happens to people who do try to face such problems? In this chapter I explore the psychological consequences for people who try to face ecological debt, comparing their journeys with that of Pip in Dickens' *Great Expectations* (Dickens 1861).

The stories that illustrate this are taken from interviews with 8 participants in Carbon Conversations groups,[1] and from contributions to a website (available at: www.whatsyourpipstory.com) set up to collect stories about ecological debt.

Great Expectations

Great Expectations opens on a windswept, late December afternoon on the bleak Kent marshes, an inhospitable landscape of fen and ditch, running to the river where prison hulks are moored. Pip, the hero and narrator, 7 years old and an orphan, is sheltering in a graveyard, puzzling over the inscription on his parents' grave, before returning home to the house he shares with his shrewish sister and her husband, the blacksmith Joe Gargery.

Out of the mist emerges the most terrifying figure Pip has ever met – an escaped convict, cursing, threatening and rattling a leg-iron. He demands that Pip should fetch him food and a file to remove the chain that hobbles him. The encounter marks Pip's life, though not in a way that is immediately apparent to him.

Those who are familiar with the story will remember that Pip appears to find favour with the reclusive Miss Havisham, who requires a boy to visit her. On these puzzling visits he meets and falls in love with her ward, the beautiful but cold Estella. On reaching adulthood he is told by the lawyer Jaggers that he has been chosen by a mysterious benefactor to receive an education as a gentleman. Pip believes that his benefactor must be Miss Havisham, that he is destined for Estella, and that the favour he finds is connected to his feeling of deserving more than the dull life of an apprenticeship to the generous and loving Joe.

The novel interests me for its description of Pip's reaction when he discovers the true identity of his benefactor and finds that person to be quite other than whom he imagined. His debt does not lie where he thought it did. He is indebted, not to some intrinsic merit in himself, not to the wealthy Miss Havisham, but to Magwitch, the convict whom he helped on that cold, harsh day on the marshes by fetching him food and a file to remove his leg-iron.

Pip's initial reactions are similar to those of many people when they discover the extent of what is sometimes called ecological debt: the moment when someone realizes that the goods, services and conveniences they enjoy do not come courtesy of their own hard work, or because they are particularly deserving, but carry a cost to others and to the rest of the natural world.

Pip, confronted with Magwitch and an uncomfortable truth, feels shock and disbelief, denies the truth and longs for flight. The journey he then goes on echoes many people's struggles as they come to terms with ecological debt. It involves revisiting developmental processes that psychoanalysis writes about richly: the young child's gradual disillusion with the grand sense of his or her own importance, the collision with the reality principle, the realization that others have given in order for him or her to receive and the achievement of the depressive position. Pip reworks oedipal dilemmas, reframes his identity, learns compassion, humility and the meaning of forgiveness. Ecological debt has a similar potential to return people to developmental processes that, if they thought about them at all, they considered resolved and finished with.

Ecological debt

The concept of ecological debt lays bare the relationship between people and the goods they consume. It is a way of understanding the connection between the lifestyles of the West and the costs to the natural world. It creates a balance sheet of who has used what natural resources and who might be indebted to whom. In the words of the economist Andrew Simms,

> If you take more than your fair share of a finite natural resource you run up an ecological debt. If you have a lifestyle that pushes an ecosystem beyond its ability to renew itself, you run up an ecological debt . . . it is a different way of understanding economic relations that grounds us in the real world of natural resources.
> (Simms 2005: 88)

Unlike the debts that drive the economy, ecological debts do not appear in the annual accounts of corporations or on the overdraft statements of individuals. The negotiation of the debt is unclear. The repayment terms are hazy. The interest rate has not been settled, and, in many cases, no arrangement has been made to pay.

Ecological debt may be owed to:

- other people, species and habitats
- future generations
- the global commons – those natural resources such as the air or the seas whose benefits cannot easily be divided up between nations.

The most obvious ecological debt at present is caused by rising CO_2 emissions, which make it clear that some countries use energy at others' expense. Per capita CO_2 emissions range from approximately 29 tonnes in the United States to 1 tonne in countries like Vietnam and Zambia. The UK figure is around 15 tonnes per capita (Hertwich and Peters 2009). A sustainable figure would be a mere 1.5 tonnes.

Another example lies in the relationship of a cheap cotton t-shirt to the devastation of ecosystems and livelihoods in Uzbekhistan, the country that provides Europe with a third of its cotton. Each t-shirt takes 2,000 litres of water to make. As a result of water extraction for cotton growing, the Aral Sea has shrunk to only 15% of its former volume, exposing 40,000 Km^2 of its seabed and wrecking the bio-systems of the area (Environmental Justice Foundation 2010).

Similarly, one might point to the products of the oil industry (the flights, holidays and commutes, the plastics and pharmaceuticals, the thousands of entertaining and ephemeral gadgets) and place them on a balance sheet with the ecological destruction caused by the oil industry in the Niger Delta (Platform 2010).

The idea of ecological debt moves away from the common notion that the services provided by the natural world are an entitlement and that people have a right to take what they want. It also stops short of the much more uncomfortable notion that Western people's relationship to the natural world might more accurately be seen as theft or crime. The idea of ecological debt emphasizes the underlying, obscured relationships between the most ordinary artefacts and the devastation of the natural world.

The fact that one is personally indebted can be hard to take in. In the eighteenth century only the minority tasted slavery each time they drank a cup of sugar-sweetened chocolate. Little has changed today. People rarely make these connections, the relationships are not apparent to them and their reaction to being shown them is often similar to that of Pip when confronted by Magwitch, that of shock and angry disbelief.

Developmentally, life is full of such surprises. Children discover that their parents do not always enjoy parenthood, that they get tired, do not enjoy their jobs, would like some time to themselves and sometimes find the children a nuisance. Gradually children are introduced to the reality that they are not the centre of the universe, that their needs do not always come first and that their demands cause pain or trouble to others. They discover that greed and selfishness have consequences, that they will not marry Mummy or Daddy, will not live forever, and must share the world with others. Gradually they come to see their parents as whole people who have given much to them. They desire to give back, start to show empathy and concern and develop a moral sense. We may, with Klein (1937), see these reactions as reparation for harm done, or with Winnicott (1963) emphasize how concern and creativity develop out of a degree of ruthlessness in the primary relationship of the baby with the mother.

If people seem unaware of ecological debt, it may be that they have never left a state of innocence, comparable to that of infants who do not yet know the personal cost to their parents of caring for them. Alternatively, they may have embraced ignorance as a defence, seduced by the collective illusion that satisfactions do not need to be paid for. A third possibility is that people are cynically engaged in or colluding in crime, aware at some level of what they are doing.[2]

Psychologically, there are three broad areas in relation to ecological debt that I would like to explore by highlighting some of the parallels and differences with Dickens' novel. The first concerns the journey that individuals go on if they allow themselves to acknowledge ecological indebtedness. The second concerns the social and political environment that disguises indebtedness as fair exchange, gift or entitlement and makes the journey hard. The third concerns the question of whether or not the journey is necessary and should be encouraged.

Facing ecological debt

I have suggested elsewhere (Randall 2009b) that theories of loss and grief can be helpful in understanding people's reactions to climate change and have used William Worden's model of the tasks of grief and their negatives (Worden 1983) to explore how people may (or may not) come to terms with the changes required of them by climate change mitigation.

There is more to facing ecological debt than mourning, however. Questions of guilt, reparation and the reframing of identity take a more powerful place. In *Great Expectations* we see Pip struggling with the nature of love and forgiveness, struggling with unresolved oedipal issues, seeking adequate ways of making reparation for the injury he has caused and the ingratitude he has shown. He has to look at the world differently, learn not to be ashamed of his origins, accept the reality of hard work and the value of reciprocity.

For the individual coming to terms with ecological debt, there are equally difficult questions of repayment and forgiveness for harm done. The reframing of identity is often significant. And the potential for depression, masochism and bitterness are all too real. The processes are both similar to and different from those that Pip goes through.

Shock and recognition

If you remember *Great Expectations*, you will know that Magwitch reappears in Pip's life, having been transported to Australia. After serving his time, he has made a fortune through sheep-farming. A stormy, windswept night brings him to Pip's lodgings to reveal that he is Pip's benefactor. The knowledge that he might be able to do something good for the child who helped him on the marshes has sustained him through a life of hardship and sorrow.

Pip's first reactions are shock, disbelief and denial, experienced as a powerful physical reaction: 'the repugnance with which I shrank from him, could not have been exceeded if he had been some terrible beast' (Dickens 1861/1946: 299). States of repugnance alternate with dejection as he struggles to take in the reality of his situation. He is 'dazed and distracted' and feels 'a frenzy of fear and dislike' (308). The gifts he has received feel tainted: 'his wretched gold and silver' (302). His thoughts turn to how to get rid of Magwitch and to dreams of running away himself: 'enlist(ing) for India as a private soldier' (315).

Most tellingly, he feels himself to be useless, 'I am heavily in debt . . . and I have been bred to no calling, and I am fit for nothing' (318).

It is clear that many people never get past the stage of shock and disbelief about ecological debt. For those who are genuinely innocent about the connections between their life and ecological damage, the charge is an affront to their sense of themselves as good people. For those, like Pip, who may be acting in bad faith, there are powerful motives for continuing to conceal the truth from themselves.

Some flee to the equivalent of India, in their own minds. Anyone who has tried to raise environmental questions with friends or at social occasions will be familiar with the establishment of a new taboo. 'Let's talk about something nicer', said an old friend. Some are repelled by ecological damage but fail to connect it with themselves or wish to disown it, complaining about the ugliness of industrial landscapes but seeing no connection to their own lives. Some try to kill the messenger, projecting responsibility onto those who have raised the alarm. This is often apparent in hostile reactions to environmental activists and climate scientists.

The triggers for recognition of ecological debt among the people I interviewed varied: seeing Al Gore's film *An Inconvenient Truth*, picking up a book on vegetarianism, talking with a family member, the oil shocks of the 1970s, a TV programme about nuclear testing, a presentation from the Stockholm Institute. Recognition was not always a single shocking moment. A number of people described a gradual development of understanding, as if the difficult knowledge was best managed by being allowed into consciousness bit by bit. Some of the strongest turning points described were from childhood, moments of being brought into contact with nature's limits or experiencing first-hand the relationship between a life of privilege and one of poverty. One woman wrote: 'I was living in Rome in the mid-1960s, and my father was short with us kids for splashing the hose over us in play in the garden. He then told us about things like not running taps while cleaning teeth, and turning off room lights. I remember feeling very sad, because so many people were not doing this and we sisters were laughed at when we mentioned it.'

Another described a childhood visit from California to Mexico that had stamped in her mind the way poor Mexicans lived literally in the waste that California discarded. A third, posted with her family at the age of 12 to a poor African country, wrote of realizing that she personally had benefited from others' deprivation and how difficult it was to come to terms with this.

For people who had made such connections later in life, the sense of shock was still raw. A man whose family values had centred on wealth and ambition said, 'It was like opening a credit card bill and finding I had spent hundreds of thousands of pounds . . . the overwhelm was too much.'

A woman told me, still with a sense of her original horror: 'I worked out that for each tonne of carbon dioxide I'm responsible for, someone elsewhere in the world loses a year of their life.'

Reconnecting

For everyone I spoke to there was a clear sense of a connection being made that, once established, could not easily be turned off. Once the obscured relationships between ecological damage and an ordinary Western life had become apparent, the knowledge would not go back in the box.

Coming to terms with indebtedness often left people overwhelmed with sadness, frightened or disorientated, as the following quotations show:

- 'It makes me feel sad, guilty and a bit hopeless. . . .'
- 'I lost my innocence and along with it my faith in authority. I remember the disbelief, anger and frustration, worsened by the fact that I was raised in a very conservative family. I remember feeling betrayed and scared'.
- 'I'd find myself in places like shopping centres, looking around and feeling like I was the only person who really "got it".'

A number of people talked of the need to experience the sadness deeply in order to come through it.

In *Great Expectations* Pip gradually attains what we might call Winnicott's capacity for concern, or Klein's depressive position. He slowly acknowledges his debt to Magwitch and his responsibility for him. He becomes frightened not of Magwitch, but of the threat to Magwitch.

> [M]y repugnance to him had all melted away . . . I only saw a man who had meant to be my benefactor, and who had felt affectionately, gratefully and generously towards me with great constancy through a series of years. I only saw in him a much better man than I had been to Joe.
>
> (Dickens 1861/1946: 417)

Unsurprisingly, the attempt to accept the painful reality of ecological debt can itself produce defensive reactions. Some people found themselves preoccupied with each terrible fact. One person compared it to '. . . trying to peer into a car crash to see every gory detail'. A number spoke of devouring information and becoming unable to stop talking about it, manically imposing the topic on whoever would (or would not) listen. This could be seen as an attempt to master trauma, or alternatively as an attempt to expel pain and responsibility and project it onto others.

In *Great Expectations*, Pip becomes preoccupied with discovering Estella's true parentage. At one level, he simply wants to know the truth. Defensively, however, he welcomes an obsession that can distract from his own sadness and guilt. As Jaggers remarks, when Pip reveals what he knows: 'For whose sake would you reveal the secret?' (Dickens 1861/1946: 387)

Becoming able to speak the truth without projecting one's own pain or blaming others seems to depend on people working through their own sense of guilt, finding a proportional and creative response, and in many cases adjusting their sense of self and their purpose in life.

Guilt, reparation and proportionality

In *Great Expectations*, the actions Pip needs to take are clear to him. The same is not true for those struggling to come to terms with ecological debt. The scale of the problem feels immense. The actions open to them feel inadequate. The division of guilt between individuals, governments and corporations – some of whom accept responsibility and some of whom do not – creates anger and confusion.

Guilt was an inevitable part for many, but not all, of those I spoke to. The following quotations are typical:

- 'I still feel deeply guilty and indebted toward all other species. . . . Doing my bit and taking responsibility have not been of any comfort here'.
- '[R]ealizing that my actions would affect my kids, that I'd be passing on a bill with interest, rather than a beautiful and bountiful inheritance'.
- '[O]ur lifestyle is causing carbon emissions that will almost certainly irrevocably damage the life chances of future generations. We've gobbled up far more than our fair share'.

Younger people were less likely to feel guilt. They were clear that they had not created this mess and were more likely to feel angry. For both groups, however, the experience of putting themselves, day after day, in contact with traumatic events was difficult to manage. For some, it felt impossible to resolve. One wrote:

- 'I feel I am in a cycle of hope and despair and action and inaction when my focus goes elsewhere.'

Another wrote:

- 'No matter what one does, it does not feel like much, and the feelings of dismay and sadness are pretty huge'.

Others had found an easier balance:

- 'When I came to accept that I couldn't change it all, I started focusing on my own lifestyle. I invested a lot of time and energy in digesting all the facts, and in finding ways of coping with the guilt, the pain and the deep sadness of it all'.
- Harsh self-criticism was a problem for some and led to defensive reactions. One woman described feeling hemmed in by the prohibitions of her activist friends. On reflection however she could not put her finger on anyone who was actually critical of her: the problem lay in her own superego.

Another woman's solution might be seen as more masochistic. She was torn between her desire for a DVD player and the knowledge that workers in third-world factories became blind through assembling electronic equipment. She bought the DVD player, but every time she watched a film, she tortured herself with images of young women thrown on the streets of China when their failing sight made them unemployable.

It is well known that guilt is a mixed motivator for persuading people to take responsibility for climate change. Reviewing the research, Suzanne Moser (2007) concludes that it should be used with caution. For some of my respondents, however, once they had engaged with the problem, the guilt would not go away. It was difficult for people to know what might constitute adequate repayment of the debt. What would be proportionate? What would be effective? One man described how fear and guilt had led him to try to take on the problem single-handed, until he had collapsed through exhaustion.

All the people I spoke to had made significant adjustments to their own lifestyle. The most common reparative action was to reduce their personal impact on the problem, and the changes many had made were significant – actions that would halve their carbon footprint. On their own, however, these personal actions could still feel inadequate. It is difficult to make reparation if no one sees and accepts your gift.

Those who managed best were those who had developed a clear sense of proportionality and placed some boundaries around their responsibility. For one person this meant protecting herself from the amount of news she read. For another it was creating a plan for the personal changes she would make. For several, it helped to see the political dimension and the power relationships clearly, to understand neo-colonialism and globalization, to contribute to a political programme, or simply to point the finger at BP or bankers and say, 'It's not all my fault.'

Where actions were intrinsically creative and had benefit to others, it was easier for people to feel that reparation might be effective. Actions with a direct connection to the rest of the natural world felt especially significant. A man who was fortunate enough to own land had planted a small wood to provide himself and his partner with firewood. He described the pleasure of looking at it and noticing how biodiversity had developed in his small patch. He then spoke of how he imagined that people in the future, after he was dead, might find the wood and be thankful that it had been planted.

Unlike Pip, those facing ecological debt face a complex struggle. Although many spoke or wrote of finding ways to make reparation, the difficulties of seeing an effect from one's actions and of receiving acknowledgment from those damaged were significant.

Identity

The struggle to come to terms with ecological debt was life-changing for a number of the people I spoke to. When Pip acknowledges the extent of his indebtedness, he is quite literally undone: 'I began fully to know how wrecked I was, and how the ship in which I had sailed was gone to pieces' (Dickens 1861/1946: 302).

He loses not just his expectations but the identity he has forged for himself as a gentleman. He loses the idea of himself as especially deserving and entitled. He is forced to confront his treatment of Joe, acknowledge his pride and reflect on who he is and who he might become in the future.

Like Pip, many of those who confront ecological debt also confront such questions. Who am I? What will I become? How should I live? For younger people still in the turmoil of making life choices about work and direction, these questions were extremely painful and confusing.

A young woman with a good degree had spent the year following graduation involved in political activity, doing poorly paid but useful work, stepping aside from the trajectory her upbringing had prepared her for. She had recently been encouraged to apply for a job in a field appropriate to her qualifications and had been offered it. She spoke eloquently of her confusion. Who was she and what did she want to be? If she followed the life of the activist, what happened to her ambition? If she took the job, how would she align her beliefs with the circles she would then move in? Was it wrong to want to be a leader? What would happen to her principles?

A man in his thirties wrote: 'It can change the core of who you are . . . there have been times over the last few years that I don't like the person I could become.' He explained how for a time he had lost his characteristic optimism. He had become preoccupied and obsessed, at risk of sacrificing the hope and creativity that made him a concerned and useful citizen. Recovering some balance had taken time.

In *Great Expectations* Pip's new identity is forged through that staple of Victorian fiction, the purification rite of fever where the old mistakes and wrongs are burned away and the new, redeemed self emerges. After Magwitch's death, Pip falls ill. The illness has a hallucinatory quality that captures Pip's struggle with the depressive position: 'I sometimes struggled with real people, in the belief that they were murderers. . . . I would all at once comprehend that they meant to do me good' (Dickens 1861/1946: 433).

He emerges from it with a renewed sense of gratitude, a longing for forgiveness and a clearer sense of who he is and what he must do. Twenty-first-century life rarely offers such convenient routes for the re-forging of identity. However, the themes of purification, the brush with mortality and the emergence of a stronger, more creative self did feature in several of the conversations I had.

Maintaining that stronger, changed self was rarely easy, and social context was mentioned by almost everyone. Marriage, friendships, belonging to organizations and appropriate work were all mentioned. Being able to talk, to share, to laugh or cry mattered to some but not to everyone. More negatively, people spoke of conflicts with old friends, family arguments and a feeling of being squeezed into silence. One woman described the casual ostracism of colleagues who would greet her by saying, 'Oh, here's Sylvia. Better stop talking about flying, girls.'

Psychotherapists see social and family groups as crucial in providing support to those whose identity is fragile or is changing under the pressure of necessity. Creating contexts where new social norms can flourish and the reframed identities of those who face ecological debt can be nurtured is essential if people are to develop a creative capacity for concern rather than a neurotic pursuit of perfection.

Vengeance and forgiveness

Questions of justice, vengeance and forgiveness may be a necessary part of understanding the psychodynamics of ecological debt. Certainly these issues appeared strongly for some of those I spoke to, and they are key themes in *Great Expectations*.

Reparation involves not just the desire to make good the wrong that has been done but the need for forgiveness. Debtors fear the vengeance of those they have wronged. The repayment needs to be accepted and seen as adequate and just. In *Great Expectations* Pip is afforded generous forgiveness. Magwitch is touchingly grateful. Joe is magnanimous. Pip has the satisfaction of seeing his reparative acts bear fruit in the flourishing of new relationships between Herbert and Clara and between Joe and Biddy.

Dickens also tells the darker side of the story, however, as the themes of revenge and justice are played out in the contrasting stories of Miss Havisham and Magwitch. Vengeance destroys Miss Havisham. The idea of justice, however crude, helps Magwitch to survive.

What are twenty-first-century ecological creditors most likely to do? Will they seek revenge, seek justice, accept repayment or offer forgiveness? Will they treat the debt as a debt or see it as a crime? These questions are not openly posed by politicians. The creditors are perhaps too weak at present to do anything at all. But I would suggest that the fear of vengeance, by people or by nature itself, is present in two contemporary phenomena: the fashion for apology and the prevalence of apocalyptic narratives.

The fashion for demanding and offering apologies for past wrongs is a recent one. In 1997 Tony Blair apologized for the Irish potato famine. In 2007 he and other politicians apologized for their countries' participation in the slave trade. In 2009 Gordon Brown and Kevin Rudd apologized for the transport of British orphans to Australia. Meanwhile the actual wrongs for which these men are responsible and for which apology and reparation might be appropriate – climate change and ecological debt among them – go uncompensated. The apologies are perhaps displaced, an unconscious acknowledgment of wrongs it is more difficult to address.

Meanwhile apocalyptic narratives of climate disaster often carry a subtext of pleasure that vengeance will be wreaked on an ignorant or uncaring human race. This is increasingly true in some of James Lovelock's writings, where he seems to enjoy the idea that the Earth's systems will find a new equilibrium without the inconvenience of people. He presents this as a neat vengeance for the hubris of the human race (Lovelock 2006). The theme of vengeance can also be found on the websites of American Christian fundamentalists who embrace the idea of the 'Rapture'. These people see climate change as an inevitable part of the disasters that presage the second coming and an appropriate vengeance on a sinful majority. Scherer (2004) gives a useful summary of these views.

Most of the people I spoke to longed to know that their actions would have an effect. They longed for their reparative impulses to bear fruit. Most were also realistic about the increasingly dark future, and this was a source of continuing pain. Some, but not all, spoke of a wish for forgiveness, worrying how they were seen by people in other countries, wondering how they would be seen by future generations. It was distressing to some to feel that there was no one who could forgive, no one who could say, 'You have done enough.' 'What would I like on my gravestone?' asked one. 'She tried.'

Boundaries and the 'no' of nature

The social and political environment in which people set out on these journeys is problematic. Ecological debt is a structural, economic problem as well as a personal one. The psychological conditions of late modernity – for example the fluidity and contingency of personal life, the fracture between human sensibility and the rest of the natural world, the encouragement of materialistic values – are reflected and confirmed in fragmented and globalized systems that can feel impervious to either individual or collective action.

There are parallels with Pip's experiences in *Great Expectations*. His history matters: it shapes and determines the context in which he can make choices. In *Great Expectations*, Pip's hopes and his blindness relate to his orphaned state. This is a novel in which all the parental figures are flawed or inadequate. Joe Gargery cannot protect Pip from the vicious Mrs Joe. Miss Havisham is embittered. Jaggers is cold. Magwitch is self-centred and demanding. There is no maternal care and no benign paternal authority.

Pip is a needy child with a vivid imagination. His conscience is extreme and punitive. He is vulnerable to flattery and to the suggestion that he is somehow, inexplicably, special. He dreams, idealizes, persuades himself that black is white and acts in bad faith. He retreats, albeit guiltily, from the depressive position and has to make a painful return.

There are parallels between Pip's world, in which parental relationships are disturbed and the responsibilities of the generations muddled, and the failures of the contemporary social environment. Just as Miss Havisham is well served in her desire for revenge by the young Pip's narcissistic vulnerability, so the needs of late capitalism for continuing markets are well served by personalities who are alienated from the rest of the natural world and who are dependent on material satisfactions to sustain their sense of self-worth and identity. As others have pointed out (e.g. Lasch 1978), we inhabit a culture that encourages narcissism and greed.

In neither world is there a sense of a strong parental couple creating the necessary boundaries. Pip lacks a clear sense of what Mollon (1993) in his writings on narcissism calls lineage: the placing of oneself in terms of gender, parentage and time. Disturbances in lineage are often oedipal disturbances, failures to recognize the passage of time and one's mortality, failure to recognize oneself as the child of one's parents' relationship, failure to deal with those basic questions of 'who am I?' and 'where do I come from?' that bring a sense of being rooted in time, space, family and society, accepting limits and boundaries.

Pip's last defensive move in his journey of redemption is to imagine that he will marry Biddy, the only person in his childhood to have shown him maternal affection. His words betray his oedipal dream. In his fantasy he imagines that she will 'receive me like a forgiven child' who is in 'need of hushing voice and a soothing hand' (Dickens 1861/1946: 442). When he arrives back on the marshes, the offer of marriage on his lips, he discovers that, unbeknown to him, Biddy is getting married to Joe. With this move, Dickens asserts the primacy of lineage, and for the first time in the novel an adequate, loving parental couple appear in its pages. Pip is forced to accept a place in the world that is both less and more than he had imagined. There is a sense of both Pip and the world around him being set to rights.

In contemporary society there is a further aspect of lineage that needs to be explicitly articulated. People need not only to understand themselves as the product of their parents' relationship, but also to see themselves as part of the hierarchies and history of the natural world, subject to its laws, subject to its finite resources, respecting their place in its systems.

In a culture of acquisition and growth people do not expect to encounter what I have come to call 'the 'no' of nature'. It is this element that needs to be restored, psychologically and developmentally. We have to enable people to embrace the reality of limits in a world that has denied that such limits should exist.

Both Pip's journey and that of people facing ecological debt take place in worlds in which truth is obscured and illusion encouraged. Establishing a realistic relationship to the rest of the natural world and the other people and species who depend on it is a difficult task in a culture that denies the need for this.

Implications

The journeys travelled by the people described here differ most markedly from that travelled by Pip in their lack of resolution. In dealing personally with ecological debt, it is extremely difficult to see the effect of the reparation one makes, to feel forgiven, accepted or comforted. The attempt can isolate people, put them at odds with friends and family and exclude them from ordinary social relationships with colleagues and neighbours. And although most of the people I spoke to refused the notion that they were involved in a crime, their awareness of ecological devastation made it difficult for some of them not to anticipate punishment or revenge and hard sometimes to prevent themselves from behaving towards others as if revenge was appropriate.

It is not surprising that many people are unwilling to embark on such a journey. The important question is whether it is a journey that people must make if society as a whole is to change its relationship to the rest of the natural world and live sustainably within its limits. Is there an easier, less painful route to making the changes needed?

Research in cognitive, behavioural and social psychology currently dominates attempts to understand human reluctance to engage with environmental problems (see, for example, Moser and Dilling 2007; Whitmarsh, O'Neill and Lorenzoni 2010; or the 2009 report from the American Psychological Association). These approaches sit comfortably with the promotion of social marketing as the best means of persuading the public to make simple behavioural and lifestyle changes (see, e.g., DEFRA 2008 or Rose and Dade 2007). The social marketing approach segments the population and tries to sell behavioural change in ways that accord with people's current aspirations. The emphasis is on small steps that do not challenge current lifestyles and on upbeat visions of the future. Such approaches sidestep the difficult questions about what is realistically possible, about the kind of society that needs to be created and about the complexity of people's unconscious and emotional responses.

These approaches are increasingly being critiqued for their potential to reinforce negative environmental behaviours in the longer term, for their focus on changes that are not commensurate with the problem and for their inability to deal with people's defensive strategies when faced with major social difficulties (see, for example, Beattie 2010; Crompton 2008, 2010; Crompton and Kasser 2009; Randall 2009b). The work of Tom Crompton on unconscious values and framing is particularly interesting in this respect. In his report *Common Cause*, Crompton argues for the need to strengthen cultural values that encourage engagement with 'bigger-than-self' problems, making a strong case for the negative consequences of focusing on behaviours that may reinforce unconsciously held materialistic values. Essentially, Crompton is arguing for the need to activate people's capacity for concern about the environment and to decrease their narcissistic investment in activities that will harm it.

The people described would mostly fall into the categories described by social marketers as 'pioneers' (Rose and Dade 2007) or 'positive greens' and 'concerned consumers' (DEFRA 2008), part of the 40% of the population mostly likely to show concern about environmental issues. That these people suffered psychologically in the process of facing ecological debt is clear. Suggesting that such suffering should be extended to the rest of the population might seem perverse and counterproductive. However, as a psychotherapist it seems to me inevitable that dealing properly with something as serious as ecological debt involves difficult emotional processes: loss, trauma, guilt, anxiety, despair and rage all appeared in the conversations and stories people shared with me. These are not surprising reactions considering the gravity of the problem being faced. It is also clear from a psychotherapeutic perspective that focusing solely on upbeat solutions and easy steps can only stack up difficulties for the future, in the form of defences that become increasingly difficult to maintain.

The journey itself, however, could certainly be made easier. The extent of the guilt, despair and anxiety felt by some of my respondents was excessive, and their social isolation was sometimes extremely painful. These extremes of feeling can mostly be attributed to the lack of a social and political context that validated what they were doing. What would help?

My shopping list would include:

- greater psychological sophistication in policy, campaigning and service delivery;
- better psychological support for environmental practitioners and activists;
- political leadership that emphasized the need for both individuals and society to make major changes;
- publicity campaigns that are truthful and straightforward, and that attribute responsibility without inducing overwhelming guilt;
- policies that provide a strong framework for personal action, validating and rewarding it;
- an emphasis on proportionality of response and boundaries for what individuals should do;
- the provision of social support and affirmation to help people feel accepted and respected for acting in pro-environmental ways.

It is clear that the great expectations held by most people in Western society need to change. Helping them do so is a challenge that should involve a sophisticated but practical understanding of the psychological processes involved. Towards the end of *Great Expectations*, Pip remarks, 'My great expectations had all dissolved, like our own marsh mists before the sun.'

He achieves a state of grace. He achieves reconciliation with those he loves and who love him. We need to dissolve our own great expectations, our aspirations, our grandiosity and our dreams of mastery so that we, too, can recover our capacity for concern and make reparation.

Notes

1 Carbon Conversations groups are facilitated small groups that bring people together to explore their responses to climate change and help them make major changes to their personal carbon footprint by working through some of the emotional factors that inhibit change. Available at: www.carbonconversations.org
2 A recently established campaign, spearheaded by lawyer Polly Higgins, demands that the UN recognize ecocide as a fifth international crime against peace. Available at: www.thisisecocide.com

References

American Psychological Association (2009) *Psychology and Global Climate Change: Addressing a Multi-faceted Phenomenon and Set of Challenges*. Available at: www.apa.org/science/about/publications/climate-change-booklet.pdf (accessed Aug. 2010).
Beattie, G. (2010) *Why Aren't We Saving the Planet?* London: Routledge.
Crompton, T. (2008) *Weathercocks and Signposts: The Environment Movement at a Crossroads*. Godalming, UK: WWF-UK.
Crompton, T. (2010) *Common Cause: The Case for Working with Our Cultural Values*. Godalming, UK: WWF-UK.
Crompton, T., and Kasser, T. (2009) *Meeting Environmental Challenges: The Role of Human Identity*. Godalming, UK: WWF-UK.
DEFRA (2008) *A Framework for Pro-environmental Behaviours*. London: DEFRA.
Dickens, C. (1861) *Great Expectations*. London: Everyman, 1946.
Environmental Justice Foundation *The Aral Sea Crisis*. Available at: www.ejfoundation.org/page146.html (accessed Aug. 2010).
Hertwich, E. G., and Peters, G. P. (2009) Carbon footprint of nations: A global, trade-linked analysis. *Environmental Science and Technology*, 43 (16): 6414–6420.
Klein, M. (1937) Love, guilt and reparation. In *Love, Guilt and Reparation and Other Works 1921–1945. The Writings of Melanie Klein, Vol. I*. London: Hogarth Press.
Lasch, C. (1978) *The Culture of Narcissism*. New York: W.W. Norton.
Lertzman, R. (2008) The myth of apathy. *The Ecologist*, 19 (6): 16–17.
Lovelock, J. (2006) *The Revenge of Gaia*. London: Allen Lane.
Mishan, J. (1996) Psychoanalysis and environmentalism: First thoughts. *Psychoanalytic Psychotherapy*, 10 (1): 59–70.
Mollon, P. (1993) *The Fragile Self: The Structure of Narcissistic Disturbance*. London: Whurr.
Moser, S. (2007) More bad news: The risk of neglecting emotional responses to climate change information. In S. Moser and L. Dilling. *Creating a Climate for Change*. Cambridge, UK: Cambridge University Press.
Moser, S., and Dilling. L. (2007) *Creating a Climate for Change*. Cambridge, UK: Cambridge University Press.

Platform (2010) *Oil Pollution in the Niger Delta*. Available at: www.platformlondon.org/carbonweb/showitem.asp?article=73&parent=7&link=Y&gp=3 (accessed Aug. 2010).

Randall, R. (2005) A new climate for psychotherapy? *Psychotherapy and Politics International*, 3 (3): 165–179.

Randall, R. (2009a) *Carbon Conversations: Six Meetings about Climate Change and Carbon Reduction*. Cambridge, UK: Cambridge Carbon Footprint.

Randall, R. (2009b) Loss and climate change: The cost of parallel narratives. *Ecopsychology*, 3 (1): 118–129.

Rose, C., and Dade, P. (2007) *Using Values Modes*. Available at: www.campaignstrategy.org/articles/usingvaluemodes.pdf (accessed Aug. 2010).

Rust, M.-J. (2008) Climate on the couch: Unconscious processes in relation to our environmental crisis. *Psychotherapy and Politics International*, 6 (3): 157–170.

Scherer, G. (2004) *The Godly Must Be Crazy*. Seattle, WA: Grist. Available at: www.grist.org/article/scherer-christian/ (accessed Aug. 2010).

Simms, A. (2005) *Ecological Debt: The Health of the Planet and the Wealth of Nations*. London: Pluto Press.

Whitmarsh, L., O'Neill, S., and Lorenzoni, I. (2010) *Engaging the Public with Climate Change*. London: Earthscan.

Winnicott, D. W. (1963) The development of the capacity for concern. *The Maturational Process and the Facilitating Environment*. London: Karnac, 1990.

Worden, W. (1983) *Grief Counselling and Grief Therapy*. London: Tavistock.

Discussion

Great expectations: the psychodynamics of ecological debt

Margaret Rustin

Exploring the concept and experience of our indebtedness to the natural world through the lens of Dickens' masterpiece *Great Expectations* struck me as a bold and imaginative idea. Rosemary Randall's reading of the novel brings out clearly a picture of Pip's pilgrimage towards realization of his own nature and of his gradual and painful understanding of what has been given to him by others, which places him in the position of a debtor. The story provides us with a very striking and moving representation of a shift from a narcissistic state of mind towards one imbued with the qualities of relationship to self and others characteristic of Klein's account of the depressive position.

Randall is especially interested in the near-breakdown this entails for Pip. So many assumptions have to be given up, and such a colossal shift in his sense of himself is required of him. She links this with the profound shock and disorientation many people feel as they become aware of what is happening to the ecosystem as a consequence of human exploitation of natural resources, and she discusses what can help us to tolerate this new awareness of the risks to ourselves and others, both present and future generations, that our way of life entails. The potential catastrophe spelt out, for example, in Al Gore's impressive film *An Inconvenient Truth*, can, she suggests, have a catastrophic effect on its audience. One might see this as akin to Bion's (1970) description of moments of catastrophic change in psychic life, in which nothing looks or feels familiar and the self must struggle with loss of identity and continuity, feelings of incoherence and helplessness, and the enormous work involved in putting things together internally in a new way. This process also requires the recognition of the provisional and shifting nature of our grasp on reality if we are to remain in touch with ourselves and not be drawn back into a complacency, which serves to shield us from facing disturbing facts.

Great Expectations offers us, additionally, some very powerful descriptions of experience at a different level which also seems relevant to our response to anxieties about the future of the planet. In the opening scenes on the marshes, both Pip and Magwitch are in a state of terror. For Magwitch the question of survival is dominant. What he needs is food, which he is unable to get without help, and the possibility of free movement, which the leg-irons impede. He thus demands from

Pip what will provide him with an escape from starvation, from the cold wet marshes (so terrifyingly depicted by Dickens and memorable in visual form in the several film versions of this book) and from the lonely contemplation of the fear of death. The violence of his threats fills Pip with such terror that he risks the all-too-familiar harsh punishment meted out at home to steal what Magwitch has asked for. Pip feels himself to be outside the known world in his encounter on the marshes, distant from the safely familiar if often unpleasant life he knows. Visions of total hunger, unprotected exposure to the cold dark night and utter isolation are projected into Pip. They have a resonance within him, which we might link with his orphan state and the nearness to death that is part of his own history. He is vulnerable to Magwitch's threats in part because of his deep identification with him: he, too, knows unconsciously the fear of abandonment and the sense of imprisonment at the hands of a powerful persecutor.

In this sense, we can see both Pip and Magwitch overwhelmed by the infantile anxieties described so poignantly by Melanie Klein (1932). This is not a world where depressive guilt has any place. It is instead one dominated by anxieties about survival and the horror of dependence on unreliable and potentially cruel others. There are no benign adults in this world, and this makes the helplessness and neediness of the infant and of this infantile state when it is evoked in later life a terrible experience. Raw unmediated cold, hunger to which there may be no end, absence of comfort or protection fill mind and body.

These feelings are like the existential terrors that child psychotherapists not infrequently encounter in their work with seriously deprived children (Boston and Szur 1983). They are also reminiscent of the states of being Tustin and others have described as lying behind some children's protective autistic shell (Tustin 1981). They are similar to the sorts of feelings we find in some deeply depressed patients whose depression expresses their doubt about any entitlement to life (Rustin 2009).

Thinking about Magwitch who is facing transportation to the fearful unknown of Australia in this light brought to my mind a patient of mine, a boy of about 9 at the time I want to refer to. He had been adopted at age 5, and his early years had included the loss of his mother, the accidental death of a younger sibling, separation from his other siblings, sexual abuse by one of his mother's partners and periods of severe neglect and hunger in his first two-and-a-half years of life before he was removed from his mother's care. In therapy, he tormented me mercilessly with physical and verbal abuse, ridiculing my attempts to understand him. But I got little glimpses from time to time of the unbearable sadness and vulnerability behind his espousal of a tough and cynical identity.

One day he told me that his class at school were doing a play about transportation in the nineteenth century. He described the scene at the docks as those to be transported as felons were forced onto the ships and the heartbroken farewells of those on the shore filled the air. He had been given the part of one of the children to be transported as a punishment for theft. He sang me the song the children would be singing at the performance of this play, which put into words and music their emotional state. They sang about the fear of cold and heat, hunger and thirst, the unknown monsters of the ocean and of Australia, and of their loss of everything and everyone they knew. It was, of course, something of a stroke of probably unconscious genius by his teacher to provide such an apt container in this drama for this boy's ruptured life experience, and the song served to provide some words for almost indescribable childhood terror. The shared singing by the group of children doubtless expressed the comfort of being able to escape the sense of isolation and the loss of identity a child plucked out of his family must endure. Becoming one of a band of lost children, like the lost boys of Barrie's *Peter Pan* or Fagin's gang in Dickens' *Oliver Twist*, is a replacement for not belonging to anyone. In his involvement with the school play, my patient found a more benign context for working through his newly discovered hopes of being a member of a group that could allow its members to experience fellowship and to recognize emotional realities.

Thus on this occasion, and with his teacher's help, my patient made use of the symbolic potential of the children's song to explore feelings of loss, fear of the unknown and states of mourning, a rare achievement for him. Much more often, the idea that he could see himself as the rejected outsider whose survival was in doubt was violently denied. Instead, it was to be my fate to be the object of humiliating revulsion.

In one session this took the form of his taking over the contents of my room to create a comfortable den for himself from within which he could mock me and pelt me with small objects. I was, he said, a homeless tramp living in a cardboard box by the Thames. That was my home. I had dirty clothes, I stank and no one wanted me. I picked up scraps of food from the ground to keep body and soul together. The vividness of this fantasy was extraordinary, and its impact on my state of mind in the session was very striking. I felt huge, clumsy, exposed and helpless as I struggled to find a place to be, both physically (a sense of having somewhere to put myself in my own room) and mentally (a space in my mind from which I could talk to my patient about this constellation and its meaning). A sense of shame was a particularly powerful component of this.

I think this clinical vignette may help to convey the quality of what I am referring to as the unthinkable infantile terrors that the awareness of global unpredictability can stir up in us. We feel catapulted from our everyday sense of being at home in the world and feel that a basic sense of security has been brutally stolen from us and we are left unprotected in the dark.

What I am suggesting is at the core of the response to ecological uncertainty and evidence of instability is this more profound level of anxiety, the anxiety perhaps most vividly imagined in our response to actual infants and in our capacity to be in touch with infantile anxieties in ourselves. This idea began to take shape in my mind when I saw, a year ago, at the Children's Literature Centre in Newcastle, 'Seven Stories', an exhibition of children's drawings related to a primary school project in local schools on climate change. Their pictures were, of course, shaped in part by what their teachers had offered them in the classroom, and I do not know what that was. But I was struck by the stark depiction of their sense that their whole known world could disappear. There were polar bears that, with no ice in which to make their home and the loss of their traditional sources of food, would not survive. Suns were so powerful that they would burn up the vegetation and burn the skin of humans, clouds of dust shut out the sun and created darkness, floods (maybe all too prescient of recent massive floods) swept away roads and bridges, piles and piles of rubbish destined to defeat the impulse to conserve and recycle: these were the images they depicted. These children of 8 and 9 linked climate change to hunger, temperatures too hot or too cold to sustain life, ruination of the known world and evidence that the human capacity to preserve Mother Earth would be overwhelmed by despoliation.

Children's drawings very often express their unconscious anxieties – this was one of the early discoveries of the pioneers of child analysis – and it is natural for young children to convey rather openly in play and drawings the feelings they have about their dependence on the world as they know it.

The everyday metaphor Mother Earth is to the point here. Infantile dependence on mother's body is where we all start from – first a protective interior womb space and later receptive arms, lap, breast and mind when we are born. This is the prototype for our dependence on the Earth's resources as well as on each other throughout life. The baby's anxieties about mother's strength and solidity, which has to be adequate to survive infantile aggression and has to be reliably supported by the wider world of father and beyond, are profound. The loss of trust in the reliable presence and durability of mother's loving care is what makes the lives of those deprived of this and the consequent fear of the overwhelming destructive power of our impulses in the early years so difficult. When we are confronted with ideas and images in relation to our planet that echo these primary anxieties, we are vulnerable to shock and terror and to attempts to defend ourselves from such realities in ways that do not help us to face things, to sort out what is realistic in our reactions, and to use our minds to try to understand what adaptations in our way of life are necessary and possible.

This is why in thinking psychologically about ecological concerns, I suggest the depressive anxieties Randall describes so clearly are only a part of the picture. More primitive and at times even psychotic anxieties lie behind them. If we bear this in mind, we can understand an important dimension of what is referred to as 'climate change denial'. The argument, for example, in the United States between the mining billionaire who claims a right to blow the tops off mountains to get at the Earth's exploitable riches and the politicians who oppose this can be heard as voices representing, on the one hand, infantile omnipotent claims to unimpeded possession of the land which represents mother's body and total rage at the idea of this being denied, or on the other hand more developed socialized perceptions of the Earth in which the right of any individual to exploit and empty it (to leave

Mother Nature in a completely depleted state) is disputed. Instead, there is an idea that we have a responsibility to share with others, perceived as siblings in the inner world, both in the present and the future. It is, however, very difficult for any of us to manage an identity as citizens of the world. It is too big a thing for most ordinary human beings to feel responsible for all mankind, and there is therefore a real problem for even the best-motivated political or scientific leaders to find ways to make the vastness of responsibility for the future of Mother Earth at all bearable. In childhood, the child needs adults to look after things. Faced with such large concerns for the Earth and the generations to come, it is easy to feel too small to take them on.

The borderline disturbances and defences we understand better in consequence of the work of contemporary psychoanalysts are an important resource in grasping our responses to this situation. The concept of attacks on linking, as described by Bion and others (Bion 1959, Rustin 2005), helps us to comprehend the apparent illogicality of some positions taken up in public discourse. The operation of Steiner's (1985) concept of 'turning a blind eye', which describes the not-noticing that allows for the failure to give meaning to known facts and to the disavowal of responsibility is also pertinent. This type of defence comes into operation not from moral failure, but from the intolerable nature of the anxiety that has to be faced. It generates too great a degree of insecurity and persecution and places too heavy a burden of guilt.

In human development the mind does, however, build up resources through experiences of care and understanding by other minds to face infantile anxieties. Most of us learn gradually, though imperfectly, to be able to recognize and name emotional experiences, to think about what is going on within ourselves and to differentiate this internal reality from external reality. When unconscious phantasy, which remains an underlying aspect of our mental life throughout our lives, can come into conjunction with our capacity to test reality, then our helplessness is modified. A book like this one aims to contribute to the development of the sort of dialogue I suggest has the potential to detoxify catastrophic scenarios of climate change and enable creative scientific and political thinking to emerge.

References

Bion, W. R. (1959) Attacks on linking. *International Journal of Psychoanalysis*, 40: 308–315.

Bion, W. R. (1970) *Attention and Interpretation*. London: Tavistock. Reprinted London: Karnac, 1984.

Boston, M., and Szur, R. (Eds.) (1983) *Psychotherapy with Severely Deprived Children*. London: Karnac.

Klein, M. (1932) The psychoanalysis of children. In *The Writings of Melanie Klein, Vol. 2*. London: Hogarth.

Rustin, M. (2005) A conceptual analysis of critical moments in Victoria Climbié's life. *Child and Family Social Work*, 10: 11–19.

Rustin, M. (2009) The psychology of depression in young adolescents: A psychoanalytic view of the origins, inner workings and implications. *Psychoanalytic Psychotherapy*, 23 (3): 213–224.

Steiner, J. (1989) Turning a blind eye: The cover-up for Oedipus. *International Review of Psycho-Analysis*, 12: 161–172.

Tustin, F. (1981) *Autistic States in Children*. London: Routledge (2nd rev. ed. 1992).

Discussion

Great expectations: the psychodynamics of ecological debt

Bob Ward

Rosemary Randall's thoughtful and perceptive contribution demonstrates the kind of insight that I think is desperately needed among a wide range of professionals who communicate with the 'the public' about climate change. Randall challenges those like me, who are part of a community whose professional reputations are based on notions of objective technical analysis of science and economics, to recognize that the efficacy of our communication with a wider audience depends more than we currently acknowledge on an ability to recognize and understand the thoughts and feelings of people about the information we generate and convey.

My colleagues and I consider ourselves to be researchers and definitely not campaigners or environmentalists. Our aim is to investigate and explore technical aspects of the science and economics of climate change and to communicate our findings in a neutral way. Our primary aim is to inform rather than to motivate. We perceive our role as providing factual inputs into rational decision-making processes by individuals, businesses and governments about climate change. We try to frame the issue of climate change in terms of costs, investments, benefits and risks and trust that decision-making is based primarily on assessing these while taking account of broader issues such as socio-economic and political factors. But while my colleagues and I have some notion of what we believe to be appropriate decisions and choices that should be taken in light of our work, we remain mostly separated from the public and their consumption of the information we provide.

Randall provides glimpses of the thoughts and views of individuals who appear to accept the information provided by mainstream researchers and have concluded that climate change is a problem that requires action. And it reveals the sometimes strong feeling of shock and guilt that they feel, akin to those experienced by Pip in *Great Expectations* when he realizes that his anonymous benefactor is the convict Magwitch rather than Miss Havisham. Randall shows how people struggle to come to terms with their share of the ecological debt, just as Pip battles with his conscience.

This strong emotional response contrasts with the detached position that researchers adopt in our quest for objectivity, even though our professional activities are often guided by the recognition that the pace and scale of domestic and international action required to cost-effectively manage the risks of climate change are currently inadequate. And while we recognize that there are many and varied reasons why action is difficult, we also see barriers that appear irrational or based on perspectives governed by commercial interests or political ideologies. This has been exacerbated recently by a series of events that appear not only to have raised doubts in the minds of many people about whether climate change even requires action, but also to have damaged trust in the technical experts who are regarded as having made the case for action.

First, the posting on the web on 20 November 2009 of hundreds of email messages from the Climatic Research Unit at the University of East Anglia (UEA) led to negative media coverage around the world and to accusations of misconduct and fraud by climate scientists. A survey carried out in early December 2009 asked the following question (YouGov 2009):

> There have been recent controversies surrounding climate change research at the University of East Anglia. In general, do you trust climate scientists to tell the truth about global warming or not?

Only 41% of the British public said yes, while 44% said no. While there is no baseline against which to compare these results, annual public opinion polls by Ipsos Mori have consistently found over the past decade that 65–70% of the population trust scientists as a profession. Inquiries into the emails have cleared the climate scientists of fraud and misconduct, while criticizing a relative lack of openness by researchers (The Independent Climate Change E-mails Review 2010; Scientific Assessment Panel 2010). However, recent surveys have indicated that levels of public trust have not increased significantly.

The controversy over the emails, dubbed by some media commentators as 'Climategate', was compounded by the admission in January 2010 by the Intergovernmental Panel on Climate Change (IPCC) that the second volume of its Fourth Assessment Report in 2007 had included a scientifically unjustifiable prediction that all of the glaciers in the Himalayas could disappear by 2035 at current rates of melting (IPCC 2010).

Not only did the 'Glaciergate' episode undermine confidence in the reliability of the IPCC's reports, regarded by most scientists as the world's most authoritative review of the evidence for climate change, but it also raised general questions about the credibility of the institution and its willingness to acknowledge and correct mistakes. Claims of further errors in the IPCC report about the likely impacts of climate change, while largely unsubstantiated, were widely reported by the media (Ward 2010a). These undoubtedly contributed to public doubts about the credibility of statements about the potential consequences of climate change. An Ipsos Mori survey carried out between January and March 2010 found that 40% of the public tended to agree or strongly agreed with the statement that 'the seriousness of climate change is exaggerated', while 42% tended to disagree or strongly disagree (Spence, Venables, Pidgeon, Poortinga, and Demski 2010).

Many researchers worry that the issue of climate change seems abstract or theoretical and so seek to draw links with events today in order to convey a sense of immediacy and magnitude about the impacts. For instance, some scientists drew attention to possible links between climate change and flooding in Pakistan and China, and extended drought in Russia during the summer of 2010, even though attribution of individual weather events to climate change is currently not possible (Ward 2010b).

Yet while some people may have responded to these speculations by becoming more aware of and/or more concerned about climate change, others may have become more suspicious of the credibility of those claiming such a link, with some highlighting the occurrence of a cold winter in the United Kingdom in 2009–10 as evidence that global warming has stopped or even that it was never happening.

Nevertheless, Ipsos Mori found that 66% of the British public were fairly or very concerned because of 'any potential effects of climate change there might be on society in general' (Spence et al. 2010).

While these survey results appear to provide a strong base from which to build public support for action on climate change, only 24% agreed that climate change is mainly caused by human activities, with a further 7% agreeing that human activities are entirely responsible. However, a further 47% thought that climate change is caused partly by natural processes and partly by human activity.

These results indicate that there is confusion about the causes and potential consequences of climate change among a significant proportion of the public. Maybe this is because of the uncertainties in the science. As the Royal Society's recent guide to climate change has pointed out: 'There is strong evidence that changes in greenhouse gas concentrations due to human activity are the dominant cause of the global warming that has taken place over the last half century'. However, it also noted: 'It is not possible to determine exactly how much the Earth will warm or exactly how the climate will change in the future' (Royal Society 2010).

Some who are opposed to action on climate change emphasize uncertainty in the science in order to promote delay or inaction over reducing greenhouse gas emissions. They are drawing on knowledge of the hugely successful way in which this tactic has been employed in the past, particularly by those who lobbied successfully against restrictions on smoking for many years by focusing on very small uncertainties about the link to lung disease and other illnesses.

Indeed, Frank Luntz, the influential US pollster, famously wrote a memo for Republican Party campaigners in which he warned: 'should the public come to believe that the scientific issues are settled, their views about global warming will change accordingly' and so advised 'you need to continue to make the lack of scientific certainty a primary issue in the debate' (Luntz Research Companies 2002).

But the fact that three-quarters of the public accept that humans are at least partly responsible for climate change perhaps explains why 63% tend to agree or strongly agree with the statement that 'I can personally help to reduce climate change by changing my behaviour'. It is important also to recognize that only 10% think individuals and their families should be mainly responsible for taking action against climate change, compared with 32% who hold national governments responsible and 30% who think that 'the international community' should lead.

These survey results provide interesting context to the exploration by Randall of the feelings of individuals who seem to have accepted their own personal share of responsibility for the 'ecological debt'. In many ways, the concept of ecological debt is a helpful way of conveying the fact that there is a cost attached to emissions of greenhouse gases, because they cause damage through climate change, which should be paid for by the polluter rather than the polluted. There is no 'human right' to pollute the atmosphere.

However, as Randall points out, guilt is not an effective way of motivating most people. Some choose to deny that there is a problem when presented with solutions that appear to limit their freedoms, such as travel in cars or planes. This is now recognized by many who are seeking to mobilize public support, epitomized by the comment that Martin Luther King did not lead the civil rights movement by declaring 'I have a nightmare' (Miliband 2009).

I think there is some evidence that climate change has been framed along broadly left-wing political lines, with the implication that the only possible solutions require some sort of penitence for profligate consumption of products and services that involve emissions of greenhouse gases. For example, flying is often portrayed as an unacceptably 'extravagant' activity, even though it is still a relatively minor, albeit important, contributor to overall emissions and brings obvious benefits to those who use it as a form of travel. In essence, this encourages the 'depressive position' highlighted by Randall.

Perhaps a more effective way to generate support and participation from a wider group of people for action on climate change is by linking it to wider benefits rather than just the repayment of an ecological debt. Many low-carbon technologies, such as electric cars, offer multiple co-benefits in addition to their value in avoiding the risks associated with climate change. Indeed, the development of these new technologies also promises potentially significant and broad opportunities for new jobs and sustainable economic growth and development in both developed and developing countries (Stern 2009).

Public opinion surveys show that the majority of the public are willing to take personal steps to reduce emissions and avoid the risks of climate change (Department for Transport 2011). They will be even more enthusiastic about these actions if they gain even wider benefits, such as financial rewards by contributing surplus electricity from household solar panels into a national grid. Being part of the low-carbon industrial revolution should generate excitement and optimism, indeed 'great expectations', and should motivate action far more effectively than the guilt associated with an ecological debt.

References

Department for Transport (2011) Public attitudes towards climate change and the impact of transport: 2010 (Jan. 2011 report). Available at: www.dft.gov.uk/adobepdf/162469/221412/221513/4387741/climatechange2011.pdf

IPCC (2007): *Climate Change 2007: Impacts, Adaptation and Vulnerability. Contribution of Working Group II to the Fourth Assessment Report of the Intergovernmental Panel on Climate Change*, ed. M. L. Parry, O. F. Canziani, J. P. Palutikof, P. J. van der Linden and C. E. Hanson (Intergovernmental Panel on Climate Change). Cambridge, UK: Cambridge University Press. Available at: www.ipcc.ch/publications_and_data/publications_ipcc_fourth_assessment_report_wg2_report_impacts_adaptation_and_vulnerability.htm

IPCC (2010) IPCC statement on the melting of Himalayan glaciers. Intergovernmental Panel on Climate Change. Available at: www.ipcc.ch/pdf/presentations/himalaya-statement-20january2010.pdf

Luntz Research Companies (2002) The environment: A cleaner, safer, healthier America. In *Straight Talk*. Luntz Research Companies. Available at: www.luntzspeak.com/graphics/Luntz-Research.Memo.pdf

Miliband, E. (2009) Speech to the 2009 Labour Party Annual Conference. Available at: www.labour.org.uk/ed-milibands-speech-conference, 2009–09–28

Royal Society (2010) *Climate Change: A Summary of the Science*. Available at: http://royalsociety.org/climate-change-summary-of-science/

Scientific Assessment Panel (2010) *Report of the International Panel set up by the University of East Anglia to examine the research of the Climatic Research Unit*. Available at: www.uea.ac.uk/mac/comm/media/press/CRUstatements/SAP

Spence, A., Venables, D., Pidgeon, N., Poortinga, W., and Demski, C. (2010) *Public Perceptions of Climate Change and Energy Futures in Britain: Summary Findings of a Survey Conducted from January to March 2010*. Understanding Risk Working Paper 10–01, Cardiff University. Available at: www.understanding-risk.org/

Stern, N. (2009) *A Blueprint for a Safer Planet: How to Manage Climate Change and Create a New Era of Progress and Prosperity*. London: Bodley Head.

The Independent Climate Change E-mails Review (2010). Available at: www.cce-review.org/pdf/FINAL%20REPORT.pdf

Ward, R. E. T. (2010a) 'Disastergate' is an excuse for IPCC critics to dig up old academic rows. *The Guardian*, 26 Jan. 2011. Available at: www.guardian.co.uk/environment/cif-green/2010/jan/26/ipcc-climate-change

Ward, R. E. T. (2010b) Communicating climate change. *Weather*, 65 (11): 309–310. Available at: http://onlinelibrary.wiley.com/doi/10.1002/wea.683/full

YouGov (2009) YouGov/Left Foot Forward Survey Results. Available at: http://today.yougov.co.uk/sites/today.yougov.co.uk/files/YG-Archives-pol-lff-climatechange-091214.pdf

Reply

Great expectations: the psychodynamics of ecological debt

Rosemary Randall

Bob Ward and Margaret Rustin share with me a desire to bring people from a state of irrationality to one where they are able to think and act creatively in response to climate change. How to arrive there is the question.

Both Ward and Rustin describe experiences from their professional lives of being on the receiving end of irrationality. For Rustin, as a child psychotherapist, this is part of her work – difficult, but not unfamiliar. For Ward, it is a new and disorienting experience. As a climate scientist, Ward is part of a profession that privileges the creativity of rational thought. Scientists are admired and trusted for their impartiality and dispassion. Recent attacks have cast doubt on their motives, questioned their integrity and portrayed them as Machiavellian schemers only interested in acquiring the next research grant. Cast unwillingly into the limelight, they have been shocked that careful reiteration of scientific knowledge has not stemmed the flow of irrational rumour, half-truth, lies and fantasy. Ward recognizes that information is of little help in this situation. He hopes, however, that both this unreason and the turmoil of painful feeling displayed by the people I describe in the chapter can be avoided by a stronger appeal to the positive.

It is important to distinguish between the grip of the irrational, which defends against reality, and the working through of painful emotion that is part of creative thought and of coming to terms with difficult truths. To be emotional and to be irrational are not the same thing. The expression of feeling, whether joyous or painful, is part of normal life. It is one of the ways through which we know the world and relate to each other. It enables and directs thought. In contrast, to be irrational is to split thought and feeling. One emotion is amplified and used to defend against another. Thought is constrained in paranoid logic. Irrationality is characterized by fantasy, violence and desperation as more and more extreme methods are needed to keep reality at bay.

Ward draws hope from the fact that the majority of the UK population say they are willing to take personal steps to reduce emissions. However, the gap between this willing attitude and actual behavioural change remains wide, as Lorraine Whitmarsh describes in the introduction to her book *Engaging the Public with Climate Change* (Whitmarsh 2011). Despite minor gains in efficiency, UK emissions continue to rise (Shrubsole 2011).

In this context it is the conflict within people that I believe we have to address. People want to change – but only a little bit. They want to stop climate change, but they also want all the things that are causing it. As psychoanalysis shows, the human mind is uniquely equipped to hold conflicting views and feelings simultaneously. Negotiating these conflicts and working through the difficult feelings can bring us closer to reality. The alternative is a descent into unreason.

Rustin is more used to grappling with the irrational. She movingly describes the unbearable sadness and vulnerability that can lie behind a child's angry and violent fantasies and points to the depths of anxiety that can be touched by the threat of climate change. Indirectly she raises the question of what climate scientists may feel as the result of their discoveries. What is it like to work day after day with this knowledge? How have they coped with the feelings of helplessness or despair engendered first by the knowledge itself and then by the attacks made on them?

In contrast to the rest of the population, the defences of denial and evasion are not available to climate scientists. Their monitoring stations, lab results and computer screens tell them day after day not just that the news is bad but often that it is worse than yesterday's. It is hard enough to bear bad news and to process one's grief, anger and confusion. It is harder still to be the messenger of this news and, like Cassandra, be disbelieved. In conversation with scientists I have encountered bewilderment, depression and despair at public attacks or indifference to the knowledge they have brought to our notice. Their solution has often been to move further into the world of reason – more graphs, tighter arguments, greater precision.

Rustin suggests a different kind of response in her description of the schoolteacher's inspired casting of her young patient as one of a group of child transportees to Australia. The play provided containment for the child to experience and express his feelings of loss and terror and to gain comfort from the solidarity of others. In this safe space, emotion and cognition are brought together. The unspeakable terrors are symbolized and embodied. Thought is integrated with feeling, rather than being abstracted. Emotion becomes the route to new understanding rather than an obstacle.

Rustin's example reminded me of the work of 'Tipping Point' (available at: www.tippingpoint.org.uk) the charity that brings artists from all art forms together with scientists to create visual, theatrical and musical experiences that can express the complexity of our responses to this desperate issue. The challenge is to create experiences that will help people to face rather than avoid the reality of climate change, to contain terror, give words to grief and symbolize our pain and disorientation. All kinds of things may form part of this containment – stories, friendship, artistic works, community projects, political leadership, for example – but they need to be underpinned by the acknowledgment of truth and the integration of feeling. It is this working through of difficult emotion that will bring the strength to make the personal, social and political changes that are needed.

This is a cultural problem that is greater than any one discipline, touching on the values, beliefs, assumptions and structures of contemporary society. The value of the conference that gave rise to this volume was precisely in bringing together people who might otherwise not have spoken and seeing how their different perspectives might integrate. More work of this kind is surely the way forward in creating the experiences that will help the public embrace rather than flee from reality. Thanks to both Ward and Rustin for their thoughtful responses.

References

Shrubsole, G. (2011) *UK's Total Emissions Set to Rise*. Available at: http://climatesafety. org/uks-total-emissions-set-to-rise-new-data-obtained-by-pirc/
Whitmarsh, L. (2011) *Engaging the Public with Climate Change*. London: Earthscan.

Chapter 6

The myth of apathy
Psychoanalytic explorations of environmental subjectivity

Renee Aron Lertzman

Introduction

'People don't care. The public is apathetic. If people cared more, or understood the threats we face, they'd be doing more.' We have all heard this refrain, in one form or another. I am reminded of Freud's reflections when he wrote about the splitting of the ego, 'I find myself for a moment in the interesting position of not knowing whether what I have to say should be regarded as something long familiar and self-evident or as something entirely new and puzzling' (Freud 1940: 275). On one level, apathy is familiar and commonplace, as a way of describing a *lack* of response or action commensurate with increasingly urgent ecological challenges we have been experiencing and face in the future. On another level, when we explore apathy through a psychoanalytic lens, the picture changes quite dramatically, and becomes altogether more complicated.

When considering psychoanalytic engagements with climate change, apathy provides a useful handle for critically engaging with common conceptions of behavioral change and 'public response' to global climate change. Its pervasiveness masks the fact that the concept of 'public apathy' itself came into being in the 1940s, when information campaigning was increasingly used to shift policy and opinions (Hyman and Sheatsley 1947). For market researchers, when the public did not respond to information campaigns in desired ways, they were deemed 'apathetic'. The label has stuck and remains an acceptable descriptor for a lack of response, action or expressed concern (or outrage, as the case may be). Apathy is presumed when 'the public' does not respond adequately to efforts to educate, inform, motivate, cajole, induce guilt or pressure them to change their behaviors in light of an array of social problems, including climate change. However, as I argue, focusing on apathy elides the complexity of potential states that can make 'action' or responsiveness difficult. As Harold Searles wrote presciently in 1972, 'The current state of ecological deterioration is such as to evoke in us largely unconscious anxieties of different varieties that are of a piece with those characteristic of various levels of an individual's ego-development history. Thus the general apathy ... is based upon largely unconscious ego defenses against these anxieties' (Searles 1972: 363). In other words, there is arguably more than meets the eye when it comes to 'apathy' and lack of response in the form of specific actions (such as political engagement, supporting advocacy groups, consumer choices). In dismantling this myth of apathy, I seek to reframe environmental subjectivity in light of prevailing assumptions regarding a unitary rational subject (i.e. the lamented 'gap' between attitudes, values and behaviors, rather than attending to potential conflicts, ambivalence, contradictions, losses and so forth), and outmoded theorizations of the 'information-deficit' model.[1]

I argue that psychoanalytic approaches – such as attention to unconscious processes, defensive mechanisms such as denial, projection and splitting, and nuanced understandings of anxiety, loss, mourning, and grief – can help us bring back into the frame the potential presence of concern, anxiety, worry, fears, desires, aspirations and hopes in how we conceptualize environmental engagement (or its lack).

Reframing subjectivity and the 'public'

I will explore not only why apathy is a problematic concept, but also specifically what psychoanalysis and psychodynamic perspectives offer towards an understanding of environmental apathy. As a psychoanalytically informed social science researcher, I want to suggest that psychoanalysis offers perhaps the most powerful tools for working with the problems confounding those in the environmental advocacy and education sectors. These problems involve how to inform without alarming and how to educate without engaging in a pedagogy of despair and disempowerment. Psychoanalysis may be perceived as not having enough 'praxis' and real-world application beyond the consulting room. However, the questions on most people's minds at all levels of climate outreach, engagement and mitigation, questions such as how do we motivate behavioral change in individuals and in organizations, can be addressed through investigating what specific issues, topics, objects and relationships mean for us, and how we are more often than not bound up in a tangle of contradictory desires and impulses. Rather than focusing on 'levers' for change, as if people and societies can be engineered, psychoanalysis offers the potential for 'deep' shifts through first asking the most fundamental, interrelated questions: what does this mean, how can we best facilitate change?

I begin with one aspect of the analytic attitude that seems most salient: the capacity to focus on relations between what is conscious and unconscious. I present a brief case study drawn from my doctoral research (Lertzman 2010) and highlight selected theoretical contributions from psychoanalysis that have informed this work. These contributions include Freud's work on transience and on melancholia; Bollas (1987) on the transformational object as a way of thinking about environmental object relations; and Klein (1937) and Winnicott's (1963) concepts of reparation and concern, respectively. I conclude with brief comments about how this work may translate in terms of practice and application in the way we communicate about these difficult issues.

Analytic attitude and climate change

In 1992, Ivan Ward convened a conference, 'Ecological Madness', at the Freud Museum in London. In bringing together environmental activists and psychoanalysts, he proposed that a psychoanalytic engagement with environmental degradation does not preclude action or praxis and suggested possible tensions between an 'analytic attitude' and environmental activism (Ward 1993). In addressing his audience of activists and analysts, he emphasized that a psychoanalytic approach is not antithetical to a political orientation – indeed, it offers the ability to inquire into motivations, desires and (often) unconscious forces that is needed for an effective political movement (Ward 1993: 179). It can do this through exploring the relations between what is conscious and unconscious, rather than on the relation between the individual and the social. This helpful distinction is useful for distinguishing how a psychoanalytic approach can work fruitfully and collaboratively to support more effective political analyses and engagements.

Following Ward, I will contextualize how certain concepts in psychoanalysis – particularly those concerned with reparation and repair, mourning and loss, and the bases for concern – may be seen to dovetail with existing concerns in environmental circles. Generally there appears to be recognition that climate change can generate anxiety in individuals, groups and culture (e.g. see Norgaard 2011 on the social production of denial). It also seems self-evident, albeit tacitly, that there are competing desires with regard to industrial development: Western industrialized societies provide pleasures, but these pleasures also can occasion fears.[2] While psychoanalysis is relatively new to the topic of climate change and related ecological threats, there are parallel and overlapping discussions taking place in psychology and communication studies concerning the role of guilt and fear-based appeals to action, and how our emotions may interfere with effective responses to climate change threats (i.e., Moser 2007; O'Neill and Nicholson-Cole 2009). These concerns regarding what makes it difficult for individuals (for it is often individuals that are being referred to) are often articulated in terms of 'barriers' or 'obstacles' to engagement or desired behavioral change. However, there is a lack of robust research and insight as to *why* fear and guilt may cause such impediments to constructive adaptive practices such as reducing carbon, changing consumption patterns, and so on. Environmental ethics also touches on these themes, in terms of how difficult issues or contradictions are negotiated. For example, Simon Blackburn writes:

> Ethics is disturbing. We are often vaguely uncomfortable when we think of such things as exploitation of the world's resources, or the way our comforts are provided by the most miserable labour conditions of the third world. Sometimes, defensively, we get angry when such things are brought up. But to be entrenched in a culture, rather than merely belonging to the occasional rogue, exploitative attitudes will themselves need a story.
>
> (Blackburn 2001: 7)

We can ask from a psychoanalytic viewpoint, what does it mean to tell stories that help maintain exploitative attitudes? What are the stories we tell to each other and ourselves? How might defensive mechanisms enable or produce certain strategies for such stories? Engaging concepts of unconscious processes, phantasies and desires, what might we learn about the psychic processes involved when facing the 'ethics' of ecological sustainability, particularly if this touches on distress, reduction of pleasure and the reminder of limits and boundaries? As Searles (1972) pointed out in writing of resistance around relinquishing our attachments to practices such as driving or flying, to what extent do we defend against the perceived threats to our hard-won technical accomplishments, such as the automobile, the plane, the luxuries provided through wealth and exploitation?

One of the most simple and powerful contributions of psychoanalysis to the way we approach climate change and the way we as individuals, societies, communities and nations respond are in the concepts of ambivalence, contradiction and conflict: that we are able simultaneously to hold conflicting desires, thoughts and impulses, even those that appear diametrically opposed. As Walt Whitman wrote, 'We contain multitudes.' Some of these 'multitudes' are more preferred than others. This seems to be a basic point that is consistently overlooked, or possibly split off, in how environmental communications and campaigns are designed. Even research methods used to understand what people 'really think' about climate or environmental threats preclude the recognition of ambivalence and contradiction through the use of polls, surveys and focus groups, as if what people say is what they feel, and that we can distill our views or feelings into a set of multiple choice questions.[3] Environmentalists are often the unwanted guests at the dinner party, spoiling the fun in pointing out the conditions that provide us with our shrimp and pineapples. From a psychoanalytic perspective, we may consider what environmentally concerned or active people are 'holding' for others, what is being projected or introjected. Might it be our anxieties? People do not want to be reminded of the dark side of our pleasures; conditions in which our food was grown, picked and shipped, our own imbrications in practices that we may on the face of it find abhorrent and opposed to our sense of ourselves as good and virtuous. And yet we are, in hundreds of small and large ways, reminded of our complicity in the destruction of our own home, our planet's ecosystems. How we manage, cope, process, reflect and respond is where psychoanalysis can help us recognize the power of unconscious desires: that we may in fact want our cars and cheap flights and also want to avoid global climate-induced catastrophes. Further, we possess both reparative and creative capacities and destructive capacities; while industrial practices may in fact involve a certain form of splitting in terms of 'good nature' and 'bad nature', what we know of human history, how we relate to nature, environment, ecology is far from straightforward and must always be contextualized socially, historically, culturally and politically.

Field study: Great Lakes and Green Bay

How psychoanalytic conceptions of subjectivity can revise our concepts of environmental engagement was made clear over the course of my fieldwork in the Great Lakes region of the United States (Lertzman 2010). I chose an ecologically troubled region on the edge of the Great Lakes in Wisconsin, home to much industry and to paper processing plants, and designed in-depth interviews with ten participants.[4] While the region has a reasonably active yet small environmental community of highly concerned scientists, advocates and educators, the city is more known for its paper industry, its football team the Green Bay Packers and the Fox River, listed as a Superfund Site by the Environmental Protection Agency (federal funds are committed for a mass-scale clean-up effort). At the time of my study there was an active campaign taking place to mobilize people to go to a website and support a new initiative to help pass legislation to protect the Great Lakes. Administered by a coalition of organizations, it was called 'Healing our Waters,' and one aspect of this campaign was through a print advertisement. This featured a girl facing a body of water, with a large sign lettering reading, 'WARNING: No more swimming. No more fishing. No more drinking water. NO MORE GREAT LAKES.' I was curious as to how well this advertisement spoke to people and whether or not it reflected their concerns; also, if the prompt to visit a website would be experienced as 'attunement' or 'mal-attunement' to their particular needs and desires.

I designed and administered an online survey to $3,024 = n$ residents in Green Bay through a partnership with a local public opinion research firm. The survey was constructed so participants could both rate their own levels of engagement and awareness – i.e. how often do you think about environmental issues, from 'never' to 'frequently' – and respond to short questions demonstrating levels of awareness and issue literacy. I selected ten participants, based largely on their self-rating (in the middle range, which includes 'occasionally' and 'depends on events', and the quality of their responses, to signify moderate levels of awareness of local and global environmental issues. None of the participants was actively involved in any form of environmental activity or 'activism.' In other words, if polled about their actions and attitudes about nature and the local environment, these participants may appear as 'apathetic' about chronic or acute ecological threats.

A more complicated story

I designed the interviews based on psychoanalytic research methodologies, such as the 'psychoanalytic research interview' (Cartwright 2004): as open-ended, free associative and narrative-based. I interviewed each participant three times, each interview lasting approximately one hour, in the participants' homes. During these interviews, I heard complicated, often contradictory accounts, containing high affective investments in the region and in specific objects (such as the river, beach, dunes, boat, fish). I also witnessed a capacity for distancing proximity to the threats facing these same objects.[5] To paraphrase Whitman, how the region was articulated itself was a 'multitude': it was spoken of alternately with affection, disgust, anger and appreciation. There was nothing monotonous about how people related and experienced their place, the environment and the degraded resources. The industry had brought thousands of jobs and made the city prosperous; it also damaged the ecosystems and, more recently, is putting the entire drinking water supply for thousands into jeopardy. The water itself was an enormous focus for the participants as sites of intense affective investments, associated with family, autonomy, love, creativity, as well as fear, threat and abjection. I began to detect narratives concerning how industrial threats and development may be negotiated affectively and seemingly in largely unconscious ways, that had little to do with more consciously expressed 'concern' or even attitudes about the environment. There appeared a surplus of affect with regard to these topics, and yet these individuals kept their emotional investments largely private and channeled in various intimate practices, from food choices to teaching grandchildren about the value of nature. It was, as one participant related to me, 'something I keep close to my person', and he said that he would never dream of becoming involved with any environmental groups or activities.

While extremely cautious about the risks of conducting 'wild analysis' (Cartwright 2004; Kvale 1999) and wary of using a psychoanalytic approach to data analysis, I nevertheless found the data powerfully suggestive of complicating issues that may produce difficulties for engaging in reparative practices, such as being involved with a local restoration project, political engagement to regulate pollution, or being involved with an environmental organization. In other words, I found high levels of concern – sadness, anxiety, loss and even grief – regarding the condition of the waters so close to home. While I had entered the project initially interested in how anxiety may inform a lack of engagement or responsiveness to environmental issues, I was struck by narratives of loss and what I sensed as an 'arrested mourning' with regard to the places and ways of life, and earlier selves, that environmental issues seemed to evoke. For example, when people spoke of specific sites (for instance a river or a beach on the Great Lakes) it was with nostalgia, as if the site itself no longer existed, it had ceased to exist. While there seemed to be longing for the reparation of these sites, at the same time they were not actively relating to them, as for instance those who are engaged in reparative practices such as clean-ups, etc. The 'environmental objects' here were often bodies of water facing chronic threats, from pollution and toxicity to invasive species, and appeared to be held in a static, idealized state. They had ceased to be alive and active for the participants.

Case study

Donald was a 69-year old man, a native of Green Bay, whose father had worked for the paper mill. He grew up with a strong connection with the region and its waters. A 'self-made man', he had started at an entry-level job at a local vegetable cannery and had worked his way up to become the president. He was not involved with any environmental activities or organizations, although he clearly had strong affective investments (demonstrated through personal narratives and activities such as caring for a small piece of private land much revered for its beauty and ecological attributes). Such concerns were to be 'held close to my person' and kept private, not to be shared in the public sphere. To understand more about this, I tracked a few themes and looked at how specific objects were invoked possibly to help maintain certain 'good object relations' with an object that had clearly also been a 'bad' object: the Fox River.

Donald lived near the Fox River, with a view of the paper mill. Two incidents in Donald's life were associated with this river. First, his father had had a serious accident, resulting in physical injury and being dismissed from the company, resulting in a severe family crisis. Second, Donald had lost a front tooth while playing with some friends on the shores of the river, resulting in a painful and shamefully visible false tooth for his entire adolescence and into early adulthood. The Fox River was hardly registered as a 'river' in the sense of a body of water used for recreation, and yet he told me in our final interview, as an afterthought, about a canoe trip he had made down the length of the river with a friend, 'just to do it'. At the same time, Donald spoke with deep affection for the region, the industry, and his affective associations with the city. I noticed there were also a few 'good objects' that seemed vital for his ability to remain positively connected with this place. One such object included a childhood book given to him by his aunt, *Paddle-to-the-Sea* (Holling 1941): an adventure story about the journey a carved wooden figure takes through the entire course of the Great Lakes.

The story presented a new dimension of analysis, in which perhaps Donald had introjected his young boy self into the adventures of this river, while remaining anchored home out of loyalty to the father (as is the case in the story, of the boy who carves the figure). The book was given to him in 1949, and he continues to read it and handle its pages. The book potentially offered Donald a 'positive' relationship with the region, as the story includes themes of resourcefulness, loyalty to family (father specifically), the love of his aunt, the kindness of strangers, and the mythic journey a boy makes in leaving home and returning a man. The second 'good object' for Donald involved a holiday home he bought with his newly wed wife: a pristine parcel of land on a river about twenty miles out of town, similar to the woods and river he played in as a child, which had since become developed and degraded. I noticed an affective investment in a new place, enabling Donald to maintain positive reparative energies, and yet not directed towards the region most in need of repair. There were a few traumatic associations with the region and the river: his father's downfall and his own loss of an adult front tooth (with potential symbolic import), but also a profound sense of affection and appreciation for what the river and the town has provided for him and his family. And yet he expressed at the end of our three interviews an intense sadness and concern for his children and grandchildren's future, and the fate of the waters he loved. Why would Donald's reparative energies not be directed actively towards the river and the Great Lakes?

The revolt against mourning: environmental melancholia

Across the interviews with the ten participants were accounts of affection and longing for the rivers and lakes of childhood. I listened to the articulations of environmental identity and also certain mantras likely inherited by family and culture, such as, 'Get on with it, one must move on, there is nothing I can do.' I began to consider more carefully a form of social melancholia that may be constituted by a lack of action or response to pressing, even urgent issues. It seemed the issue was not so much a lack of affect or concern, as is often assumed in environmental advocacy circles, but a static set of relationships with the lost or damaged object: in this case a body of water or a way of life. Building on the fundamental psychoanalytic insight concerning splitting, the topic of loss and mourning is central to a consideration of the affective and psychic dimensions of contemporary ecological issues. I have found Freud's work on mourning and melancholia particularly fruitful, including his short essay 'On Transience' (Freud 1916). While the essay speaks to modes of response to an awareness of loss through change – in this case, the seasons and the transience of nature and indeed of life – I feel they can be extended to provide a powerful lens onto how we might manage encountering environmental degradation. He begins with an account of how an awareness of loss leads to a withdrawal of affect and engagement:

> Some time ago I took a walk through a blossoming summer landscape in the company of a silent friend and a young and already well-known poet. The poet admired the beauty of the nature around us, but it did not delight him. He was disturbed by the idea that all this beauty was bound to fade, that it would vanish through the winter, like all human beauty and everything beautiful and noble. . . . All the things he would otherwise have loved and admired seemed to him to be devalued by the fate of transience for which they were destined.
>
> (Freud 1916: 179)

He added, 'We know that such absorption in the susceptibility to decay of all that is beautiful can produce two different impulses in the mind. One of these leads to the painful world-weariness of the young poet, the other to revolt against the asserted fact' (Freud 1916: 179). That is, we can either withdraw affectively from the world, or we can deny the prospect of loss (reality).

While Freud was writing in a different historical and ecological context, he articulated one of the fundamental aspects of the experience of industrial change and ecological threat: anticipatory mourning and the risk of withdrawing affect from those damaged objects (what can appear as 'apathy'). The vignette speaks to dilemmas of experiencing and encountering environmental issues, the way our experience of our material world and invested objects can be mediated by the sense of impending loss or change. Freud's walk in the summer landscape, with the devastation of the First World War on the horizon, is not unlike a walk through a surveyed forest, or viewing a mountaintop slated for mining, or perhaps watching a nature documentary about rare creatures whose very existence is in peril. There is the turning toward or away from the risk of loss, from the sense of unpleasure Freud writes about, or as the 'silent friend', not engaging directly with what we see before us.

The essay suggests how environments and affectively invested objects may be experienced through (imagined or actual) loss and impending threat. He presents a parable of three modes of being: one in suspended engagement, the poet who cannot be fully present, who is arrested by an anticipatory mourning that is neither active nor inactive and a silent witness. The mourning experienced by the poet is not 'worked through': objects in the garden were transient, fated to extinction: mocked by its own frailty, beauty was eclipsed by its negation and had no value and no meaning. The other mode (the narrator, presumably Freud) reflects a capacity to appreciate what is, to be present to it; the fleeting quality of existence increases, not diminishes, appreciation of value and beauty and potentially mobilizes the desire to engage and *connect* (we can think of environmental activists who, while being aware of the ecological threats, are avid outdoors enthusiasts, with a keen appreciation for nature, wildlife and recreation). Freud describes the mode of being his friend the poet manifests as a 'revolt in their minds against mourning'. The knowledge of loss so disturbed him that he could no longer appreciate beauty except as something already lost (von Unwerth 2005: 3). Freud considered it must have been the psychical revolt against grief that devalued the pleasure of beautiful things and gave 'a foretaste of mourning its decease, and since the mind instinctively recoils from anything that is painful, they felt their enjoyment of beauty interfered with by thoughts of its transience' (Freud 1916: 306).

Freud writes that the war

> broke out and robbed the world of its beauties. It destroyed not only the beauty of the countrysides through which it passed and the works of art which it met with on its path, but it also shattered our pride in the achievements of our civilization, our admiration for many philosophers and artists, our hopes of a final triumph over the differences among nations and races . . . In this way it robbed us of so much that we had loved, and showed us the fragility of much that we had considered stable.
>
> (Freud 1916: 307)

Freud presciently notes the way such an affected society tends to cling 'all the more intensely' to that which remains in the aftermath of such loss, including a renewed passion for nationalism, kin and pride on what is held in common. (This echoes Randall's work on loss, identity and climate change; see Randall 2009.) In what appears to be an articulation of reparative capacities, Freud notes that mourning does, indeed, come to an end, and our libido is 'free' to become attached to new objects. What has been lost can be mourned but does not damage the capacity to love again:

> As long as we are still young and active, it is also able to replace the lost objects with objects that are, where possible, equally precious, or with still more precious new ones. . . . Once mourning is overcome, it will be apparent that the high esteem in which we hold our cultural goods has not suffered from our experience of their fragility.
>
> (Freud 1916: 200)

In the poet's stance towards the garden and his affective withdrawal (unable to take pleasure or even be present to the surroundings), we recognize what appears and is often labeled as 'apathy' or complacency. While it is impossible to know what may be taking place for those who withdraw from the world for a variety of reasons, we must also remain open to the possibility of a form of psychic revolt as described by Freud, if we seek to understand what may appear as apathy or a lack of 'engagement'.

Toward an environmental object relations theory

The interviews I conducted in Green Bay led to the second theoretical construct so helpful in thinking about environmental object relations. The phenomenon of loss, particularly of specific objects – such as a clean lake, a woodland, a bit of river-bank behind the house to enjoy, the ideal of clean air and water – is both a subtext of environmental issues and a topic engaged with in psychoanalytic work pertaining primarily to the loss of human (object) relations. To view ecological, nonhuman objects, or at least to allow for the ways in which we imbue our object world with associations that may involve human others, sensations, memories or desire, calls on a different way of approaching environmental 'objects' (and thus, to try to understand the potential meanings of their losses). Bollas (1987, 1992) developed in his 'transformational object' relations theory (in addition to and building on Winnicott's theory of the 'transitional object', 1971: 86–94) the notion that things and events have psychic resonance, and how we relate and respond to them potentially presents another language, one of desires, longings and unconscious wishes. It is not to say objects are 'only' a construct of our imagination, but to acknowledge place of subjectivity in the human-non-human object world.

To illuminate the significance of certain environmental object relations, in terms of how certain places or objects contain resonances or meanings (i.e. what is the Fox River to a participant? Or the shores of Lake Michigan, enjoyed as a child?) I created maps for how participants related to and articulated specific 'objects' and began to trace potential lines of affective associations. For example, as discussed, for Donald the river was a site of a traumatic accident (losing a front tooth), his father's trauma (an injury leading to job loss) and ecological degradation (a perception of the river as an abject object). I could see how he potentially channeled his reparative energies into a different object – a holiday home nearby on a different river, a more pristine and 'wild' site. As also discussed, Donald also introduced (literally and figuratively) a childhood book about the Great Lakes

(*Paddle-to-the-Sea*) and spent much of one interview telling me about the story, and the aunt who had given it to him (the same aunt who took him hiking in the woods at age five). I was fascinated how this object helped him perhaps maintain a 'positive object relation' with the region that had created great distress and crisis in his family, as well as with his beloved aunt who had first taken him into the creek – literally, as they both fell in on their walk – as a child.

The theory of the 'transformational object' is based on the premise that in adulthood we seek out objects – relationships, things – that offer the potential to alter our internal mood as our mother once could. It is the endless quest for a reconnection, the ability to re-experience 'an uncanny fusion with the object, an event that re-evokes an ego state that prevailed during early psychic life' (Bollas 1987: 16). It would seem that this orientation to environmental object relations could be fruitful for understanding the complex binds we find ourselves in. Our worlds are often full of objects that are, in fact, connected with ecologically degrading practices, whether or not we are conscious of this. Once these connections are made visible or at least felt through awareness or literacy, dilemmas arise of how we may shift modes from consumptive to reparative. To seek the transformational object in adult life is to recollect an early object experience, to remember not cognitively but existentially – through intense affective experience – a relationship identified with cumulative transformational experiences of the self. The object itself is being identified with specific states of being, with affective relations. Bollas is thus conveying the often unconscious and mysterious – or not so mysterious – attractions and longings expressed for certain places, things, events, as transformational objects. As Bollas points out, the concept of the transformational object brings us to transference and countertransference, the more operationally relational aspects of psychoanalytic practice (1987): 'Transformational-object-seeking is an endless memorial search for something in the future that resides in the past,' Bollas writes. 'I believe that if we investigate many types of object relating we will discover that the subject is seeking the transformational object and aspiring to be matched in symbiotic harmony within an aesthetic frame that promises to metamorphose the self' (Bollas 1987: 40).

Guilt, loss and ambivalence

Finally, it is of no minor significance that the concept of reparation itself is a central topic for both environmentalists and psychoanalysts. Klein addresses the process by which reparation – the desire to repair, make right, restore – arises out experiences of guilt, loss and ambivalence. Our ability to experience (tolerate) ambivalence toward that which we have harmed (mother, nature, lakes, sibling, etc.) enables the desire to repair others and our environment (Klein 1937; Segal 2003). It is the inability to tolerate ambivalence (socially and psychically) that can lead to splitting and manic defenses (Segal 1997). Object relations theory has been applied and discussed primarily in the context of clinical treatment (Anderson 1992), with rare forays into social and political topics (e.g. Ben-Asher and Goren

2006). However, object relations theory also provides persuasive and compelling theoretical schema for approaching human–environment relations, specifically concerning ecological environments and human treatment of nature.

As Joseph Mishan (1996) wrote, it is the avoidance of these feelings of loss, guilt, and subsequent mourning that acts as the greatest barrier to reparative capacities. On the other hand, when ambivalence can be recognized, aggression is felt as damaging an object that is also needed and desired (e.g. the mother, or our natural resources) and brings in its wake not more hatred but a mobilization of loving impulses and the desire to repair and restore. This is referred to as 'reparation' and is seen to exist in dialectical relationship with aggression and hate; that in order to be moved to repair, we must be able to tolerate and acknowledge our destructive capacities. As Segal points out, 'the recognition of ambivalence, guilt and fear of loss is extremely painful, and powerful defenses can set in, manic defenses, paranoid defenses, all necessitating some degree of regression to more primitive forms of functioning' (Segal 1997: 159). Segal explicitly makes this point in considering the ability to move from destructive to constructive modes of being. It is essential to differentiate the fact of the existence of ambivalence, which is there from the beginning, from the achievement of knowing one's ambivalence, accepting it and working it through. Such working through is accomplished primarily through the recognition of guilt and loss brought about by ambivalence, which leads to the capacity to mobilize restoration and reparation. This does not mean that aggression is absent; but it becomes proportional to the cause, as does the guilt attached to it (159).

Psychoanalytic theory has a unique contribution to make towards the understanding of contemporary social and political problems, in this case specific to human–environment relations and current crises in the various formations of public response. Because of its focus on the experience of conflicts between constructive and destructive attitudes, the psychoanalytic approach is well placed to shed light on some of the destructive forces taking place socially (Segal 1997: 157). While a central problem as articulated in environmental sectors concerns a lack of public responsiveness or what appears to be apathy or inertia (e.g. the 'attitude–behavior gap' and 'barriers to action' discourses), psychoanalytic and psychodynamic thought has for decades engaged with problems of anxiety, defenses, and the phenomenon of resistance. To be precise, psychoanalysts and psychotherapists have had to develop strategies for working with impaired and neurotic processes that present barriers for engaging with reality more effectively and competently. Such resistance has close parallels with the manifestations of 'resistance' observed in relation to climate change and other ecological degradations, such as the increase in consumption and enjoyment of toxic goods (Randall 2005), denial of the problem, aggressive belief in technological fixes and rescue schemes, scapegoating and blame and forms of disavowal and rationalizations.

Situating psychoanalysis within environment, social relations and human subjectivity

Placing psychic analysis within broader social, political, economic and ideological contexts has been a notorious weakness in psychoanalysis. The tendency is to focus with a fine grain on the interior worlds, with some neglect to the forces beyond that arguably help shape affective experience. Therefore, rather than focus exclusively on the content of in-depth interviews in my research, I endeavored, with varying levels of success, to take account of the place as having its particular circulations of stories, mythologies, legacies and identities. Thus when participants told me what a wonderful place Green Bay is to raise a family, or the fact that industry has provided such resources for the community, I considered the meaning and function of such tropes in terms of community identity, historical mythologies and specific meanings in individual biographical lives. The constellations produced are therefore place-based, affective, social and cultural. Guattari's political philosophy of the 'three ecologies' – the (ecological, biotic) environment, the social, and subjectivity is concerned 'with visible relations of force . . . but also take into account molecular domains of sensibility, intelligence and desire' (2000: 28). This is an approach that refuses to compartmentalize and parse out these relations, which are in fact mutually shaping one another dynamically, although within clear asymmetrical power relations (e.g. the species of frogs under threat from human activity are arguably with less power than, say, those capable of either ruining their habitat or poisoning the waters in which they live).

Guattari sought to acknowledge the paradox we find ourselves in on these various levels:

> Wherever we turn, there is the same nagging paradox: on the one hand, the continuous development of new techno-scientific means to potentially resolve the dominant ecological issues and reinstate socially useful activities on the surface of the planet, and, on the other hand, the inability of organized social forces and constituted subjective formations to take hold of these resources in order to make them work.
>
> (Guattari 2000: 31)

It is important to note that he does not articulate these observations through the language of a 'disconnect' or the 'gap' between attitudes, values and practices, for the similar reasons psychoanalysis would never do so: because it would ignore the mutuality and systemic nature of these processes (e.g. Bateson 1972; Trist and Murray 1990). In fact, the notion of a 'gap' between values, actions and attitudes would be incoherent and unproductive. Thus, paradox is a term for this apparent gridlock between awareness, recognition, and action. If we can replace apathy with paradox, contradiction, grief, shock, loss and other affective processes, we may start to get somewhere.

Reframing the myth of apathy: contributions from psychoanalysis

An analytic attitude – afforded by a psychoanalytic perspective – privileges an emphasis on the relations between conscious and unconscious processes, making space for the presence and influence of psychic negotiations with conflict, distress, contradiction and ambivalence. Further, in exploring our relations with the natural world and human impact on ecological systems, an analytic attitude would recognize the integral phenomenon of loss, mourning and grief in human experience and seek to insert such sensitivities into how we understand the (often) painful confrontations with ecological issues. It is an attitude – or, perhaps more accurately, an underpinning epistemology and ontology – that assumes the constitution of human subjectivity as conflicted, anxious and ambivalent, but also creative, reparative and capable of great concern. Seen in this light, it is possible to rethink conceptions of apathy, not as a clear lack of concern but, rather, as complicated expressions of difficult and conflicting affective states. If we can approach apathy through this perspective, we may start to see how in fact messages and vehicles for transmitting environmental issues may in fact do more harm than good. If we appreciate and are sensitized to the myriad ways we may respond to distress, anxiety and potentially frightening information, such as the extreme fragility of the Great Lakes or the prospect of eating fish contaminated with PCBs – depending on our respective social and biographical contexts – we may think twice before alarming the public into swift action. Further, messages of moralizing and admonishment of poor response or action may also reify self-states or self-concepts of an 'apathetic subject' which do not necessarily help mobilize reparative energies.

How does this translate into practice? As my work, professionally and academically, has been concerned primarily with environmental communications and engagement, I consider how a particular campaign can be made both to *acknowledge* and *offset* anxieties, guilt and ambivalence. I believe this has traction for the various ways climate change issues are communicated, across sectors and contexts (i.e. education, outreach, campaigns, media, entertainment). Such work requires research and piloting to support its efficacy. There is a profound need for investment in further research and pilot projects in the domains of affect and emotional attributes of contemporary environmental subjectivity and politics. An approach that manages to integrate the lessons outlined here – how to acknowledge and provide space for contradiction, ambivalence, loss and mourning – avoids the simplifying and patronizing tone of many environmental messages and the manic emphasis on 'solutions,' as if the messiness of our situation can be avoided and glossed over. Acknowledgement of the painful dilemmas we grapple with can have a potentially disarming effect, ideally softening defenses and sparking creativity and concern (Winnicott 1963). If we frame our communications presuming a presence of care and creativity, rather than an absence, as is often the case, we may see some radical reframing of public engagement.

It is my hope that in presenting these particular contributions from psychoanalysis, a field that is generally considered to tend towards being too esoteric and insular to have real-world effects outside the consulting room, we can begin to appreciate how a psychoanalytic conception radically shifts the ways in which environmental issues and responses are played out. There remains much work to be done. I believe a psychoanalytic engagement with environment and climate change is not only productive, it is vital. It is up to all of us to consider the most effective ways in which this can be carried out. The portability of clinical work into social and political arenas is not at all clear and is rather fraught with potential pitfalls, such as the ignorance of socio-cultural and historical contexts, the over fixation on the psyche and internal processes, and an inability to move outside a rarified esoteric language to build bridges with other communities of practice. The best antidote to this tendency is actively to interface with multiple sectors dealing with these issues: climate scientists, artists, poets, social scientists, engineers. It is time for us to have humility in our limitations of knowledge and at the same time, be forceful and strong in advocating for a place for these dimensions. This is the challenge and the opportunity that faces us.

Notes

1 The 'information-deficit' model refers to the theory that if people knew more about climate change, had the facts and the information, there would be more action and response towards mitigation and general acknowledgement. This theory has been consistently proven to be otherwise (e.g. Norgaard 2011; Lorenzoni et al. 2007).
2 In an interview conducted with geographer Yi-Fu Tuan, Tuan comments, 'We have finally managed to regulate nature, and after we have done so, tend to worry, instead of feeling contented. We feel uneasy and wonder why we are doing this. Why? Could it be ignorance of history?' (Lertzman 1997).
3 For example, see the Yale Project on Climate Change and Communication report, *Climate Change in the American Mind*, Nov., 2008.
4 My interview methodology was based largely on the work of South African psychoanalyst and researcher Duncan Cartwright (2002), who had created an approach to the 'psychoanalytic research interview' as a mode of exploring highly sensitive and possibly charged content, and psychosocial methodologies innovated in the United Kingdom (e.g., Hollway and Jefferson 2000; Walkerdine 2002; Wengraf 2001).
5 For more background and information about the research methodologies used and developed, see Lertzman 2010.

References

Anderson, R. (1992) *Introduction*. In: R. Anderson (Ed.), *Clinical Lectures on Klein and Bion*. London: Routledge.

Bateson, G. (1972) *Steps to an Ecology of Mind: Collected Essays in Anthropology, Psychiatry, Evolution, and Epistemology*. Chicago, IL: University of Chicago Press.

Ben-Asher, S., and Goren, N. (2006) Projective identification as a defense mechanism when facing the threat of an ecological hazard. *Psychoanalysis, Culture & Society*, 11: 17–35.

Blackburn, S. (2001) *Being Good*. Oxford: Oxford University Press.

Bollas, C. (1987) *Shadow of the Object: Psychoanalysis of the Unknown Thought*. London: Free Association Books.

Cartwright, D. (2002) *Psychoanalysis, Violence, and Rage-type Murder: Murdering Minds*. London: Routledge.

Cartwright, D. (2004) The psychoanalytic research interview: Preliminary suggestions. *Journal of the American Psychoanalytic Association*, 52: 209–242.

Freud, S. (1916) On transience. In J. Strachey (Ed.), *The Standard Edition of the Complete Psychological Works of Sigmund Freud, Vol. XIV*. London: Hogarth Press.

Freud, S. (1940) Splitting of the ego in the process of defence. In J. Strachey (Ed.), *The Standard Edition of the Complete Psychological Works of Sigmund Freud, Vol. XXIII*. London: Hogarth Press.

Guattari, F. (2000) *The Three Ecologies*. London: Athone.

Holling, H. C. (1941) *Paddle-to-the-Sea*. Boston, MA: Houghton-Mifflin.

Hollway, W., and Jefferson, T. (2000) *Doing Qualitative Research Differently: Free Association, Narrative and the Interview Method*. London: Sage Publications.

Hyman, H., and Sheatsley, P. (1947) Some reasons why information campaigns fail. *Public Opinion Quarterly*, 11: 412–423.

Klein, M. (1937) Love, guilt and reparation. In *The Writings of Melanie Klein, Vol. I, Love, Guilt and Reparation and Other Works 1921–1945*. London: Hogarth Press.

Kvale, S. (1999) The psychoanalytic interview as qualitative research. *Qualitative Research*, 5 (1): 87–113.

Lertzman, R. (1997) At home in the world: Interview with geographer Yi-Fu Tuan. *Terra Nova*, 1 (1): 98–105.

Lertzman, R. (2010) *The Myth of Apathy: Psychoanalytic Explorations of Environmental Degradation*. Unpublished PhD thesis, Cardiff School of Social Sciences, Cardiff University.

Lorenzoni, I., Nicholson-Cole, S., and Whitmarsh, L. (2007) Barriers perceived to engaging with climate change among the UK public and their policy implications, *Global Environmental Change: Human and Policy Dimensions*, 17 (3–4): 445–459.

Mishan, J. (1996) Psychoanalysis and environmentalism: First thoughts. *Psychoanalytic Psychotherapy*, 10 (1): 59–70.

Moser, S. C. (2007) More bad news: The risk of neglecting emotional responses to climate change information. In: *Creating a Climate for Change: Communicating Climate Change and Facilitating Social Change* (pp. 64–80). Cambridge, UK: Cambridge University Press.

Norgaard, K. (2011) *Living in Denial: Climate Change, Emotions and Everyday Life*. Cambridge, MA: MIT Press.

O'Neill, S., and Nicholson-Cole, S. (2009) Fear won't do it: Promoting positive engagement with climate change through visual and iconic representations. *Science Communication*, 30 (3): 355–379.

Randall, R. (2005) A new climate for psychotherapy? *Psychotherapy and Politics International*, 3 (3): 165–179.

Randall, R. (2009) Loss and climate change: The cost of parallel narratives. *Ecopsychology*, 3 (1): 118–129.

Searles, H. (1972) Unconscious processes in relation to the environmental crisis. *The Psychoanalytic Review*, 59 (3): 361–374.

Segal, H. (1997) From Hiroshima to the Gulf War and after: Socio-political expressions of ambivalence. In: H. Segal and J. Steiner (Eds.), *Psychoanalysis, Literature and War: Papers 1972–1995*. London: Routledge & Institute of Psychoanalysis.

Segal, H. (2003) From Hiroshima to 11th September 2001 and after. *Psychodynamic Practice*, 9 (3): 257–265.

Trist, E., and Murray, H. (1990) *The Social Engagement of Social Science: A Tavistock Anthology*. Philadelphia, PA: University of Pennsylvania Press.

von Unwerth, M. (2005) *Freud's Requiem: Mourning, Memory and the Invisible History of a Summer Walk*. New York: Riverhead.

Walkerdine, V. (2002) *Challenging Subjects: Critical Psychology for a New Millennium*. London: Palgrave.

Ward, I. (1993) Ecological madness, a Freud Museum conference: Introductory thoughts. *British Journal of Psychotherapy*, 10 (2): 178–187.

Wengraf, T. (2001) *Qualitative Research Interviewing: Biographic Narrative and Semistructured Methods*. London: Sage.

Winnicott, D. W. (1963) The development of the capacity for concern. In *The Maturational Processes and the Facilitating Environment*. London: Karnac, 1990.

Winnicott, D. W. (1971) *Playing and Reality*. London: Tavistock Publications.

Discussion

The myth of apathy: psychoanalytic explorations of environmental subjectivity

Irma Brenman Pick

'Not I'

I am pleased to have this opportunity to think about Renee Lertzman's rich and stimulating paper. She introduces us to many other interesting contributors too, and I shall single out two: I was particularly grateful to be introduced to the work of Harold Searles and also that of Simon Blackburn, both of whom she quotes. As early as 1972, Searles said,

> The current state of ecological deterioration is such as to evoke in us largely unconscious anxieties of different varieties that are of a piece with those characteristic of various levels of an individual ego-development history. Thus the general apathy is based upon largely unconscious ego defenses against these anxieties.
>
> (Searles 1972: 363)

Blackburn much later wrote,

> Ethics is disturbing. We are often vaguely uncomfortable when we think of such things as exploitation of the world's resources, or the way our comforts are provided by the most miserable labor conditions of the third world. Sometimes, defensively, we get angry when such things are brought up. But to be entrenched in a culture, rather than merely belonging to the occasional rogue, exploitative attitudes will themselves need a story.
>
> (Blackburn 2001: 7)

I too am interested in the way that ruthless exploitation becomes entrenched in a culture, rather than belonging to the occasional rogue, as well as in the disowning of personal responsibility. This kind of disowning, which accompanies the exploitation, is so well expressed in the words of Samuel Beckett's (1984) 12-minute verse play on the death of a baby: there we see only a mouth recalling the event and re-iterating, in the title of the play, 'NOT I' – that is, it is Not I who will feel the loss, nor I who will bear the guilt (of this ruthless exploitation).

Lertzman draws our attention to the views of Christopher Bollas (1987) that things and events have psychic resonance – and what more so than Nature, Mother Earth, onto which, perhaps in different ways, we may transfer both our earliest love and appreciation of the beauty and nourishment provided by the good mother/ breast, as well as our – notably in the modern Western world – destructive rapaciousness.

If we look at this narrative, as Blackburn suggests, we might ask, what is the narrative, and where does this begin? Freud spoke of His Majesty the Baby, and many analysts since have stressed how in their view the infant is governed by a wish to have it all and be it all. Klein, in rather graphic language in the 1930s, speaking of the infant's (unconscious) phantasy of an inexhaustible breast, wrote of 'the infant's wish to totally possess not only the breast but the mother's whole body, to scoop out the contents, attack all her other babies, etc.' (Klein 1935: 282). The ruthlessly exploitative links to the body of the Earth and its degradation were not made at that time.

But of course Mother Nature, as well as being, even sentimentally, equated with something good, also represents violent forces – floods, storms, earthquakes, droughts – in keeping with the infant's phantasies of his own nature and also his fears of retribution or even primitive parental violence. Just as we now think about what comes from the baby and what comes at the baby, we may want to think about what humans do to so-called nature, and also what nature does to humans? And so we may, for example, experience global warming as the work of a retributive, punitive superego. So we may not only be angry when this is brought up, as Blackburn suggests, but also fearful of what may be experienced as retribution from Mother Nature.

In the course of healthy personal development, the child's growing concern for the mother and her other babies is supported by the father, and the infant gradually modifies his demanding behaviour, becoming more 'civilized', but only up to a point. Psychoanalysts argue that these primitive wishes, then, are never entirely given up. One way of gratifying them would be to split them off and project these wishes into others, and then vicariously identify with characters who are indeed endowed with being able 'to have it all and be it all'. I have in mind the adulation of, and wish to emulate, say, the royal family, Hollywood stars, footballers and other 'celebrities', to name but a few.

So we split off and distance ourselves from our rapaciousness, such that it is BP or Walmart who exploit the Third World and the Earth itself; it is NOT the responsibility of an I, as a middle-class, car-owning, holiday-going, cheap-flight seeking, etc., individual who wants cheap food, petrol, clothing, etc. And indeed NOT I who does not want to have to give anything up. Yet there are situations where we do willingly give things up, in times of war and for our loved ones; and perhaps we need to give more thought to the particular circumstances that mitigate for or against this.

Lertzman, in her study of the Great Lakes, emphasizes the difficulty of mourning the loss that industry brings to what is then remembered as an earlier, idyllic world. While I agree with her, I think the difficulty in mourning may be exacerbated by the fact that, like the infant, we want it all. We want the benefits and comforts brought by industry, and we want the untainted idyllic world; I think the nostalgia she describes goes together with a disowning of the wish to have it both ways or, like the infant, to be able to have it all.

I notice this, for example, when looking at a younger generation, some of whom may feel very strongly about the dangers of global warming yet may in our culture be part of a group where they absolutely MUST HAVE the latest fashions, the most up-to-date technology, etc. How do our psyches and the times we live in interact? When I arrived in London in 1955, we did not have, nor expect to own, central heating, washing machines and dishwashers, all now considered to be ESSENTIAL! And, once we have them, it is very difficult to give them up.

As Lertzman says, very many of us want our cheap flights and want to prevent global catastrophe. We also want all our wants satisfied and want to be morally self-righteous about the greed of others too; perhaps we are like our patients who both want and do not want insight, want to change and want to be able to maintain the status quo, like the saying, 'God, make me virtuous, but not yet.'

Winnicott (1969) famously said that the first duty of the analyst/mother is to survive. It becomes intensely anxiety-provoking when we are faced with a picture of a damaged Mother Earth or her 'babies', even in far-away places. These are the animals threatened with extinction, massive groups of people wiped out by floods, and so on. These sights provoke such anxiety not only because of the current environmental reality, about which we may indeed feel guilt but also, I believe, because it touches off our earliest guilt about damage we have done much closer to home, to our earliest and most essential – indeed, life-giving – relationships.

Psychoanalysts, among others, tend to assume that at a primitive level we feel threatened, then, not only by the external catastrophes that may befall us, but the catastrophe of retribution from a primitive superego, which makes us feel, as Lertzman says, so vulnerable and helpless and so persecuted by guilt that we can only turn a blind eye and become apathetic.

What might be the relevance for politics of the problems we think about in analysis: namely, how does the infant make the move from, in Klein's terms, the paranoid-schizoid position, where the infant is at the mercy of the persecutory superego, to the more depressive 'position', where the infant can begin to bear that he cannot have it all and begin to take some responsibility for his destructiveness?

It seems to me that the capacity of the infant to make this move is very much allied to the presence of a 'good' realistic parental couple who share responsibility, support him to take his responsibility for damage done, to bear the guilt for what cannot be repaired and to make appropriate reparation where possible; in other words to do the best that can be done under the circumstances.

What would a government akin to this model look like? Work, for example that of Rustin (1991), already exists thinking about the question of the link between the psychic and the political and, more specifically, the work of Weintrobe. In her paper on 'Runaway Greed and Climate Change Denial' (2009) she has sought to address the question of the way an attitude of ruthless exploitation, often unconscious, may become entrenched in a culture.

When we feel vulnerable and helpless, we do depend on realistic 'parental' leadership. Why is this is so hard to come by? So often leadership, even that which starts out by presenting itself as concerned for others – say, the Church or the Communist Party – quickly becomes corrupted. The leaders, while preaching moral self-righteousness, become again the ones who have to have it all and be it all. A member of Mugabe's tribe once 'explained' to us that Mugabe was not to be criticized because in tribal culture the Chief is entitled to have it all. So the very processes that may motivate leaders to wish to make things better seem to revert back to infantile rapaciousness.

Lertzman asks us to think about what might help people to move away from the apparent apathy she has described. I believe that facing some truths about ourselves may strengthen our capacity to think about and deal with these very complex problems. The more we avoid facing the conflict, the more we are at the mercy of relentlessness, which makes human understanding worthless.

So, I return to my earlier point: Do we at some level put or keep in place 'leaders', whether appointed by heredity or elected by democratic process, whatever may be the conscious rationale, also to carry both our unacknowledged moral self-righteousness and our greed – that is to say, to carry parts of ourselves that we find unmanageable, and which we cannot bear to acknowledge? And, because our 'leaders' carry split-off, unacknowledged parts of ourselves, we may become excessively vulnerable to their machinations and helpless to deal with their excesses, just as we were unable in the first place to deal with our own.

In conclusion, once again I want to thank Renee Lertzman for addressing some of the underlying causes of 'apathy'.

References

Beckett, S. (1984) *Collected Shorter Plays*. New York: Grove Press.

Blackburn, S. (2001) *Being Good*. Oxford: Oxford University Press.

Bollas, C. (1987) *Shadow of the Object: Psychoanalysis of the Unknown Thought*. London: Free Association Books.

Klein, M. (1935) A contribution to the psychogenesis of manic depressive states. In *Love, Guilt and Reparation and Other Works 1921–1945. The Writings of Melanie Klein, Vol. I*. London: Hogarth Press.

Rustin, M. (1991) *The Good Society and the Inner World: Psychoanalysis, Politics and Culture*. London: Verso.

Searles, H. (1972) Unconscious processes in relation to the environmental crisis. *Psychoanalytic Review*, 59 (3): 361–374.

Weintrobe, S. (2010) On links between runaway consumer greed and climate change denial: A psychoanalytic perspective. *Bulletin Annual of the British Psychoanalytical Society*, 1: 63–75. London: Institute of Psychoanalysis.

Winnicott, D. W. (1969) The use of an object. *International Journal of Psychoanalysis*, 50: 711–716.

Discussion

The myth of apathy: psychoanalytic explorations of environmental subjectivity

Erik Bichard

How sustainable change agents can adopt psychoanalytic perspectives on climate change

Renee Lertzman's essay is a valuable and welcome addition to a growing volume of work that seeks to understand the human response to the implications of climate change. She successfully argues that the debate should be expanded beyond the social and cognitive psychological descriptions of barriers, gaps and values, and the social marketer's focus on environmentally friendly behaviour. The chapter offers evidence on 'how humans cope with and manage anxieties, and how these strategies may inform or impede constructive responses'. This is important to sustainable change workers who come from other backgrounds, such as ecology, urban regeneration or corporate responsibility, for example. Much of our focus to date has been on trying to influence policymakers who fund evidence-based policy campaigns. Thus far these have failed to increase the volume, frequency and potency of the public's sustainable response to climate change. The main tools have been fear and apocalyptic narratives and a combination of exhortation, education and awareness. Some limited economic subsidies have been targeted at vulnerable groups, but none of these approaches has worked very well so far.

A behaviour change strategy that targets people who do not care, when actually they care too much, will have very little effect and may be counterproductive. This may explain the disconnection between the belief that responding to climate change is a personal responsibility, and the failure to address the threat in a timely manner (Bichard and Kazmierczack 2009). If a more tuned approach could be adopted based on coaxing people into believing that some form of action will make a difference, this could not only ease levels of anxiety, but it could mitigate the more severe effects that climate change is predicted to have on vulnerable populations. Proposals on how psychoanalytic methods can be translated into public policy could lead to valuable new approaches with which to foster the 'mobilization of reparative energies' that Klein referred to over 70 years ago.

It must be tempting for strategists who have been relying on more and varied types of education and awareness, or stoking worries about future well-being, to blame their lack of success on public apathy. Lertzman places the onus firmly back onto the policymakers and campaigners by arguing that, far from a lack of concern, people are wrestling with inner conflicting tendencies where the winner is invariably inaction, the default state of the cautious and the confused. While facing some formidable challenges in moving these ideas into an effective motivating strategy, Lertzman's essay deserves to be read widely outside her own discipline.

Psychoanalytical perspectives have the potential to influence policymakers, but there are also difficulties associated with making these observations operational when seen through a political lens. It would be impractical to seek to understand the individual needs and anxieties of the entire population or even a neighbourhood, in order to shape policy around personal histories. But this does not undermine the importance of the psychoanalytic perspective, and the work needs to resonate beyond the discipline and into the wider world of the sustainable change agent.

Aspects of the language and theory expressed in Lertzman's work may be inaccessible to other disciplines, and the psychoanalytical perspective on climate change responses may benefit from being located within a wider list of influences (Swim et al. 2009). Specifically, the affective response (how emotional responses to climate change are influencing concern) needs to be considered in relation to other potential influences, including:

- Coping appraisal: if the threat occurs, what is the severity of its impact, and how long will this last?
- Motivational processes: how much priority should be placed on acting in a timely manner, and who is behind the warnings to act?

In her Great Lakes field work Lertzman is able to colour in some of the conflicts and anxieties of people who are responding to a landscape that has been degraded within living memory. While this is helpful to explain individual reaction, it prompts many questions about whether this approach could also assist with the understanding of collective reactions to climate change. It is understandable that the psychoanalytical approach concentrates on the individual, but work on communities reveals that collective and norm-based influences are also a key element of the way a community will respond to an environmental threat.

The Swedes are a good example of this. In *Positively Responsible* (Bichard and Cooper 2008) the authors identify Sweden as the country most associated with internalizing the importance of nature and sustainable living. Swedes seems to have an advanced sense of deliberative democracy (they like to move forward by consensus), and they have a deep appreciation of natural renewal (perhaps brought on by the experience of long cold winters). Their history has also taught them that resources are finite, and there is a fear that resources could run out if they are not managed in a sustainable manner. A famine in 1867 and the subsequent mass migration to the United States of over a million Swedes may have contributed to a collective duty of care towards the environment from the remaining population.

One of the ways this manifests itself is in the concept *Allemansrätt*, the public right of access to land. The anthropologist Gudrin Dahl (1998) explains that the Swedish right to roam is considered by Swedes as a human right, which symbolizes the values of freedom and equality. These are basic human desires and, as such, it becomes much clearer how the denial of access to Nature looms so large in the Swedish psyche. Referring to a sub-set of the legal right to roam – the right to take resources from the countryside – she says 'it is hard to see why the right to pick something of such limited economic value has to be granted by the constitution, if it were not for the symbolic value. Being allowed to pick berries, mushrooms and wild flower stands as a metaphor for having access to Nature' (Dahl 1998: 296). These cultural collective outlets to action may temper the powerlessness and isolation that individuals feel when they think they are fighting against global trends on their own. It may be one route to the agency that appears out of reach by those reacting to the same changing conditions in other cultures, but it may also be possible to transfer the factors that are present in Swedish society to others in a way that resonates with their own identity.

A further dimension uncovered by Bichard and Cooper concerns the collective cultural reaction to a specific threat. Cultural tendencies can overcome the feeling of powerlessness in the face of a threat to the sea, for example. In 1995 there was widespread condemnation of plans by Shell to dispose of an obsolete North Sea oil platform by sinking it rather than dismantling it on land. The country that showed the most active opposition to the proposal, including a nationwide boycott and some violent attacks on Shell filling stations, was Germany, even though it has one of the smallest coastlines in Western Europe. The timing was right for a combination of religious and political influencers to take up the cause. However, Jochen Vorfelder, head of Media at Greenpeace Germany at the time, had a theory about why the Germans cared so much. His view was that Germans elevate the North Sea from a minor extension of the Atlantic to a romantic entity (personal communication, 15 July 2007). This stems from a general tendency of Germans to idealize nature, but they also have a specific interest in the sea, and the North Sea in particular. Some 90% of Germans have very little contact with the sea, and this may be why some have a greater sense of appreciation and very positive feelings when they do have a chance to come down to the coast. Vorfelder speculated that this love of the sea may be associated with childhood memories, reinforced by a large body of German romantic poetry and literature. Heinrich Heine's *Heimkehrcycle, Die Nordsee* (or North Sea Cycles) is a prime example of this. Vorfelder thought he understood, as a German as much as an environmentalist, why the public were so outraged by Shell's intentions over Brent Spar.

This anecdotal evidence of overcoming inaction and ambivalence through a collective identity or experience goes some way to addressing possible ways by which those affected by climate change can foster reparative actions. It may be possible that the responses of people living in Wisconsin could lead to different behaviours depending on the magnitude and significance of their experience. Those who lose their sense of place as a life-long resident may differ from those who experience change in an adopted area. Those living through the slow decline of a fishery may react differently to those who see at first hand the result of a fish kill incident after a chemical spill. The reaction of an individual to a threat to a local park may be different depending on the presence or absence of a local green group, regardless of whether the individual was active in that group.

The proposition that some sections of society care too much about environmental loss clearly needs more investigation. Some may be waiting for the right set of explanations before they take action out of fear that their status could be undermined if they do the wrong thing. Others may worry that they will be identified as being gullible or foolish for taking action based in information that later is discredited, or committing time and resources while others do nothing. This is exemplified in a Joel Pett cartoon showing a man standing up in a climate change conference and saying, 'what if it's a big hoax and we create a better world for nothing?'

However, the really interesting test-bed for the theory of caring too much may be the corporate sector, where the norm-based pressures from peers, employees, regulators and the constraints of fiduciary duties may be intertwined with individual responses to climate change, which are the more familiar ground for psychoanalysts. One way of tackling this is to read business observers' descriptions of what they think is hindering pro-environmental and adaptive behaviour through the psychoanalytic filter.

Llewellyn (2007), at the time senior policy advisor at Lehman Brothers, described four different ways in which he thinks business leaders manage to avoid taking action on climate change. First, there are the 'ideological contrarians'. Llewellyn says that 'if these people have an intellectual belief, it is that they are smarter than the crowd. More often, to them, it is just a game of attracting attention by attacking the majority'.

He called the second category the 'grey conservatives', who like to appear reasonable, say they are neither 'pro' nor 'anti' things like climate change but also say that there is not enough evidence to support action. 'Do more research, collect more data and continue the debate, they counsel sagely.' Next are the 'non-sequiturians', those who produce a range of different arguments that all share a common structure. These people highlight all possible explanations of why the Earth is warming, other than man-made influences. Llewellyn explained that they often wrap up their statements by saying, 'Therefore, it cannot be caused by mankind.' He pointed to the 'therefore' as the giveaway, 'the delicious non sequitur: just because the Earth has warmed for one reason in the past is no reason why it cannot warm for a completely different reason in the future.'

Llewellyn's last category is the 'busy executive'. He said that their argument is loftier and more pragmatic than the others'. They are unmoved by the scientific evidence, preferring to wait until they know what the policymakers are going to do. This allows these busy people to avoid the facts and simply keep a weather eye on the implications for their business. Llewellyn wondered if, when we are 'confronted by a troubling issue, we seek out some territory in which we feel intellectually comfortable and are surrounded by friends'. A comparison of Lertzman's findings to Llewellyn's description could reveal some new dimensions to the understanding of corporate inaction and may inform the tactics adopted by sustainable change agents.

Finally, Lertzman's work raises some timely questions for those attempting to understand how to direct pro-environmental behaviour change. Two examples of this are briefly presented here. The first is the use of behaviour theory to understand how different people respond to a range of influences when faced with a decision. These influences, set out in the 'theory of reasoned action' (Ajzen and Fishbein 1980), can be difficult to understand for those outside the disciplines of psychology or psychoanalysis. I have sought to interpret the barriers as questions that weigh differently in each individual including:

- Do I understand that there is a problem?
- Do I care about the problem?
- Do I know what to do about the problem?
- Will my solution work or make a difference?
- What will others think of me if I act?

While many of these questions may not be consciously considered when individuals are asked to act in response to the threats of climate change, they do offer a useful guide to policymakers during the design stage of a campaign. Reasoned action has been criticized by some as being over-reliant on rational decision-making processes, and the psychoanalytical experience suggests that this may be justified. Looking for consensus in this area might lead to a synthesis of these different approaches which could help to build better policy.

The second example is a values-based method that segments the population terms of their needs and desires. Developed by Cultural Dynamics (available at: www.cultdyn.co.uk) this is founded on the Maslow-based research into the hierarchy of human needs. The segmentations falls into three main types of people: inner-directed 'pioneers', outer-directed 'prospectors' and security-driven 'settlers'. Settlers like to meet people like themselves and people they know. They connect through clubs and family and like to be associated with tradition. Their reaction to a problem is to look for somebody to do something about it, and they search for brands that make them feel secure. 'Prospectors' like to meet important people and connect through big brands and organizations. They like to be associated with success and don't like threats to the things that they have worked for. Their reaction to threats is to organize, and they search for brands that make them feel good. 'Pioneers' like to meet challenging and intriguing people and connect through their own networks. They like to be associated with good causes where they can put their values into practice. Their reaction to threats is to do something about it themselves, and they search for brands that bring new possibilities. Rose (2007) explains that these three segments can be sub-divided further into four grades or 'value modes' for each segment.

Values are a further influence that may have origins in early experiences and relationships. The Cultural Dynamics team developed a system that segments people according to their psychological needs, as opposed to the usual lifestyle or shopping behaviour, or class and wealth demographics. Understanding why people hold these values and identifying likely value trends in neighbourhoods could help policymakers to frame campaigns in a way that would result in better levels of pro-environmental behaviour.

As climate change inexorably continues to impact the health, safety and well-being of global populations, psychoanalytic insight into the effects that this has on people will be very important, but particularly if this can be translated into effective public policy.

References

Ajzen, I., and Fishbein, M. (1980) *Understanding Attitudes and Predicting Social Behavior.* Englewood Cliffs, NJ: Prentice-Hall.

Bichard, E., and Cooper, C. L. (2008) *Positively Responsible: How Business Can Save the Planet.* Oxford, UK: Butterworth-Heinemann.

Bichard, E., and Kazmierczack, A. (2009) *Resilient Homes: Reward-based Methods to Motivate Householders to Address Dangerous Climate Change.* Project Report, Environment Agency. Available at: http://usir.salford.ac.uk/11276/5/report_FINAL_160909-2.pdf

Dahl, G. (1998) Wildflowers, nationalism and the Swedish Law of the Commons. *Worldview: Environment, Culture Religion,* 2: 281–302.

Llewellyn, J. (2007) In a confusing climate, I think the scientists are probably right. *The Observer,* 2 Sept. Available at: www.guardian.co.uk/business/2007/sep/02/politics.greenpolitics (last viewed 4th May 2011).

Rose, C. (2007) *Sustaining Disbelief: Media Pollism and Climate Change.* Accessed Aug. 2007. Available at: www.campaignstrategy.org

Swim, J. et al. (2009) *Psychology & Global Climate Change: Addressing a Multifaceted Phenomenon and Set of Challenges.* A report of the American Psychological Association Task Force on the Interface Between Psychology & Global Climate Change. Available at: http//:www.apa.org/science/about/publications/climate-change.aspx

Chapter 7

Unconscious obstacles to caring for the planet

Facing up to human nature

John Keene

Introduction

This exploration of some difficulties in our psychological relationship to the planetary ecosystem grew out of two challenging conversations. The first was with my grandson, who worries about the possibility of a Third World War; the second was with a politician, who questioned whether we will be able to do anything in time about climate change. Children are acutely aware of their dependence on adults for their safety and survival, and so they can be sensitive barometers of the pressure of anxiety about keeping the world safe for human beings. Keeping the world safe for human beings looks increasingly difficult, as the actions needed to prevent global warming from exceeding 2°C have widely been opposed or not implemented. Given that so many of our inherited adaptive patterns were developed to manage problems on a family and local scale the challenges of cooperating on a planet wide project are daunting and require the acknowledgement of many difficult aspects of our individual and collective behaviour.

I suggest that when it comes to how we see ourselves, we live in a curious world of doublethink. In spite of Darwin's contribution linking mankind with its biological heritage and Freud's account of the disowned operations of the mind, our public discourse tends to follow the Enlightenment view that rational thought now predominates, and there is recurrent surprise on finding so frequently that this is not the case. One might say that the problems potentially posed by significant global warming tick all the wrong boxes as far as our evolved, individually learned and group responses to our environment and to danger are concerned. The plasticity of human behaviour and the power of language, which have been such an advantage in the development of the species, mean that human individuals have to develop their own models of the world and their relationship to it. These models, which operate to a considerable degree outside awareness, are profoundly affected by experiences in infancy. These partly unavailable and partly disowned assumptions, which powerfully affect our behaviour, are not just the domain of psychoanalysts but are well recognized in folklore, myth and in our literary and dramatic heritage. Sadly, rapid and magnificent technological advances have had little impact on these fundamental processes, which restrict our capacities to comprehend and to deal with external reality and to restrain our capacities for self-destruction. For seemingly wish-fulfilling reasons the existence of anxious pessimistic scenarios in the past is taken by sceptics as reason to ignore the problem of climate change.[1] This is poor logic, as even hypochondriacs can get seriously ill. The argument that climate change is just another mistaken apocalyptic vision does not fit well with the readily available evidence of humankind's poor record in dealing with other large-scale problems such as the destruction of habitat, the widespread deterioration of water supplies, the elimination of wild food stocks, mass extinctions of species, the reduction of bio-diversity and the pressures of a growing world population.

My approach here is to emulate the struggles of the ego (covering the organizing and deciding functions in our minds) to wean itself away from reliance on magical and wishful thinking and painfully attempt to face what really is the case (Freud 1911). This chapter considers influences on our attitudes to the environment, problems in our relation to facts, evidence and change, and the unconscious forces operating in groups and organizations that amplify these difficulties. These factors interfere with our ability to protect ourselves and others from harm. They include cultural values, which undermine protective responses to our living space. Finally, I examine some proposals as to how these dangerous tendencies in our individual make-up and collective behaviour might be mitigated.

Evolutionary and developmental factors

Two major hindrances to effective management of planetary resources follow from survival responses that evolved long before the present-day challenges.[2] Early humans survived if they could make an immediate response to a sharply defined threat: Is it a predator, friend or foe? (See, for example, Bowlby's discussion of man's environment of evolutionary adaptedness in Bowlby 1969.) By comparison, a diffuse, slowly evolving but potentially serious threat remains easy to ignore. Our attention prioritizes what we can currently see, smell and hear. 'Out of sight' can easily turn to 'out of mind' if the subject is uncomfortable. Hence we are highly attuned to 'weather', but our grasp of 'climate' is far more emotionally elusive in the way that Jared Diamond (2005) uses the term 'landscape amnesia' to describe our problems in registering slow changes in our environment. The second evolutionary preference for immediate gratification over longer-term needs is linked to the first. When it comes to the basic survival of the individual, it is 'now' that counts. This tendency is moderated through experiences in childhood, but it is exacerbated by the culture of consumption and it informs the emotional logic of the contention that there are far more urgent challenges than climate change.

Beyond these fundamentals, our attitudes to the external world grow out of our earliest experiences. The baby's earliest relationships with the world centre on the need for love and the meeting of bodily needs for food, comfort and the excretion of waste. The schemas, attitudes and expectations that grow from these basic needs remain unconsciously active throughout life, although they are often obscured or rationalized by later, more sophisticated ways of thinking.

The feeding situation provides a model based on bodily experience for how we take in and form ideas about the physical world. Objects are tasted, and those that taste good are consumed and the others rejected. This earliest love is ruthless (Winnicott 1958) and orientated towards immediate survival needs. It is only later in favourable external and internal circumstances that the capacity for concern for the mother and others tempers the demandingness and early sense of entitlement. Like the mother, the Earth – or, so aptly, 'Mother Earth' – is experienced as utterly enormous in relation to our individual activities and therefore often believed to be quite immune to our puny demands on her.

In earliest infancy, maternal provision for urgent needs and a holding environment is taken for granted unless it lapses (Freud 1911; Winnicott 1965). I see this 'environment mother' as contributing to a sense of the world as sustaining and there for us to use without undue concern. She may be seen as the bountiful and limitless sleeping mother whom we can forever take for granted. These fantasies of the infinitely bountiful breast-mother may underlie repeated beliefs that particular fish are bountiful and need no protection, until they are rendered almost extinct.

Where infant care is generally sensitive and responsive, a sense is built up that wishing makes things happen. In these circumstances the infant can feel a sense of optimism, hope and confidence in relation to his surroundings and for the future. Where the opposite is true, the result may be a pervading experience of a frustrating, vengeful mother and a pessimistic and fearful attitude to the world. The ordinary infant has to deal with varying balances of good and bad experiences in a state of maximum psychological vulnerability. The earliest way of managing this is for the infant to regard the good and satisfying experiences as coming from a wholly good person who is quite separate from, and has to be kept well apart in the infant's mind from, the bad person who is the source of the infant's pain and frustration. This separation or 'splitting' of good and bad helps to avoid the anxieties that the good mother will be destroyed by the bad mother or by the infant's own needs or demands.

Unmanageable anxiety is in phantasy evacuated into someone or something else in the way that the infant evacuates its waste. The 'good-enough mother' (Winnicott 1965) takes away baby's 'poos' and 'wees', but, more importantly, by identifying with the infant's anxieties and soothing the baby, she is able to detoxify these too. As a result, the baby gains confidence that helps it to deal with both anxiety and its bodily waste. I believe that these repeated encounters contribute to the complementary belief that the planet is an unlimited 'toilet-mother', capable of absorbing our toxic products to infinity. This belief figures frequently in arguments against human impact on climate. Many people find it impossible to comprehend the aggregate impact of millions of similar actions on the planet, whether of consumption or waste discharge. For much of the last century it was believed that the oceans could absorb whatever toxic waste we put into them. The millions of tons of rubbish circulating in the Pacific show its limitations as a detoxifying toilet, but few are there to see it. The perception of pollution is also mediated through familiar evolved cues of smell and appearance. If it is slimy brown, sticky and smelly like faeces, its presence in the back garden or beach is an outrage, and compensation will be demanded. If the pollution is dubious assets well presented by smart professionals, then this aspect is ignored. A recent comparison comes in the huge demands for BP to compensate the Gulf region of the United States for its leaked oil. There has been no similar demand made to the United States to compensate the rest of the world for the fraud perpetrated by its financial sector. Pollution is taken seriously mainly if it affects people and places to which we feel connected. Union Carbide's Bhopal disaster probably killed between 4,000 and 15,000 people and caused generations of birth defects; 20 years later, the compensation offered is tiny compared to the billions of dollars demanded from BP for pollution that caused few deaths. Carbon dioxide, the major climate-forcing agent, is colourless and odourless and naturally occurring – we breathe it every day. This makes it easy for sceptics to argue that it should not be regarded as a pollutant and its effects charged to the companies that generate it, regardless of its destabilizing effect on the global climate.

Attitudes to the environment are further complicated by old attitudes to the mother's body, to rivalry and to loss. The infant's dependency needs are painful and may be hated, which can lead to wishes to punish, control, empty out or destroy the mother who is felt to be the wilful source of the infant's frustration. The child's passionate attempt to understand and master the world can similarly be aggravated by sadism. Pleasure in destruction provides quicker and more immediate satisfaction than the painstaking matter of the creation or repair of things. This is sadly a frequent gratification for politicians and managers where the glee in inflicting pain can be only too obvious. It is particularly worrying where the environment is the unconscious target.

Reality testing is difficult: ideologies and culprit hunting are preferred

The search for truth and the evaluation of evidence involve hard emotional work. They involve facing doubt and uncertainty, which rapidly expose the thinker and any group to profound anxieties. These appear to recapitulate the anxieties of the infant who is totally dependent on adults whose benevolence cannot be taken for granted. These anxieties arouse fear, suspicion and a sense of persecution, which group situations tend to amplify (Bion 1961, 1962a). Bion (1962b) sets out three ways by which the mind manages anxiety. When anxiety is completely intolerable, it is evacuated by projective identification – someone else ends up experiencing it. Where there is a large degree of tolerance of anxiety, thinking and therefore reality testing is possible. Sadly the option so frequently found in our social discourse is not a nil, but a minimal tolerance of anxiety, which is managed by taking a position of moral superiority in place of knowledge and is followed by the search for who is to be blamed and punished. This seems to be the default position for much of the media and a proportion of the public at large. Witch-hunting and conflict are more exciting and satisfying than the painstaking evaluation of evidence, which requires a capacity to bear uncertainty and depression. Even in adulthood there is a recurrent pressure for a return to the defensive strategies of early infancy. The preferred response is to treat every new challenge as a repetition of something familiar and already mastered until that proves untenable. Keeping things the same is a major source of our sense of safety. In this context the early need to split the inner world into clearly good or bad people and things recurs, expressed through the construction of mutually exclusive classes, frequently pushed towards extreme values. This leads to the frequent polarization of positions with regard to disputes, people, theories, and ideologies and rapid moves to either catastrophization or complacency. Attention to complex interrelationships (and the necessary imperfection of proposed solutions) is despised as muddle, weakness, and a failure to make a proper choice. Joined-up thinking is largely aversive and difficult to achieve. It is emotionally much easier to live in a world of simple certainties and the voyeuristic pleasures of scandals and personal triumph or weakness.

This splitting into ideally good and bad persecutory figures is alluring because the illusory clarity it promises is much prized. It is, however, inherently unstable because only one bad element changes the ideally good into the unmitigated bad. The primitive nature of this transaction is readily observed in recent 'climate-gate' scandals in which a few incompletely explained modifications to data and email evidence of personal feelings in the scientists were seized on by some to invalidate the whole scientific endeavour. Ultimately the reviews of the behaviour of the scientists concerned found little to criticize in their science. However, many critics found them guilty of the grossest misconduct and deceit, whether for alleged personal gain or in pursuit of their fanaticism. The extremity of the splitting required academics to function in a totally idealized manner, quite unaffected by the complications of being human beings working in the real world.

Splitting promotes paranoia, and conspiracy theories like this can be very stable. This is because their believability is reinforced rather than reduced by the absence of evidence. If there is no evidence, then the alleged perpetrators are felt to have been extremely clever in concealing their true motives, while the conspiracy theorists are even cleverer to have detected the 'truth'. In addition, they probably gain emotional force from an unconscious phantasy of triumphantly reversing the childhood experience of exclusion from the parents' bedroom and working out (often incorrectly) what the grown-ups have been up to.

Stability and the minimizing of emotional work are readily achieved by modern variants of 'shooting the messenger'. The effects of these tropes in human nature are simply summed up in T. S. Eliot's telling observation, 'Humankind cannot bear too much reality' (Eliot 1944).

Group functioning is constantly under threat from regressive pulls and the demands of 'sentience'

While thinking is hard enough for an individual in quiet contemplation, thinking clearly and acting in a group setting generates anxiety rapidly as the size of the group increases above 6 or 7 (Bion 1961; Kreeger 1975; Menzies Lyth 1988,1989). Here the individual may be exposed to the risks of shame and criticism, isolation, fears of loss of identity (Turquet 1975) or, at worst, losing his or her mind. Freud (1921) emphasized how groups deliver security by creating a 'horde' of equals with the leader carrying the burden of the group's ideals.

Without capable and sophisticated leadership, groups and organizations unconsciously collaborate to produce some stable configurations – which Bion (1961) called *Basic Assumption* activity – whose basic unconscious premise is that the group should be emotionally absorbing, but nothing really novel should take place. One basic assumption is organized around the issue of dependence, and it can be seductive for both leader and followers. Here all moral and practical responsibility is invested in the leader who feels admired and powerful but subject to unattainable expectations, while the followers feel like dependent children. They will be taken care of and are relieved of responsibility but will end up feeling psychically diminished. Our political parties seem to find it very hard to break out of these assumptions in addressing the electorate, and the media's need for dramatization and scapegoats reinforces it. When disappointment sets in, the standard responses are either to find someone to blame and fight with (Basic Assumption: Fight-Flight), or else attention is devoted to some symbolic idea or couple (in psychoanalytic terms representing the parental intercourse) whose activity promises to solve everything in *due course*. (This is Basic Assumption: Pairing.)

Governments and organizations face innumerable conflicts of interest and priority. It is helpful to separate the declared task of the organization (the normative primary task) from two others: the existential primary task and the phenomenal primary task. The existential task covers the conscious and unconscious strategies focused on the psychic and functional survival of the individual, the sub-group or the organization as a whole. Our early dependence on our caregivers initiates attachment patterns that can be extremely durable. Maintenance of these affectional bonds to people, groups and ideas frequently unconsciously take priority over task performance and rational considerations. Each individual may thus have his own view of what he should be doing, but this may be dominated by acting in a way that ensures his economic or psychic survival regardless of the impact on the organization. This may be quite explicit – for example, 'to keep our jobs this department needs a crisis to show it is needed' – but it may also include fears such as upsetting authority figures and the need to sustain a favoured picture of the self, which may put others or the enterprise in jeopardy.

This survival or existential task also explains why 'sentience' (the loyalty that a group or 'tribe' expects and receives from its members) is a more dominant factor in group and organizational performance than more distant or more abstract elements of the normative task or even evidence and facts. As a poignant example, David Clark, Robin Cook's special adviser, describes[3] how Cook's diaries contain insights about the mind-set of cabinet colleagues and the way they responded to events in the run-up to the Iraq War. They show a government for whom the real nature of the threat posed by Iraq was subsidiary to other considerations: for the Prime Minister the imperative was sticking close to Washington, while for most of his colleagues it was about loyalty to the Prime Minister. Some cabinet members admitted to swallowing private reservations in order to stand by him. However, there should be no illusions that those with an understanding of group and organizational dynamics are immune to these pressures. To quote Gordon Lawrence, a highly experienced group consultant: 'I find myself continually perplexed by the capacity of . . . (organizational training conference) . . . staffs to create lies that they come to believe in order to preserve the staff group and its relationships' (Lawrence 2000: 150).

The policymaking of governments and other large organizations is therefore frequently dominated by the existential primary tasks of individuals (for example, their ambition, envy and rivalry), in tribal configurations such as subgroups, departments, professions, ministries, and so on. If climate-friendly policies add costs to a department's budget and make life easier for another department, how could they possibly be adopted? Many of the problems derive from inherent and legitimate conflicts of interest: will a government that imposes extra costs on individuals and business get re-elected? Governments wish to retain electoral support as well as do what they believe is right. The media may wish to focus on drama and catastrophe to ensure sales rather than present a balanced and reasoned account of uncertainties that attracts less interest.

More perversely, groups can be set up in such a way as to ensure failure, to pursue a divide-and-rule policy and subvert other tasks, to delay, to exact revenge, and as a result of other unconscious impulses. Demanding consensus, for example, gives everyone a veto on action. Other familiar devices to postpone action or responsibility are to set up working parties, enquiries, royal commissions and so on. This is the domain of the *phenomenal primary task*, which is the task the group appears to be undertaking although unaware of it. James Hansen (2009: Ch. 9) has suggested that the whole structure of carbon 'cap and trade' has this kind of basis, since it functions like the mediaeval selling of indulgences. Those who can afford it have little incentive to stop sinning, and anyway there is money to be made from the creation of a market.

Protective mechanisms and culture

Any attempt to deal with worldwide problems, therefore, has to manage these universal human modes of functioning on a grand scale. Positive actions have to be initiated and sustained in the face of additional difficulties to do with national attitudes to cooperation with others. Our moral functions (superego functions in psychoanalytic terms), which push us to act in accordance with our ideals and guard us from self-harm, operate largely out of awareness but become conscious as the voice of conscience or a sense of anxiety or alarm. However, from infancy onwards such restraint to the individual's desires for satisfaction is resented, and this may live on powerfully in the conscious and unconscious mind as a resistance to authority, duty or responsibility. The cultural expectations that surround us are the medium in which our individual superegos swim and develop.

Howard, Orlinsky, and Lueger (1995), putting forward a general model of how psychotherapies function, called the first stage of any therapy *re-moralization*. By this they meant the process at the beginning of therapy that restores to patients some hope that they may be able to recover from their problems and heal themselves. This focus on moral values resonates with two impressive texts, one on the success or failure of societies and the other on an analysis of good and bad power. Diamond (2005) noted that past societies that survived their environmental crises had been able to re-examine their core values. Mulgan (2006) argued that in spite of the pressure of immediate challenges, any state that only tries to maximize the well-being of today's citizens would betray its deeper responsibility to the interests of the community and the ecological systems on which human life depends: 'The ideals of trusteeship require us to become servants to the future and leave the world better than we find it' (2006: 306).

Since the world economy and its dominant business models drive the present surge towards growth with increasing pressure on the Earth's resources, this would seem a necessary place to start looking to generate hope for the recovery or protection of the world patient. However, reviewing developments over the last thirty years, one can only recall the Irishmen's advice to the traveller asking for directions: 'If I were you, I wouldn't start from here.' My sense is that rather than experiencing a sense of increased morality and responsibility we have wittingly or unwittingly been through a period of amoralization in Western culture. In Britain, from the war-time period, when the welfare state was envisaged to provide care for the population after the ravages of war and when austerity was the order of the day, we have been through a period when individual and social superego functions have been treated very oddly, dominated by splitting and moves between extremes. Demonization or idealization has regularly shifted between capital and labour (currently represented by those on welfare) and the state versus the private sector. Debate can often appear reduced to the question, 'Who is holding the country to ransom?' First it was the trades unions and, for a brief period, the bankers and their minders. However, this latter reality is being cleverly side-stepped and massaged out of the public discourse. Why the super-wealthy and their tax havens have escaped this role so far may be a source of some bewilderment, until we factor in some of Mulgan's observations, described below. The old music-hall song shows how familiar this is: 'It's the rich what gets the gravy, and the poor what gets the blame.'

During the post-war period of austerity and re-building, the state was seen as the good object with the provision of welfare and security its duty while the markets had barely recovered their credibility from the crash and depression of the 1930s. From the early 1980s, this was reversed, and the social message came that greed was good, competition better than collaboration and that there was no such thing as society. Governments, too, were divesting themselves of responsibilities for managing their economies in a way that would properly benefit their citizens by projecting responsibility into the supposedly infallible markets, on the basis that as long as inflation or the money supply were controlled, only good would follow if business could proceed unfettered. Other entities to whom responsibility was delegated included news media proprietors, editors, focus groups and the stock and bond markets. (The seriously flawed idea of markets as fundamentally and automatically guided by rational processes is discussed in detail by Tuckett 2011). The role of primitive splitting involved in this exercise can be detected in the fact that the total trust given to market forces was accompanied by the evacuation of untrustworthiness and venality into anyone who was *not* a trader. Teachers, doctors, lawyers, civil servants, everyone in the public sector were supposedly all on the make, exploiting their jobs for personal gain and sucking the state dry. To deal with the projected corruption and incompetence of everyone else, governments came to see themselves as the only people who could be trusted to know right from wrong and to dictate change from the centre. The personal authority of individuals derived from knowledge, experience, responsibility and integrity was replaced by a culture of management by checklists.

Two psychoanalytically inspired investigations of the social psyche in the postwar period (Lawrence 2000; Miller 1993) discussed how this change in the social contract led to an experience of failed dependency, with a resulting withdrawal from reality into the virtual worlds of film, literature and, later, the Internet. They also noted a withdrawal from collective action into smaller groups of twos and threes in the workplace. At its extreme, responsibility for others disappeared, and the only reality to be attended to was that of the individual and his survival. This is a culture of selfishness in which individuals appear only to be conscious of their own boundaries. These they have to protect against incursions from attack from those who are feared to contain all their own repudiated envy, greed and violence.

A world order that follows these trends is reminiscent of the internal world of narcissistic and borderline patients. Here, weakness of the ego is unable to integrate activity or prevent the eruption of primitive impulses that are likely to be greedy, sadistic or self-destructive. These primitive impulses are also frequently combined, as Fairbairn (1952) and Rosenfeld (1971) have described, to form organizations within the self, within a society or between nations, which mock and attack the loving, caring, protecting parts of the self. These parts sustain belief in love, goodness and relationships. In their place the organization argues that it is better to trust triumph, narcissism and sadism. Such dynamics are powerfully visible on the international scene. Power and money (which, as well as their inherent desirability, are also aphrodisiacs) exist in powerful networks, while the regulating authorities, which are the carriers of the protective superego functions of restraining and policing, are usually underfunded or compromised in their roles. This situation powerfully affects two major worldwide challenges. The first is how to restrict the frankly bad behaviour of those who will defy the law for personal gain. The second is that it remains rational to grab whatever you can as fast as you can if you cannot guarantee that your restraint will not be taken advantage of by others. (This is the group of strategy problems known widely as 'the prisoner's dilemma' – Flood and Dresher 1948.)

For most of the world's population, the threats of financial collapse, terrorism or climate change are now more pressing than the threat of invasion (Mulgan 2006: 296–297). However, our inherent dislike of controls makes it hard to get enforcement taken seriously. It is on these grounds that Mulgan (2006) and Hansen (2009) are pessimistic about global attempts to control the emission of greenhouse gases. Having let the genie out of the bottle that it is all right do what you want even if it is not morally right – as long as you can get away with it – it is very hard to get it back in again. The global capital markets remain voracious in a way that is insatiable even in a crisis. International collaboration on bank reform or planetary protection remains difficult because historically nations have seen themselves as closed sovereign islands that in moral terms are sufficient unto themselves. Concern for what is good for the nation – or, more precisely, even in democracies, the ruling elites that hold power and wealth – trumps what is good for the world as a whole. Neither China nor the United States likes to be constrained. By the third decade of the century, CO_2 levels in the atmosphere may be reaching levels that will be impossible to reverse, and both China and the United States will be contributing some quarter of the world's total.

Precisely because the actions needed to arrest climate change will have an uneven distribution of costs and benefits, it remains unlikely that consensus can be readily achieved. Any attempt to curtail the developing world will be viewed by it as just another 'con' to deprive it of chances that others have had. On the other hand, even dominant nations will need people to trade with them, which offers the rest some leverage if nations can cooperate to use it. Those who hoped that the recent financial crash would usher in a re-evaluation of core values and inspire international cooperation on climate have been disappointed. Two psychological issues seem important here. First is the fact that the crisis threatened to affect all the major economies at once. It was therefore a common and sharply defined threat, while the effects of global warming will be patchy and uneven until far advanced. Second, the responses to the financial crisis have been similar to that following a serious car crash. For those close to people who are killed or maimed there is major anguish, and the world is changed. For those who escape unscathed, there may be a few miles of careful driving, but surviving when others do not contributes to a sense of omnipotence and immortality and there is a rapid return to 'business as usual'. Some will be able to benefit as competitors will have disappeared. Howard Davies, then Director of the London School of Economics, observed (2010) that once the fear of total collapse of the world economy was past, the need for concerted action receded; governments returned to the priorities of what suited them best. On both sides of the Atlantic there is a reluctance to empower international regulatory bodies combined with the tendency of special interests to try to get all regulation watered down.

Restraint evokes unconscious phantasies aroused by weaning, which is the prototype for managing loss and is complicated by feelings of unfairness, feelings that may be revived by inequality in adult life. It seems to me that avoidance of guilt and pain at what we may have done at a global level to other people and to the planet through our exploitation adds its force to an argument propounded at the Seattle Convention in 1999. This is that in the absence of better alternatives, the present economic system of providing global enrichment through continued growth had to be sustained, while chillingly describing as 'zones of sacrifice' those whose environments or communities are destroyed in the process – I would add here, as long as they can remain out of sight and so out of mind.

Servants of the future

It seems probable that the evidence of mankind's amazing achievements and mastery of nature feeds the fantasy that more and greater benefits can be used to avoid guilt and depression, not just about present and past damage (the zones of sacrifice), but also the pain of facing unfairness in a growth-driven world. Therapeutically, hope that is not manic or hallucinatory comes from a realistic assessment of the damage we have caused and the adoption of realistic plans for reparation. How individual, organizational and national responsibility for past and present damage to the environment is assessed is complex and is likely to be resisted because it will cause pain and guilt, and no one wants to have to give up anything.

This connects with the view expressed by Lawrence (2000) that in the West a healthy future cannot be brought into being until we experience and consciously call to mind the meaning and significance of tragedy, both as private trouble and as a public issue at our point in history. Tragedy refers to all the factors that are beyond our control, from unhappiness and misfortune to death. As a result of our successful mastery of so much of nature we have come to believe that life should be trouble-free, and we have poor means of integrating tragedy into our lives. We split tragedy off into characters in films and television dramas and into people 'not like us'. These include the weak, the underclasses, strangers and foreigners. Tragedy readily comes to be felt by people as an intrusion into their lives, as an impertinence of fate. For those who are relatively privileged, there is always a tendency to bring that good fortune into the realm of personal omnipotence as something earned or deserved. Humankind is powerfully programmed to attribute personal outcomes to moral virtue, or its lack, and not to structural societal factors.

Until reconnection is made with the depth of our species' dependence on the natural world and the inevitable precariousness of individual lives, there can be no proper engagement with these tragic elements as a public issue. Instead, when tragedy happens, politicians often offer foolish promises that 'we must act so that this can never happen again'. This challenge returns the focus to the interdependence of leaders and followers. Apart from natural tragedies that no one can prevent, much tragedy in the world is brought about through our 'mindless' acting regardless of consequences. Societies are particularly vulnerable to the acts of immature narcissistic leaders who promise to relieve all anxiety but, being out of touch with elements of their internal world, only attempt to satisfy their 'I want' wishes and desires. Such narcissistic people beget tragedy, for they enter into a course of action unable to consider the consequences except on their own terms. In contrast to the drama of tragedy, there is no recognition of hubris or ultimate self-knowledge. Sadly, the 'me-ness' stance, coupled with withdrawal from reality and the increased insecurity that has arisen in the past decade or so, has led to an increasingly fearful mode of social functioning.

In trying to enliven our capacity to think and dream of a better future and to reverse the withdrawal from engagement with the unconscious life of groups, there remains the problem for citizens of affecting the policies of nations and organizations. Like the loving part of patients held hostage by a mafia in their minds, the healthy impulses of our populations are frequently outflanked by the operations, even in democracies, of ruling elites or particular concentrations of power and self-interest within them. I believe it is the problem of how to influence policy, more than apathy or individual greed, that can make individual impulses to care for the planet seem hopeless or futile. In the United Kingdom hundreds of thousands of protestors against the Iraq war, probably representing many more, had no impact on the decision. Al Gore (2009) cites the vision that sustained over centuries the construction of the cathedrals of Europe as a demonstration of our species' capacity to embrace goals far beyond the lives of individuals. I do not think such aspirations are absent among the current population of the world, but the sustaining philosophy that led to the cathedrals was very different from the doctrines of maximizing share-holder value and the pursuit of short-term returns.

Diamond (2005) and Mulgan (2006) have each proposed strategies to counter the sense of powerlessness that regularly affects members of the professions, company boards and members of parliament, as well as individual citizens who wish for their voice to be taken seriously. Diamond pointed out that Kennedy completely altered the 'kitchen cabinet' approach to government between the Bay of Pigs fiasco and the Cuban Missile Crisis. He recognized that 'groupthink' had guided decisionmaking during the former crisis. 'Groupthink' occurs where personal doubts and contrary views are suppressed. With the Cuban Missile Crisis, Kennedy ordered his groups of advisers to think sceptically and to raise all the objections they could think of in a free-wheeling way. He insisted that his advisers should regularly meet without him to avoid undue conscious and unconscious pressure on them to say what they thought he wanted to hear.

Mulgan argued that every society, including the emerging world society, needs a 'party for the future'. This would involve institutions inside and outside government devoted to countering the gaps between the interests of the people and the interests of states and their ruling elites. Such a party would need to integrate the idealism of youth with the knowledge of mortality of the older generations. The idea of such groups evokes the 'specialist work group' function described by Freud (1921) and Bion (1961) for the Church and the Army whereby groups or institutions carry out essential functions on behalf of society as a whole, which would here extend to the future of the planet. This is an enlivening idea, but such movements would constantly have to be on guard against their marginalization by those with more powerful competing interests. They require stimulation and contributions from every level of organization in society from the individual upwards. For each level there would need to be an assessment of the dominant state of mind of the group: whether it lacked awareness of the problem, was complacent or was paralysed by anxiety. This could not be a once-only assessment but would need to be something akin to a psychoanalyst's ongoing monitoring of the patient's state of mind during a session.

Movements that want to influence states have to learn how to argue not only for the welcome benefits of their proposals and provide positive narratives for change, but they also need to concentrate their forces on the ruling groups' pressure points, such as their electoral majorities, tax receipts, company profits or party funding. Shame is a powerful motivator, and some major companies are well aware that environmental awareness is good for business. Public pressure crucially can reinforce this, although it has so far had little success in bringing the environmental and social costs of business activity (described by economists as 'externalities' or more vividly as the 'zones of sacrifice' referred to above) on to companies' balance sheets.

Mulgan emphasized ways in which the mental models required for such a work group are very different from those needed for quick decision-making, rationalization and dramatic sound bites. They require openness to the unexpected, respect for the time it takes to become conversant with a complex system, familiarity with many disciplines and the mental toughness needed to escape the tyranny of the status quo. They require counterbalances to the current emphasis on the tactical and the contingent, which includes the fear of leaks that crushes honest debate, the insecurity that prevents rigorous self-scrutiny and the wishful thinking that prefers not to contemplate unpleasant possibilities. Governments have to wean themselves from their need for *certain* forecasts of what the future will bring and develop, rather, methods that prepare them for both more and less likely possibilities. Mulgan observes that smaller countries seem to do this better than those with a greater sense of their global significance.

These are challenging but not impossible tasks for individuals and states that frequently use the excuse that there are higher priorities for time and attention. Yet, contrary to the widespread fantasy, in group life *not* to act or speak is not to do nothing. Rather, it constitutes collusion with whatever is happening. To paraphrase an earlier slogan, quoted by Segal (1987) in her work on the threat of nuclear weapons, 'silence remains the real crime'. Individuals and societies that avoid the challenge will prove correct Yeats' dark view of leaders – and, by implication, of followers too:

Mere anarchy is loosed upon the world,
The blood-dimmed tide is loosed, and everywhere
The ceremony of innocence is drowned:

. . .

The best lack all conviction, while the worst
Are full of passionate intensity.

(Yeats 1920)

Fortunately, this is not the total picture. Melanie Klein (1959) observed how some children by being predominantly friendly and helpful improve the family atmosphere and have an integrating effect on the whole of family life. Klein emphasized the influence of people with integrity, sincerity and strength of character on others around them. Even people who do not possess the same qualities are impressed and cannot help feeling some respect for integrity and sincerity, 'for these qualities arouse in them a picture of what they might themselves have become or perhaps still might become. Such personalities give . . . some hopefulness about the world in general and greater trust in goodness' (Klein 1959: 14–15). A reconsideration of what is needed for a good and sustainable life on the planet depends on social and national policies that foster such qualities and reinstate the values and practices that provide security for the development of loving relationships and creativity and respect for the planetary environment.

Notes

1 For earlier examples see Freud (1915, 1930), Bion (1991), Fromm (1974), Hobsbawm (1994).
2 The creation of excess greenhouse gases in the atmosphere is just over two centuries old, a by-product of the industrial revolution, while our evolutionary history as a separate species is perhaps one million years long, and our adaptations to city life began 5,000 years ago.
3 *The Guardian*, 3 Feb. 2010.

References

Bion, W. R. (1961) *Experiences in Groups*. London: Tavistock.
Bion, W. R. (1962a) *Learning from Experience*. London: Heinemann/Karnac.
Bion, W. R. (1962b) A theory of thinking. In *Second Thoughts*. London: Heinemann/Karnac.
Bion, W. R. (1967). *Second Thoughts*. London: Heinemann. Reprinted London: Karnac, 1984, 1987.
Bion, W. R. (1991) *Cogitations*. London: Karnac.
Bowlby, J. (1969) *Attachment and Loss. Vol. 1: Attachment*. London: Hogarth Press and the Institute of Psychoanalysis; Penguin Books.
Davies, H. (2010) Don't bank on global reform: When Lehman crashed world leaders vowed to change the system. Why haven't they? *Prospect* (Sept.): 20–21.

Diamond, J. (2005) *Collapse: How Societies Choose to Fail or Survive*. London: Penguin Books.

Eliot, T. S. (1944) Burnt Norton. In *Four Quartets*. London: Faber.

Fairbairn, W. R. D. (1952) *Psychoanalytic Studies of the Personality*. London: Tavistock.

Flood, M., and Dresher, M. (1948) *A Game Theoretic Study of the Tactics of Area Defense*. RAND Research Memorandum. Santa Monica, CA: Rand Corporation.

Freud, S. (1911) Formulations on the two principles of mental functioning. In J. Strachey (Ed.), *The Standard Edition of the Complete Psychological Works of Sigmund Freud, Vol. XII*. London: Hogarth Press.

Freud, S. (1915) Thoughts for the times on war and death. In J. Strachey (Ed.), *The Standard Edition of the Complete Psychological Works of Sigmund Freud, Vol. VIII*. London: Hogarth Press.

Freud, S. (1921) Group psychology and the analysis of the ego. In J. Strachey (Ed.), *The Standard Edition of the Complete Psychological Works of Sigmund Freud, Vol. XVIII*. London: Hogarth Press.

Freud, S. (1930) *Civilization and Its Discontents*. In J. Strachey (Ed.), *The Standard Edition of the Complete Psychological Works of Sigmund Freud, Vol. XXI*. London: Hogarth Press.

Fromm, E. (1974) *The Anatomy of Human Destructiveness*. London: Penguin.

Gore, A. (2009) *Our Choice: A Plan to Solve the Climate Crisis*. London: Bloomsbury.

Hansen, J. (2009) *Storms of Our Grandchildren*. London: Bloomsbury.

Hobsbawm, E. (1994) *The Age of Extremes*. London: Michael Joseph.

Howard, K. I., Orlinsky, D. E., and Lueger, R. J. (1995) The design of clinically relevant outcome research: Some considerations and an example. In M. Aveline and D. A. Shapiro (Eds.), *Research Foundations for Psychotherapy Practice*. Chichester: John Wiley.

Klein, M. (1959) Our adult world and its roots in infancy. *Envy and Gratitude and Other Works: 1946–1963* (pp. 247–263). London: Hogarth, 1975.

Kreeger, L. (1975) *The Large Group: Therapy and Dynamics*. London: Constable.

Lawrence, W. G. (2000) *Tongued with Fire: Groups in Experience*. London: Karnac.

Menzies Lyth, I. E. P. (1988) *Containing Anxiety in Institutions: Selected Essays*. London: Free Association Books.

Menzies Lyth, I. E. P. (1989) *The Dynamics of the Social: Selected Essays*. London: Free Association Books.

Miller, E. (1993) *From Dependency to Autonomy: Studies in Organization and Change*. London: Free Association Books.

Mulgan, G. (2006) *Good and Bad Power: The Ideals and Betrayal of Government*. London: Allen Lane.

Rosenfeld, H. A. (1971) A clinical approach to the psychoanalytic theory of the life and death instincts: An investigation into the aggressive aspects of narcissism. *International Journal of Psychoanalysis*, 52: 169–178.

Segal, H. (1987) Silence is the real crime. *International Review of Psychoanalysis*, 14: 3–12.

Tuckett, D. (2011) *Minding the Markets: An Emotional Finance View of Financial Instability*. London: Palgrave Macmillan.

Turquet, P. (1975) Threats to identity in the large group. In L. Kreeger, *The Large Group: Therapy and Dynamics*. London: Constable.

Winnicott, D. W. W. (1958) *Through Paediatrics to Psychoanalysis*. London: Hogarth.

Winnicott, D. W. W. (1965) *The Maturational Process and the Facilitating Environment*. London: Hogarth.
Winnicott, D. W. W. (1971) *Playing and Reality*. London: Tavistock.
Yeats, W. B. (1920) The second coming. In *Michael Robartes and the Dancer*. Churchtown, Dundrum, Ireland: The Chuala Press.

Background reading

Bollas, C. (1989) *Forces of Destiny: Psychoanalysis and Human Idiom*. London: Free Association Books.
Hinshelwood, R. D. (1987) *What Happens in Groups: Psychoanalysis, the Individual and the Community*. London: Free Association Books.
Symington, N. (1986) *The Analytic Experience: Lectures from the Tavistock*. London: Free Association Books.

Discussion

Unconscious obstacles to caring for the planet: facing up to human nature

Michael Brearley

I would like to open the discussion of John Keene's excellent chapter by underlining and elaborating on his central point: the difficulties, general and particular, of following the reality principle with regard to the topic of climate change. Keene sums up one of Freud's (1911) main claims as follows: the task of the ego (is) to wean itself away from its early reliance on magical and wishful thinking and painfully attempt to represent to itself what really is the case. This is a lifelong struggle. And, as Keene shows, there are particular obstacles to reality-principle functioning when it comes to climate change. I see the whole of my contribution as a discussion of what lies behind these difficulties.

I will begin with another battle, the battle over smoking, and hope to draw out from this some similarities and differences from the battle over climate change. From the 1950s, it has been known that smoking is bad for your health. It was also known that secondary smoking is bad for us. Evidence for all this was widely suppressed by tobacco companies.

Of course, smoking has its attractions. The nicotine and the psychological addiction ease tension. Cigarettes offer something for restless hands. There may be worse ways of dealing with anxiety or low-level depression. It is a hard addiction to give up. My own tastes in this matter involved seeking out the non-smoking carriages on the London Tube trains (in those days, two out of seven on the District Line). As a boy I was excited by what felt like the manly atmosphere of the bridge evenings my father had with three male friends, where cigars would be smoked and the room carried the fug for days afterwards. But, except for a few weeks at university when I briefly smoked a pipe in retaliation against a friend whose smoke seemed to be used to supplement his arguments in debate, I never smoked.

As I grew older, I resented more and more having the stuff blown into my face. It gave me a slight allergy – a sort of physiological reaction to add to my psychological one. I believed that we would always have to submit to this tyranny of the smoker. I thought that the force of destructiveness – the damage done by smokers and the connivance in this by Society at large – would prevail. I had no trust in the capacity of Society to overcome the inertia that allowed us to accept it, no hope that rational decisions to save people from lung cancer and other dreadful diseases would be taken.

And yet change has happened: one of the most significant social changes in my lifetime. Smoking is now banned from all indoor public places in Britain and in many other countries. Wonderful! One can enjoy one's meal without this pollution; fewer young people will take up this noxious habit; lives are already being saved, as is the financial cost to us all in Britain via the National Health Service.

The massive, long-term, multi-faceted campaign against smoking, with its small but incremental shifts, is an example of what Keene is suggesting we need to do on the crucial issue of climate change. Across many countries people got together to combat the attractions and the lure of smoking, the pernicious assumptions and lies of the powerful tobacco lobby and the general inertia. They forced through restrictions that gradually led to the current, healthier situation. No doubt there is further to go. No doubt too there will be difficult lines to be drawn between freedom and enforcement.

If it was difficult to drive through change in our attitudes to smoking, how much bulkier and more powerful are the obstacles to thinking clearly and taking appropriate action in relation to the much larger issue of climate change! The implications of the reality principle in relation to climate change are more complex, harder to assess, and more challenging to our narcissism.

First, the demand that people restrict their smoking meant that only smokers (and manufacturers) had to give something up. The rest of us did not. The rest of us stood to gain, both in the short and the longer term. And, as Keene says and Harrison's chapter 10 in this volume makes clear, the threats of climate change are patchy: not everyone is equally affected in the short term. With climate change, everyone has to give up something, now and in the future. Second, cigarette smoke is visible and unpleasant. CO_2 and other greenhouse gases are invisible and apparently harmless. Third, the consequences of climate change, as of the financial crisis, are vast, and much more difficult to hold in mind and deal with than a relatively isolated arena of conflict and controversy. More radical and more ramifying changes are called for. As Keene says, 'so many of our inherited adaptive patterns were developed for challenges on a family and local scale', and 'early man survived if he could make an immediate response to a sharply defined threat'. Opposing smoking did indeed call for recognition of long-term damage; but how much harder to rethink all our attitudes and behaviours in the light of threats to the Earth that are large-scale, distant (relatively) from us in their impact and in the long term so all-encompassing, frightening and difficult to predict. What might, for instance, be the consequences, in terms of famine, migration and violence, if climate change does bring rapidly escalating drought in Africa? What would be the economic and social consequences of a possible flooding of the London Underground system with salt water from the Thames, or of the rapid transformation of the UK climate to something like that of Labrador if the Gulf Stream were to cease to warm us? Moreover, while we are so afraid of disaster scenarios that we cannot bear to think of them, less disastrous scenarios fail to trouble us enough.

Thinking according to the reality principle means challenging one's narcissism, as Keene spells out in many detailed ways. We cannot have all that we want. I find persuasive his linking of our attitude to the Earth, seen as Mother Earth, to our persisting attitudes (ruthless, entitled, and indifferent) to our actual mothers or to the mothering we received. He rightly adds that we are not only indifferent but also cruel and punitive to our mothers; as he says, how much quicker destructiveness is than repair! The point is beautifully expressed by Homer; he had this to say about Sin and Prayer:

> Destructiveness, sure-footed and strong, races around the world doing harm, followed haltingly by Prayer, which is lame, wrinkled, and has difficulty seeing, and goes to great lengths trying to put things right.
>
> (*The Iliad*, Book 9, ll 502ff: my translation)

Keene also makes cogent comments about groups, about the ideals of trusteeship and about failed societies. As members of groups, people are liable to behave like lemmings (Bion 1961). Trusteeship: the less-narcissistic person is concerned for future generations as his or her arc of concern goes beyond the limit of personal death. And those societies that have been unable to rethink their central values at times of threat and enforced change are more likely to fail, as Diamond (2005) has illustrated. Keene importantly adds that the culture of consumerism encourages our wishful thinking and militates against our facing the facts.

I think that there is a danger of oscillation between opposing values from one generation to the next. As the philosopher John Wisdom wrote:

> In ethical effort people take note of the voice or prick of conscience – of the immediate response, 'O no, mustn't do that.' But they do not always take this as final. They say, 'But there's no harm in it really, it's only my puritanical conscience', and a small Dionysian voice grows louder, 'It's foolish but it's fun.' They join in the frolic of the Restoration. And then they turn again and say, 'The Puritans had something after all', and take to driving in a Victoria round Balmoral – only to leave it for a faster car and the dancing twenties and so on.
>
> (Wisdom 1953: 107–108)

Similarly, we moved from over-valuing dependence and superego obedience in the 1950s to over-valuing competition in the 1980s. Keene is particularly keen to emphasize the 'me-culture' that became more predominant in the 1980s.

He calls on us to have different attitudes, both as leaders and as followers. We have to struggle with the lack of a good superego and the lack of a strong ego, lacks that both create and live off our sense of entitlement to unlimited growth. Projecting our responsibility, we bask in passivity. Internationally, if we risk taking measures against global warming, we fear (partly realistically) the rapacity and mockery of others. Individually, too, we are liable, as he says, to hand over power to elements – 'internal organizations', in the helpful notion familiar to psychoanalysts – that mock our own inclinations to restraint and cooperativeness.

Keene's picture of our current society is richly drawn. He has important things to say about the role of tragedy in life (psychoanalysis has underlined our universal capacity for damaging what we value and need), about the need for grieving (and the danger that this tips over into grievance) and about infantile ways of mistaking hyper-sensitivity to unfairness for fairness.

Keene also has some suggestions for change. One practice he refers to that I particularly admire was J. F. Kennedy's fostering, as President of the United States, of rigorous criticism of his ideas. We need non-narcissistically to encourage the willingness of others to 'tell truth to power' (in the Quaker phrase). We need to foster that quality in ourselves. Gordon Lawrence's (2000) 'specialist work groups' – think-tanks on climate change – are another attempt to build what Bion called 'work-groups', which work to oppose short-termism and subservience to the status quo.

There is always the risk that such healthy challenging may degenerate into oppositional stances driven by envy, cantankerousness, self-righteousness or triumph. Narcissism, as we know from our work as psychoanalysts and from our own analyses, creeps back in all sorts of ways – and we have to be on the lookout for such tendencies on an occasion such as this: we may slip into self-righteousness and superiority, or become excited by catastrophe-scenarios.

Keene starts his chapter with his conversation with his nine-year old grandson, and one of the questions this leads on to is how we should educate our children and grandchildren to be more deeply involved in protecting the planet than we have been. Daniel Barenboim was asked by a sceptical questioner whether children should be taught Beethoven sonatas when they cannot understand the range of emotions expressed. His response was that there are two dangers: one of pushing children to be adult too soon, to force on them things they cannot understand, while the other is of babying. When it comes to Beethoven, he preferred to take the former risk rather than the latter. No one can fully understand these works, he went on; he himself has been playing and studying them for 50 years, and he does not. Familiarity, he said, need not breed contempt. Keene and Barenboim would, I think, be on the same side, encouraging children to take up challenges with whatever level of emotional and intellectual understanding they are ready for rather than protect them too much from difficulties.

Keene ends his chapter as he starts it by talking about children, those mentioned by Klein as having 'an integrating effect on the whole of family life', who, 'by being predominantly friendly and helpful, improve the family atmosphere' (Klein 1959: 261). So it is not only a matter of educating children, but also being open to being improved by them, 'for these qualities arouse in people a picture of what they might themselves have become, or perhaps still might become'.

Perhaps this framing with references to children is a clue to one of its central messages: that it is our children (and theirs) that we need to focus on and rely on when it comes to fighting against the pressures to ignore the risks of climate change.

References

Bion, W. R. (1961) *Experiences in Groups*. London: Tavistock.
Diamond, J. (2005) *Collapse: How Societies Choose to Fail or Survive*. London: Penguin Books.
Freud, S. (1911) Formulation of the two principles of mental functioning. In J. Strachey (Ed.), *The Standard Edition of the Complete Psychological Works of Sigmund Freud, Vol. XII* (pp. 218–226). London: Hogarth Press.
Klein, M. (1959) Our adult world and its roots in infancy. In *The Writings of Melanie Klein, Vol. 3* (pp. 247–263). London: Hogarth, 1975.
Lawrence, G. (2000) *Tongued with Fire: Groups in Experience*. London: Karnac Books.
Wisdom, J. (1953) *Philosophy and Psychoanalysis*. London: Blackwell.

Discussion

Unconscious obstacles to caring for the planet: facing up to human nature

Bob Hinshelwood

Goods and bads

John Keene's chapter is extraordinarily rich in offering us an understanding of *unconscious* aspects of humans. It shows us the intersection of the unconscious with conscious thinking and, moreover, indicates the unconscious aspects of the individual intersecting with group and social dynamics. It also links more biological factors that are connected with human survival with the intense and painful dependency of a baby on its mother. Climate change issues provoke similar intense feelings of dependency to survive biologically as individuals and as a species. It is important to recognize how those baby-like feelings have a role in powerful cultural and commercial forces, self-seeking interests, and politics.[1]

At all these levels, Keene shows the conflicts, and conflicts of interest, that form the heart of human affairs. We may wonder how, with all this complex variation among individuals, anything collective could emerge at all – and yet it does. Keene shows how individuals *do* line up with specific social issues, though not necessarily *why* they do. From Freud (1921, 1930) onwards psychoanalysts have puzzled about how social order seeps across this individual diversity. If individuals collectively constitute the social, they do so with an implicit cooperation only partially explained by conscious negotiation and agreement. Beyond the conscious motives there are implicit and unconscious coordinating influences as well. Keene implies, and I agree, that without a knowledge of those unconscious influences we are culturally and individually at their mercy.

I should like to use this space to discuss how individual experiences are swept together by a culture, and then a particular type of group dynamic that ensues.

Cultural icons

One of the organizing principles in society is iconic cultural entities. The display of the national flag, or the chords of a national anthem, call people to a solidarity, a sense of belonging to a nation, whatever the mosaic of differences it otherwise displays.

For example, in an earlier paper I explored cultural icons that represented the countryside (Hinshelwood 1993). I argued that, historically, attitudes appear to have changed radically. In Shakespearean times, the countryside was seen within a dominant cultural form – that of literature – as the domain of highwaymen, of madmen (just as the three witches of *Macbeth* exemplified that sinister and all-powerful quality). Known as the heath, the countryside was seen as a dangerous place, in contrast to the safety of the hearth, as the warmth of civilized life. These opposing sets of views, which place nature and civilization at opposite ends of a spectrum of safety, are foreign to ways of thinking in the twenty-first century. In recent times, that dimension seems to have reversed. Nature is now seen as a sad and threatened victim of civilization. A contemporary icon might be the Disney cartoon of Bambi the baby deer whose mother was shot by human hunters. Today civilization seems to be the sinister villain armed with murderous technology. So, I argued, the experience of nature has moved from being a fear of its danger to a concern for a forlorn and sentimentalized Disney caricature. Neither is perhaps valid, and *both* are one-dimensional. Fearfulness versus concern appears to be a defining feature of the Shakespearean/Disney pair of icons (although with very different means of expression).

If the cultural icons Shakespeare and Disney purvey express certain latent and available human emotions, at the same time they coordinate those individual perceptions within a culture. The Ancient world has handed down its versions of such coordinating iconic signals, as psychoanalysis has consistently proclaimed. The Oedipus story was extremely popular in Greek theatre two and a half millennia ago. It captured some profound response in individuals through the cultural form of a drama. The extraordinary Greek discovery that tragedy is entertainment now seems commonplace, but it is difficult to explain. How can fear and pity be 'enjoyed'? Aristotle found that he could give only an analogical explanation on the basis that the body humours need purging from time to time, and similarly the emotions do as well (see also Lear 1992; Nussbaum 1986; Nuttall 1996).

These icons energize a two-way response – the inner emotional life of a person's imagination, and a cultural form that can bring out those imaginary configurations *en masse*. It is this coordinated interaction between individuals and social culture that I think needs to be added to the psychoanalytic account. The point of turning to psychoanalysis is to find some explanation of what drives these cultural icons (though it says little about the *nature* of cultural forms in themselves).

Idealization and demonization

One extraordinary principle of group life is the 'us-and-them' dynamic. It is the enhanced capacity in groups to make either over-valuations or under-valuations and, moreover, to believe intensely in those distorted evaluations. Freud characterized this as 'the narcissism of minor differences' (Freud 1930: 114). One could say that groups are narcissistic. But it is more that groups bring out and support the narcissism of the individuals who make up the group. So, groups maximize the individual's belief that 'we' are right and good. At the same time, this superiority is welded with the certainty that 'they' are wrong and bad. So, experiences at multiple levels – personal, group, societal – cohere, and they do so around the axis of good–bad, right–wrong. Individuals employ the divisive processes of idealization or of demonization and when those processes cohere at the group level, they create the familiar us-and-them pattern.

In a psychoanalytic account, idealization and demonization are not merely descriptive terms. Idealization is a defence against the hatred of demonization. The belief that something is 'all good' (idealization) is selectively emphasized in order to obliterate awareness of dangerous things. To quote Melanie Klein, 'The idealized breast forms the corollary of the persecuting breast; and in so far as idealization is derived from the need to be protected from persecuting objects, it is a method of defence against anxiety' (Klein 1952: 64).

Defensive idealization is necessary to cope with the bad intentions and destructive elements of self and others. However, in groups a demonization of the 'other' is licensed, and possibly our species evolved an us-and-them destructiveness to survive biologically through eliminating rivals for the food supply – a brutal strategy that nature seems to adopt rather readily. However, the brutality of nature, of the Shakespearian 'heath', is not incompatible with a cooperativeness – within a group, or even between species in an ecological niche. Reality is a pretty mixed bag.

Nothing is perfect, as everything has pros and cons. The perception of ideal persons, however comforting, distorts realistic perceptions, excludes intermediate evaluations, and consigns us merely to a world of oppositions. For instance, industrial exploitation is not simplistically destructive. It is also beneficent in some measure, providing health and wealth. It is complex: exploitation is neither all bad, nor all good. Making fine distinctions between the actual benign and malign influences is not easy, especially on a global scale. Instead, we may relax into easy polarized thinking and feeling, such as the Shakespeare/Disney icons.

Good/bad knee-jerk reactions avoid assessing the real balance, especially when a group of colleagues support easy, minimalist thinking. Adding the us-and-them narcissism to the avoidance of difficult thought produces a potent pressure to mis-evaluate others. The various groups arguing about nature and climate are not immune from these instant reactions.

Nature is our sustenance. We will still plant seeds in the good earth and depend on climate for them to grow. At the same time, the destruction of large areas of Japan and its tragic inhabitants by the earthquake and tsunami in 2011 make nature double-edged. Tsunamis, tornados, and natural disasters remain to terrorize us. We are, every one of us, vulnerable until we die, when nature finally triumphs over our puny efforts to survive. Nature and climate are a very mixed bag. As Keene says in this chapter, the complexity of dependency is always with us. We are needy and we are concerned, we hate and we fear. This multi-valent but realistic dependence is hard to keep fully in mind. Zoos and circuses are perhaps icons for simplifying our attitudes to dependence by showing our hoped-for control.

Like the Disney stories, cultural icons grab us deep in our souls, at the place where we were once children.

That does not mean that the notion of climate change as an evil done to nature by human beings is not true. In part. But layers of meaning need to be unpicked, otherwise we lose the fact that at least in some respects there is a two-way mutual dependence. Humans are deeply dependent on nature and its arbitrariness, as many Japanese families must be pondering. But nature and the climate are increasingly vulnerable to human industrial production, car use, deforestation and so on. Sometimes humans are good to nature and sometimes bad, according to our purposes. And sometimes nature is good to us and sometimes not, according to conditions.

The role of the climate change activist

Psychoanalysts and psychotherapists may slot the climate automatically into the role of a 'patient' to be cared for. And a range of views on that therapeutic power relation may then be unthinkingly activated. For others, different roles and attitudes may spring up with an equal lack of reflection, as if similarly self-evident. For instance, for the owners of shares in Rio Tinto Zinc, exploiting the Earth's resources is a vital necessity, so that cautious reflection threatens a number of things – their identity, their way of life, and awareness of a potential guilty responsibility.

The two groups I have just characterized – the 'therapists' and the 'exploiters' – may exemplify the us-and-them group dynamic. Their very perceptions may form on the basis of attitudes arising from their separate social locations. With such a mindset, therapists will tend to see the exploiters as greedy and self-seeking, oblivious to Bambi-like nature; and the exploiters will tend to disparage the therapists as do-gooders manufacturing the guilt and blame they spread liberally around. Such perceptions winging back and forth enable the two groups to establish convincingly for themselves that the other is wrong-headed, maybe even maliciously so. And therefore 'they' are beyond the pale of understanding and sympathy.

'Us', the therapists (climate carers), who wish to *do something* about climate change, can be identified simply as do-gooders and disparaged as such. It is a complicated place to be; we are marginalized but also, at a very unconscious level, we represent that caring side of society in a rapacious culture. Even the most avid stock-market follower has had to disown his uneasy conscience in order to remain in line with his group, and he does so by leaving others to have the uneasy conscience on his behalf. The complex point is that group dynamics allot to carers the role of care and 'good sense' *on behalf of* everyone else. We are *needed* to represent the conscience of an exploitative society. But located as a do-gooder group, sufficiently denigrated, the social conscience is rendered both marginal and ineffective.

This unconscious strategy of making a smallish group of people the *sole* representatives of one function of human thoughtfulness, in order to immobilize it, can play out with other groups. If the scientists represent that aspect of society devoted to reality-testing, it means that we can rely on them to do that thinking-work. But the function, too, can be reduced to impotence, as were the climate scientists at the University of East Anglia in the so-called 'climategate scandal' (e.g. Adam 2010). At the same time, wealth-creators who keep us warm, housed, fed and entertained can be disparaged as simply greedy, callous, and the carriers of all *our* guilt.

The importance of these group dynamics is that they seriously inhibit everyone's capacity to see the full picture. We end up thinking in partial terms, locked in a restricted cultural location, and trapped with everyone else into simply allotting good versus bad evaluations to ourselves and others. We, of all people, who study these impelling and unconscious processes, should draw back a little from simplistic and polarized thinking and shake free some of our hard-earned capacity to understand others and our understanding of ourselves *with* others. Since we do have that understanding, maybe we must avoid becoming merely do-gooders and take responsibility for recognizing the range of others' positions, even if they seem not so good.

If we engage in polarizations about nature and climate, or about other groups' attitudes to them, we only engage in defensive postures and functions. Politics may be the art of the possible, but it will only effectively realize the possibilities if it addresses the unconscious dynamics as well as the thoroughly conscious issues.

Note

1 See also Averill (2007).

References

Adam, Daviad (2010) Climategate scientists cleared of manipulating data on global warming. *The Guardian*, 10th July 2010.

Averill, K. (2007) Englishness, the country, and psychoanalysis. *Psychoanalysis, Culture & Society*, 12: 165–179.

Freud, S. (1921) *Group Psychology and the Analysis of the Ego*. In J. Strachey (Ed.), *The Standard Edition of the Complete Psychological Works of Sigmund Freud, Vol. XVIII* (pp. 67–143). London: Hogarth.

Freud, S. (1930) *Civilization and its Discontents*. In J. Strachey (Ed.), *The Standard Edition of the Complete Psychological Works of Sigmund Freud, Vol. XXI* (pp. 59–145). London: Hogarth.

Hinshelwood, R. D. (1993) *The Countryside*. Paper presented at Freud Museum Conference, 'Ecological Madness'. Published in *British Journal of Psychotherapy*, 10: 202–210.

Klein, M. (1952) Some theoretical conclusions regarding the emotional life of the infant. In M. Klein, P. Heimann, S. Isaacs and J. Riviere. *Developments in Psycho-Analysis* (pp. 198–236). London: Tavistock.

Lear, J. (1992) *Kartharsis*. In A. O. Rorty (Ed.), *Essays on Aristotle's Poetics*. Princeton, NJ: Princeton University Press.

Nussbaum, M. (1986) *The Fragility of Goodness: Luck and Ethics in Greek Tragedy and Philosophy*. Cambridge, UK: Cambridge University Press.

Nuttal, A. D. (1996) *Why Does Tragedy Give Pleasure?* Oxford: Oxford University Press.

Chapter 8

How is climate change an issue for psychoanalysis?

Michael Rustin

I take as a given that the risks from climate change, as these are being explained by scientists across the world as primarily the consequence of human activity, are both real and exceptionally serious. Nothing that I have to say about the different perceptions of this situation, from a psychoanalytic point of view, should be taken to call into question the facts and probabilities themselves.

Many different disciplinary perspectives throw light on climate change and its possible consequences, which include:

- The physical sciences, which track the effects of carbon and other emissions on the climate, and the associated effects of temperature change, rising sea levels, rainfall patterns, extreme weather effects, etc.
- The impacts of climate change on life forms, which include risks of species extinction, and changes in plant and animal ecologies with many implications for food supply, health and illness.
- Consequences for human geography from rising temperatures and sea levels, changing rainfall patterns and severe weather effects.
- Technological issues involved in response to these changes, for example means of reducing energy consumption, moves to non-carbon producing energy production, and more speculative or fantastic 'fixes' of a technological nature, such as mirrors in space, sowing the oceans with iron filings to increase carbon-storing algae populations, etc.
- Economic dimensions, including what would be the costs of measures to keep climate change within acceptable bounds, and how could these be shared? The Stern Review (2006), for instance, proposed that relatively small investments to avoid the most damaging effects of climate change would be much less costly for the economy than doing nothing.
- The sociological perspective: How far does the impending threat of peak oil and global warming to the carbon economy put in question our entire social order? Is catastrophe the most likely end of this story? (See Szerszynscki and Urry 2010.)
- Political economy and political science: the obstacles to achieving agreement and effective action in response to these perceived problems, and their

explanation in terms of conflicts of interest among corporations, states, electorates, social movements, etc.

- Issues of cultural representation: How are these issues mediated to publics, and with what effects? For example, there are disagreements within scientific communities, and media interventions that seek to discredit mainstream scientific opinion.

All of these approaches are relevant. Each field of 'effects' is interlocked with many others.

It was James Lovelock's contribution, in his 'Gaia hypothesis' (Lovelock 1979) to demonstrate that the Earth's climate was a bio-physical phenomenon, in so far as plant life was responsible for sustaining its atmosphere and thus its life-sustaining temperatures and rainfall. We now understand this as a bio-physical-social phenomenon, as human beings have acquired the power to influence the climate through their own activities.

But the question I explore in this chapter is not what is known or what can be done about climate change in relation to all these relevant perspectives and methodologies; rather, I ask whether psychoanalysis has anything distinctive to contribute to the debate – and, if so, what might that contribution be?

Psychoanalysis and the public sphere

I have argued elsewhere (Rustin 2010) that psychoanalytic perspectives on public issues where they are illuminating are also likely to be experienced as disturbing and unwelcome. This is because psychoanalysis is essentially concerned with unconscious mental processes, usually repressed or split off from recognition. Just as in its clinical practice, therefore, where psychoanalysis has something valuable to say, its contribution will often seem unexpected or even paradoxical and will meet resistance. Relevant to this is Freud's understanding of the pleasures gained from wit and humour, which, he suggested, came from the 'safe' or contained expression and recognition of desires and thoughts that are normally forbidden.

Perhaps the leading example of a powerful psychoanalytical insight into a public issue was Hanna Segal's contribution during the 1980s to the debate about nuclear weapons. Segal (1987) argued that the system of nuclear deterrence was sustained by a structure of paranoid-schizoid anxieties, in which unconscious desires for destruction and death were on each side denied and projected into the other. Each alliance claimed itself to have constructed its vast armament of destruction as an instrument of peace ('Peace is our Profession' was stencilled on to the fuselages of the aircraft of the US Strategic Bomber command) but asserted that its capacity to annihilate millions, and even civilization itself, was made necessary by the malevolence of its enemy. Fortunately some capacity for reason remained within this socio-technical system, and after the near-catastrophe of the Cuban Missile Crisis the two sides took some practical steps[1] to avoid an inadvertent outbreak of war and concentrated their many exercises of violence in areas of the world from which escalation of local wars to nuclear conflict was a lesser risk.

The depth of Segal's understanding was demonstrated when she predicted, after the collapse of the Soviet Union and the end of the Cold War, that the established paranoid-schizoid structures of mind would retain their potency, and that new objects of fear and enmity would be chosen to sustain them. Segal (1995) argued that a compelling explanation of the first Gulf War lay in the redirection of paranoid-schizoid hostility in the United States and its allies towards the Iraq of Saddam Hussein. Even though the force of Segal's argument might be qualified by the other motives there were for the conflict with Saddam Hussein, following Iraq's invasion of Kuwait, the insight of her analysis became clear as later developments unfolded. The panic over weapons of mass destruction, the second invasion of Iraq, the 'war on terror' and the fear of fundamentalist Islam revealed the potency of unconscious structures of mind dominated by destructiveness and anxiety. These involved massive projections onto and from the imputed enemy.

How far is Segal's analysis of the catastrophic anxieties of the Cold War applicable as a model to the dangers of climate change? How far can we identify powerful unconscious motivations as major causal agents in the environmental crisis, and how far are these shaped by the same psychic forces that Segal perceived as sustaining the Cold War and the subsequent 'war on terror' and on disparate enemies in the Islamic world? There are some similarities. Modern global capitalism legitimizes the pursuit of individual and corporate self-interest as notionally contributing, according to economic theory, to the universal benefit. But on what actual motivations does this system depend? On the one hand, there is a widely diffused appetite for possessions, which can amount to greed and in whose pursuit regard for the harmful consequences of much economic activity is disregarded. But there are other motivations in play too, which bring Segal's hypothesis of paranoid-schizoid mentalities and unconscious destructiveness into closer proximity. Competition involves conflict, which can be more or less regulated by laws and shared values. Its motivations include the will to triumph over competitors, to be the strongest and to triumph over one's rivals or enemies. The reason for the widening gap between the wealth and income of those in top positions and that of all others is not that economic elites wish merely to consume more but, rather, that they wish to assert their power, relative both to their immediate rivals and to everyone else. At these levels, even consumption becomes mainly a signifier of competitive success, as in the theory of positional goods set out by Hirsch (1977). In so far as corporate ruthlessness is a significant factor impeding actions to limit environmental risk, the environmental crisis becomes caught up in a dynamic of destructiveness related to the dynamics of unconscious conflict analysed by Segal.

Linked to these dynamics is the way that the fear among national leaders of losing competitive advantage leads them to disregard what they know to be the risks of climate change, as they defer taking measures the necessity of which they have previously recognized. It is also reasonable to suggest that the potential exhaustion within only a few generations of the planet's fossil fuel resources, which had been accumulated over millennia, might be understood in part as an unconscious attack on the young and still-unborn. Might the dominant culture of self-interest and individualism, a state of narcissism of a kind (Rustin and Rustin 2010), be connected with a weakened sense of commitment and obligation towards future generations? Might there be a link between this disavowal of the needs of future generations and concurrent disavowal of the value of past legacies? After all, the term 'conservation' signifies respect for heritage and its continuities, in the spheres of both nature and culture. The idea being enacted in current reforms in the United Kingdom – that the young should take entire financial responsibility for the funding of their own higher education, rather than education being conceived not as an individual investment in oneself but, rather, as a gift between generations intended to safeguard the future of society – embodies such a change of mentalities. Some psychoanalytic discussion of climate change reasonably pursues arguments like this kind. There are good reasons for holding the moral deficiencies of capitalism as in part leading to environmental risk.

But while such arguments capture some elements of the present situation, they are incomplete as a psychoanalytic perspective on these issues. This is because over the past three or four decades climate change has become a very widely debated and contested issue in many different circles. There is now a broad scientific consensus on the risks of global warming. There are considerable activities by governments, corporations, social movements and individual citizens, insufficient as they still are, to try to limit or avert its dangers. The extent of openly expressed concerns about these issues makes it questionable whether the primary motivations and anxieties in this field *are* unconscious ones that can only be recognized through psychoanalytic insight. While one may reasonably see the 'death instinct' and considerable unconscious destructiveness involved in the drift towards environmental catastrophe, there are also countervailing life-instincts and widespread creative impulses in play in the growing realization of the problems and in the efforts being made to respond to them.

Distinctively, a psychoanalytic perspective searches for the existence of unconscious anxieties and defences against them, and also for various forms of 'group psychology' (Freud 1921, 1929) where individuals project their desires and fears into larger collectivities or belief systems, and by doing this weaken their capacity to discriminate and think rationally. Such formations are likely to emerge in the context of an environmental crisis that has now been in the public mind for several decades. Psychoanalytic attention needs to be given to the various aspects of this, certainly including the pathologies of unconscious destructiveness, resistance and denial. But one should note that the mechanisms of splitting, idealization and denigration are likely to manifest themselves on each side of a major social conflict. Environmentalism and its objects can be also become idealized, at the expense of recognizing and negotiating unavoidable complexities of motive and situation. Hinshelwood (2002), writing about the defences against the fears of nuclear war, suggested that the activities of peace movements could sometimes sustain a destructive social system rather than effectively challenging it. Its virtuous example of idealism and self-sacrifice could, Hinshelwood suggested, reinforce the majority in their complacent acceptance of the necessity for violence, while nevertheless assuaging its conscience by their existence. Environmentalists must beware of being drawn into projective dynamics of this kind.

Contrasting 'structures of feeling' towards the environment

How are we broadly to understand relations between human society and the natural environment? One view is that the present threat of climate change is the culmination of the inherent destructiveness of humankind towards Nature. But one can identify two opposed belief systems in this sphere, which one can also think of in Raymond Williams' terms as 'structures of feeling' (Williams 1978: ch. 9).

One such view focuses on 'modernization' as a process that has brought about a deep transformation in the relations of humankind to nature. According to this, the world-view of modernity introduced deep splits in human relations to the world, substituting, for an earlier relation of reciprocity, damaging polarities and antagonisms. The separation of reason from emotion, of individuals from society, and the conception of Nature as an object of 'conquest' by human powers are versions of these oppositions. Marxism, as Raymond Williams pointed out in his early reflections on these questions (Williams 1980) absorbed much of this way of thinking from bourgeois or capitalist forms of thought.[2] A forceful and critical statement of this perspective was given by the Frankfurt School theorist, Max Horkheimer, in his essay, 'The Concept of Enlightenment' (1944). An omnipotent idea of human reason has engulfed all other spheres of life, Horkheimer argued, expunging all scope for creativity and autonomy.

Zigmunt Bauman's argument in his *Modernity and the Holocaust* (1989) is also close to this view in its argument that the Holocaust – in its industrial extermination of a whole category of human beings – far from being an exceptional anomaly of modern societies, was the culmination of a transformative outlook and programme, in which the powers of reason, science and technology were deployed without moral limits in pursuit of whatever purpose those in control chose to adopt. In *Legislators and Interpreters* (1987) he contrasted an approach that saw nature and society as appropriate objects for transformation in accordance with rational plans of various kinds, with one which would confine governmental and social intervention to one of interpretation and clarification of the different purposes of human agents.

From a psychoanalytic perspective one might ascribe to this modernist, trans-formative, conquering spirit a paranoid-schizoid character, in Melanie Klein's terms (Klein 1935). This 'position' is characterized by its radical splitting between loved and hated objects, between an idealized inside and a denigrated outside – the good self or 'us' and the bad other or 'them'. Such splitting involves the projection of negative impulses outwards. Hostile enactments against 'the bad other' often follow. Those engaged in these projections at some point have to face the question of what has happened to the objects that are thereby being damaged, in reality and/or fantasy. Can the damage be faced and reparation attempted, or will unconscious guilt be too great? Will retribution be feared as the return of the aggression and hatred that has been projected outwards? This situation can lead to a cycle of escalation of these projections, in which an enemy is felt to be more dangerous as a consequence of the hatred directed towards it and the injuries thereby caused. Perpetrators as well as their victims can suffer psychological damage from the hatred they project outwards, though this is usually less recognized.

Until the emergence to more widespread visibility of the ecological crisis in the 1960s and 1970s, we have perhaps been more aware of the construction of other human beings as the objects of antagonistic splitting than of seeing Nature itself in this way. The miseries of slavery and factory labour (William Blake's 'dark satanic mills') were more often, understandably enough, the major objects of criticism of industrialism than the fate of the natural environment itself. But these environmental dimensions have been present in many dystopian contrasts drawn between the city and the country (Williams 1985) and in representations of the mechanical devastation brought about by modern wars. Raymond Williams, in his *Culture and Society* (1958), identified an aesthetic dimension to the critique of industrialism and capitalism as mechanical, ugly and destructive of beauty, for example in the writings of John Ruskin, William Morris and D. H. Lawrence.

Paranoid-schizoid states bring about the inhibition or destruction of mental function, since the discriminations and differentiations that are necessary to thought are made impossible by the emotional drive to categorize objects as wholly good or wholly bad, and by the denial that they possess elements of both.[3] A further development of this theoretical frame has drawn attention to the disavowals and denials of reality, the 'psychic retreats' into narcissism or self-sufficiency, which can be responses to the pain of recognition of the harm caused to and the needs of loved objects. Not-seeing and not-noticing is the most widespread response to a psychic situation in which objects are felt to have been damaged and where little hope exists that reparation can take place. Moving out of the paranoid-schizoid into more depressive ways of thinking and feeling can be found too painful to endure, if there are no internalized good objects to sustain a belief in the existence of good objects outside the self (Steiner 1993).

In the light of the contemporary environmental crisis, it is tempting to see what Benton (1991) has described as this 'Promethean' version of man's relation to nature as the dominant, hubristic and ultimately destructive historical story. But there is a contrasting historical narrative of human relationships to nature, which was set out in Thomas's *Man and the Natural World: Changing Attitudes in England 1500–1800* (Thomas 1983), and is also implicit in Elias's thesis of the 'civilizing process' (Elias 1994). Thomas described the emergence in the early modern period of attitudes that began to question and modify an earlier conception of nature that had been wholly anthropocentric and exploitative, and not at all the state of benign harmony between mankind and the natural world sometimes imagined by critics of industrialism. Christianity, Thomas points out, had claimed the authority of God to justify the subordination of all other species to the service of human needs (or indeed the subordination of 'primitive' to supposedly 'civilized' peoples). Early science retained these assumptions. For Bacon, the purpose of science was to restore to man that dominion over the creation which he had partly lost at the Fall, while Robert Boyle was egged on by his correspondent John Beale to establish what Beale called 'the empire of mankind'. To scientists reared in this tradition, the whole purpose of studying the natural world was 'that, nature, being known, it may be master'd, managed and used in the service of human life.' Descartes argued that animals were 'mere machines or automata, like clocks, capable of complex behaviour but wholly incapable of speech, reasoning, or in some interpretations, even sensation'. 'Although for Descartes the human body was also an automaton, the difference was that within the human machine there was a mind and therefore a separate soul, whereas brutes were automatons without minds and souls. Only man combined both matter and intellect' (Thomas 1983: 33).

Thomas here describes the foundations of an anthropocentric and rationalist world-view, which is now being challenged as threatening to destroy the entire planet. But his primary purpose was to show that the founding principles of this cosmology were being challenged and modified even while they were being elaborated. Rather than attitudes to nature, to other species and to members of other human communities becoming exclusively exploitative and indifferent during the early modern period, Thomas argued that it was at this time that contrary ways of thinking were beginning to be heard. He put it thus:

> moralists urged that the beasts should be treated with kindness and consideration. Aesthetes saw the earth as an object of beauty and contemplation, rather than as a mere resource to be plundered. By 1800 there had been generated feelings which would make it increasingly hard for men to accept the uncompromising methods by which the dominance of their species had been secured.
>
> (Thomas 1983: 33)

Thomas described the changing language of natural history, the greater responsibility taken by farmers for the well-being of their animals, the growth of pet-keeping, the spread of tree-planting and flower-cultivation, the origins of vegetarianism and admiration for the wilderness as aspects of this change in sensibility. In the following century came Darwin and his definitive challenge to the idea of man's created difference from and superiority to other species. *The Origin of Species* memorably concluded: 'from so simple a beginning endless forms most beautiful and most wonderful have been, and are being evolved'.[4] More inclusive and respectful conceptions of human relations were also being advanced, which were critical of slavery, the subjection of women, indifference to children, and which led on to modern conceptions of universal and inclusive human rights.

Elias's account of this historical process described the gradual inhibition in everyday life of brutish and selfish human instinctual impulses, and their regulation and sublimation in more sociable directions. Elias located the beginnings of these inhibitory conventions (the rise of 'manners' as he put it) in court society, but observed their downward transmission through the social hierarchy. In effect, as Bauman (1979) pointed out, Elias gave an interpretation of Freud's (1929) *Civilization and its Discontents* as a historical narrative of the development of civility and restraint.

Psychoanalytically, one can think of this more responsible conception of the relations between human beings and the natural world, and human beings with one another, in the Kleinian framework of the depressive position, in contrast to the paranoid-schizoid vision of the conquest of nature and the imposition of civilization on the realms of the primitive. The depressive position, in this psycho-analytic perspective, is understood as enabling loved and hated attributes to be recognized as belonging to the same object. The capacity to integrate rather than split conflicting feelings is the precondition of rational discrimination and thinking. This is conceived in the Klein–Bion theory of child development as an aspect of maturation.

Conflicting perspectives on the crisis

How do we choose between these contrasting historical narratives, noting as we may the different 'internal' states of mind or psychological configurations ('paranoid-schizoid', 'narcissistic', or 'depressive') to which they seem to give a public form? The reality is that each of them embodies a substantial element of the truth, each describing a different major aspect of our history. In fact, the different tendencies represented in these narratives remain in contention in contemporary society and are competing elements in the responses to environmental danger.

It is instructive to map the ongoing debates about the environment through these contrasting psychoanalytical categories. Where environmental destruction is proceeding apace, with massive investments continuing in carbon-producing and carbon-burning technologies and few efforts being made to reduce prevailing patterns of energy use and consumption, one can readily see evidence of a paranoid-schizoid splitting between positive human agency and resistant but expendable nature, and of pathological denials of reality – or even, as some believe, an unconscious destructive desire to deny the resources of the planet to future generations.

Naomi Klein's article, 'Gulf Oil Spill: A Hole in the World' (*Guardian* 19 June 2010), set out such a psycho-political critique in vivid terms. She pictured the inside of the world being penetrated and pillaged, as millions of gallons of oil spilled out of the seabed. There was a feminist aspect to her description, drilling for oil being made to seem like a particularly brutal rape of Mother Nature. One does not need to look far to find apt objects of such a critique, as, for example, Sarah Palin's 'drill, baby, drill' approach to the problems of American energy supply.

And, for an argument that showed these conflicting perspectives in fierce opposition, there was the debate in Charleston, Virginia (*Guardian* 23 Jan. 2010) between US 'coal baron' Don Blankenship and Robert F. Kennedy Jr on the issue of 'mountaintop removal mining'. This technology blows the tops off mountains to get at thin seams of coal, and Blankenship is a notorious promoter. Kennedy described this type of mining as, 'the worst environmental crime that ever happened in our history. It is a crime, it is a sin, it is our moral obligation to stop this from happening.' Kennedy attacked Blankenship's company for its anti-unionism, its destruction of jobs, and for its breaches of the law. Blankenship replied that 'it's a bunch of rhetoric and untruths. This industry is what has made this country great. If we forget that, we are going to have to learn to speak Chinese. Or expect early deaths, noting that life expectancy in Angola is 39 years.' Blankenship is a climate change denier: 'Global warming is a hoax. Anyone who says they know what the temperature of the earth is going to be in 2020 or 2030 needs to be put in an asylum because they don't.'

The irrationalities of Blankenship's position are scarcely obscure. 'Coal is what made the industrial revolution possible. If windmills were the thing to do, if solar panels were, it would happen naturally', he said. But excess is not only on one side. 'Companies such as Blankenship's are exploding the explosive equivalent of Hiroshima every week,' Kennedy said, even though it is evident that the monstrosity of Hiroshima was not so much the scale of its explosive energy, but its object.

There are many instances of this kind of 'denialist' argument, and also of morally outraged responses to them. It is tempting to position those expressing most concern about the environmental future as having the most enlightened and mature psychological orientation, while those in apparent denial of such concerns as being possessed by the most pathological states of mind.

But the reality is that unconscious phantasy can shape the imaginative constructions both of an 'industrial' mentality that seeks to subordinate Nature to the rational will, and of a conservationist state of mind that identifies with Nature against human exploitation and cruelty. The environmentalist side of the argument can merely turn on its head the 'modernist' split between man and nature, ascribing all value to the latter and withholding it from the former.

A view of modernization as a narrative of destructiveness may deny the broad improvements in the conditions of human life that industrialization has brought about. Arguments in favour of the continued global advance of the economic system now extrapolate this progressive historical story to developing parts of the world. They hold that the populations of China, India and 'the south' are entitled to seek similar low levels of infant mortality, extended life expectancy and access to education as those achieved in 'the north', even if a great deal of change is needed if sustainable modes of material production are to be achieved.

On the other side of this dualistic argument, there are difficulties with the views of nature, which are held by some conservationists when they oppose economic development. In reality, nearly all of what we conceive as the natural world in developed societies is already a 'hybrid' entity created through the interactions of human activity and nature and has been so for hundreds of years. The Highlands of Scotland perhaps have their beautiful scenery because their trees were once deliberately destroyed, and because patterns of animal husbandry have not permitted them to regenerate naturally. The habitats of downlands, fenlands, broadlands and brecklands in southern and eastern England seem to need nearly as much careful management to sustain them in their desired 'natural' condition as the growing of arable crops. Although there are large expanses of the globe – the remaining areas of rainforests for example – which are still little affected by human activities (and which need to remain so), there are many others whose state can no longer be described as pristine or 'natural'. In fact, the terms 'nature' and 'natural' are frequently deployed to defend landscapes that are in fact the inheritance of one epoch of cultivation against new human interventions that threaten them.

The antithesis of a pristine nature and a destructive modernity is a conceptual cul-de-sac in this debate, which obscures the approaches that are necessary to the urgent problems of climate change.

An alternative way of thinking about these issues, which avoids the antithesis set up by the advocates and opponents of 'modernity', has been developed by Latour (1993). Latour calls into question the distinction between the categories of nature and culture. He argues that the very idea of nature as a sphere separate from humanity and human agency was always an ideological one, framed to uphold a certain kind of dissociated rationalism. But this split between the natural and the human does not in reality exist. The title of one of Latour's books proclaims that '*We Have Never Been Modern*', because mankind has always necessarily been a part of nature, not separate from it and since the 'nature' we experience has been continually reconceived and reshaped through human agency. The world that we see and interact with is full of 'hybrid' entities, such as atoms, electrons, gravitational forces, bacteria, viruses and genes and, one could add, unconscious minds, which only ever became visible entities as a consequence of actions by scientists within and upon nature. This conception of humankind as an integral element in a larger system within which it has evolved with certain powers of understanding and reflection is a valuable one, and may help us to resolve some misleading antinomies and misconceptions in the environmental debate. Latour contends that mankind lives in a continuing interaction and interdependence with the rest of nature and needs to accept its responsibilities within the whole system of which it is a part. He has even argued (Latour 2004) for a system of governance in which elements of nature, such as rivers or forests, would have advocates or 'voices' of their own. This is not because Latour ascribes some mystical authority to the sphere of nature, but because there are many elements of this interdependent human–natural system that social actors, in their hubristic pride, are liable to discount or overlook, even though they retain immense causal potency. The phenomena of climate change are a pressing instance of these effects of systemic interdependence.

Latour does not, however, take the 'social constructionist' position that to all intents and purposes nature is whatever human beings conceive it to be, or have made it, through their transformative powers. His argument is that the relations between human beings and nature are a continuing interaction, 'nature' having causal powers and imposing limits that human action cannot transcend. Human powers, though great, are far from infinite, as the threats of climate change and of the possible exhaustion of the resources of the planet for sustaining both human life and the diversity of life-forms now demonstrate. The need is for a realist kind of responsibility to be taken by human societies for their interactions with the non-human material and organic spheres. There is no pre-industrial Garden of Eden to which mankind can or should now return, nor can the limits that the properties of nature impose on human desires be denied.

One part of nature of which psychoanalysis offers an understanding is human nature itself. Here there are also limits to human powers, set by limited life-spans, the inevitability of disease and unavoidable differences of gender and generation[5], as well as by the permanent coexistence in human nature of the conflicting impulses of love and hate. The capacity for rationality and for concern for the well-being of other human beings is, in the psychoanalytic frame of reference, a precarious achievement in every lifetime and every society, not a 'natural' condition of life to be taken as a given. 'Sociable' dispositions are always liable to be disrupted by more aggressive impulses and often exist in a precarious equilibrium with one another. In particular, psychoanalysis draws attention to the role of anxieties, both conscious and unconscious, in disturbing rational mental function and in pushing human beings towards the aggressive and irrational end of their innate spectrum of motivations.

Evolutionary explanations throw some light on these conflicting aspects of human nature. Human beings first evolved as hunter-gatherers to live in relatively confined family groups, among whom it was functional for survival to regard outsiders and strangers as potential enemies competing for scarce resources (Hrdy, 1999).[6] The extension of human sympathies and identifications to wider groups – eventually to the idea of an identification with the human species as such – was a long, gradual and continually interrupted historical process. Probably, as Marx suggested, human societies only pose problems in thought to which there have already emerged potential solutions in practice.[7] Thus it was only as broader social identifications became a realistic source of benefit that universal claims on behalf of humankind came to be conceived and proclaimed.

This argument suggests that in the face of acute anxieties about material or social survival, regression from more inclusive to more divisive and exclusionary modes of thought and action is liable to occur. One possible outcome of a serious crisis of global resources is the regression of threatened societies to conditions of antagonism and conflict. This would resemble the 'war of all against all', described by the seventeenth-century political philosopher Thomas Hobbes, in his warnings about the consequences of an absence of sovereign power, which, he held, entailed severe dangers to life and security. Unconscious as well as conscious anxieties would surely have a major influence in such a crisis. Not only would 'rational' forms of competition and conflict take place, as always, but fantasy, delusion and misrepresentation would exercise increasing sway, allowing the needs of others to be disregarded and seizing on scapegoats and enemies to explain away ills. Whenever individuals and collectivities are faced with serious threats to their security and well-being, such perverse reactions are common occurrences. Such unconscious dynamics of group psychology are essential to understanding the catastrophe of Nazism in Germany and connect its defeat and humiliation in the First World War and the severe disruption of its economic and social life in the years following it to the perversions of the Nazi regime, with its extreme forms of splitting and its addiction to violence and pain.[8] There are unconscious psychodynamic elements in the emergence of fundamentalisms of all kinds. The fears and anxieties aroused by global economic competition are even now obstructing agreements on initiatives to reduce carbon emissions.

Problems and solutions

The real difficulties of the situation lead many to take a pessimistic view. They cannot see how the world can or will make the transition to a low-carbon economy in the limited time available, given the entire dependence of the current economic order on the excessive consumption, over mere decades, of energy stored beneath the earth's surface over millennia. Urry (2010) has recently pointed out the widespread currency of catastrophist accounts of the present situation. This view gains plausibility if one holds innate destructiveness, or its embodiment in capitalism, to be the source of the problem. But a different view is that the problems of climate change have a more contingent origin, that they are the unforeseen and unintended effect of developments that, while they can cause great damage, have also achieved much good.

Specific environmental threats have sometimes been successfully met by remedial action. Smallpox, having once been a scourge across the world, now exists only in a few test-tubes in two nations' research laboratories. Organochlorine pesticides, which decimated many animal species, have been banned in many countries, and some threatened species have recovered. It was recently found that an anti-inflammatory drug administered to cattle in India to relieve suffering was rapidly destroying the huge population of vultures essential to India's ecological equilibrium as its top scavenger species. This drug has now been banned, in a much shorter time than it took to achieve the prohibition of DDT, and it looks likely that the vulture population may recover.

But, of course, climate change is a much larger order of problem than these specific threats. The socio-technical changes that are required are the equivalent of the largest industrial revolutions of the past – for example, the introduction of coal and steam to power mills, factories and the means of transport, the development of electrical power and petroleum to create usable energy and, more recently, the rise of electronic means of communication and control. The systems associated with each of these technologies took many decades to evolve. Most of these technologies had pathological side-effects. The problem with climate change is that its damaging effects are likely to be general and calamitous to all, whereas, as Anthony Giddens (2009) has pointed out, the difficulty with global warming has been to generate motivation for drastic changes before it was apparent to most people that they were urgently needed.

An implication of a psychoanalytic understanding of this crisis is that if solutions are to be found, they must be inclusive of the interests of all human beings and must allay unconscious anxieties to a degree that makes rational action possible. 'Solutions' that demand the defence of 'nature' at the expense of human societies or of human societies at the expense of 'nature' are bound to fail. In the first case, people will resist them in their own self-interest and, second, natural forces are essential to human well-being and not its enemy. Nor do solutions that require that major sections of the world's population, whether 'developed' or 'undeveloped', have to see their basic interests sacrificed for the benefit of others stand any chance.[9]

The question is whether any solutions to these threatening problems exist which are consistent with this criterion of inclusive well-being. One such solution was put forward in economic terms in the Stern Review (2006). It argued that the costs of investment in the reduction of carbon emissions were now affordable and, if made in time, would avert much larger costs in later years. The argument is valid, although it leaves unanswered the question of whether there are potential investments available that are technically capable of averting the pressing dangers. This is a key issue, since if an 'inclusive' solution is to be found, then it must be one that enables the global economy to continue to function at something like its present level of productivity, even though with many changes in its goals and using technologies that halt ongoing alterations to the earth's climate.

There are some grounds for hope. More than enough energy to satisfy current and predicted economic needs could be generated from current inflows of solar energy and its effects on the earth, in the form of radiation and the movement of winds, waves and tides. It is technologically possible to base a global economy not on the exhaustion of existing energy *stocks* but, instead, on the use of continuing energy *flows*. In other words, the earth *could* live on its 'energy income', rather than continuing to deplete its 'energy capital'.

It seems likely that the use of the world's hot deserts to produce electricity from solar radiation is the most promising technology now being developed (Wolff

2011). Quite a small proportion of existing hot desert environments (in North Africa, the Arabian Peninsula, the south-western United States, south-west Africa, and Australia) could generate sufficient energy to meet the world's needs, and from terrains where few other valuable activities would be displaced.

Such transitions are very difficult to achieve. Many changes are required, beyond means of energy generation – for example, towards zero net energy consumption in building design and use, the reduction in carbon-intensive forms of manufacturing and transport and conceptions of human well-being that are responsible and restrained in their use of finite material resources. But we can see many of these developments already being anticipated and pioneered. Such adaptations are readily imaginable and do not require unacceptable (and therefore unachievable) sacrifices of human well-being for any major part of the world's population.

The sun, as some earlier civilizations recognized, is perhaps the largest force of nature of which human beings need to take account. Survival requires understanding, and working within the limits of nature, rather than disavowing them. Freud saw human respect for the 'reality principle', during psychic development, as a precarious precondition of maturity and sanity. In this situation of global danger, both non-human and human dimensions of 'reality' must be respected. These are the limits imposed by physical nature on how much human societies can change their environments without jeopardizing their own survival; and the limits of human nature itself, especially in its capacity to respond in reasonable and ethical ways to survival anxieties. The contribution that psychoanalytic understanding can make is in understanding the nature of these anxieties and the irrational responses to which they are liable to lead.

The 'reality principle' is relevant to both material and psychological conditions. Thus, on the material side, if feasible solutions to environmental problems are absent, it becomes reasonable to expect the worst. Equally, if there are insufficient concerns for the well-being of all human beings and for the continued diversity of life forms, there is little ground for believing that the actions necessary for meeting this crisis will be taken.

'Technical' solutions do exist, and are being worked on by many people with skill and imagination. And there is some understanding that what is at stake is the future of a global society.

Notes

1 Robert McNamara's strategic doctrine of Mutual Assured Destruction (M.A.D.), developed during 1960s, was paradoxically a step towards greater safety, in its logic that neither side should be allowed to develop the capacity for a successful 'first strike' on the other.

2 Ted Benton (1991) provided valuable clarification of the different ideas within Marx's and Engels' writings on relations to nature.

3 The emphasis on mental function in psychoanalysis has come especially from the work of W. R. Bion (1967).

4 Darwin's reverence for the beauty and complexity of nature is as much to the point as the misappropriation of his ideas by social Darwinists seeking legitimation for ideologies of conflict or competition.
5 Ted Benton (1989) argued for the necessity to recognize biological constraints on human action, against over-ambitious forms of social constructionism.
6 Jim Hopkins (2000) has argued that these evolutionary origins explain why the inner world of infants and mothers is as full of latent conflict and violence as Melanie Klein controversially described it to be.
7 'Mankind thus inevitably sets itself only such tasks as it is able to solve, since closer examination will always show that the problem itself arises only when the material conditions for its solution are already present or at least in the course of formation' (Marx 1859: 2).
8 Adorno (1951) provides an exemplary analysis of the mass psychology of fascism, as represented in its propaganda.
9 Ulrich Beck (2010) argues that a kind of 'cosmopolitan solidarity' is needed to combat these problems, but also that well-being needs to be conceived in less material and more egalitarian terms.

References

Adorno, T. W. (1951) Freudian theory and the pattern of Fascist propaganda. In G. Roheim, (Ed.), *Psychoanalysis and the Social Sciences, Vol. III* (pp. 408–433). New York: International Universities Press. Reprinted in J. M. Bernstein (Ed.), *The Culture Industry: Selected Essays on Mass Culture*. London: Routledge, 1991.

Bauman, Z. (1979) The phenomenon of Norbert Elias. *Sociology*, 13 (1): 117–125.

Bauman, Z. (1987) *Legislators and Interpreters*. London: Polity Press.

Bauman, Z. (1989) *Modernity and the Holocaust*. Cambridge, UK: Polity Press.

Beck, U. (2010) Climate for change, or how to create a green modernity? *Theory, Culture and Society*, 27 (2–3): 254–266.

Benton, T. (1989) Marxism and natural limits: An ecological critique and reconstruction. *New Left Review*, 178: 51–86.

Benton, T. (1991) Biology and social science: Why the return of the repressed should be given a (cautious) welcome. *Sociology*, 25 (1): 1–29.

Bion, W. R. (1967) *Second Thoughts*. London: Heinemann.

Elias, N. (1994) *The Civilizing Process* (rev. ed.). London: Blackwell.

Freud, S. (1921) *Group Psychology and the Analysis of the Ego*. In J. Strachey (Ed.), *The Standard Edition of the Complete Psychological Works of Sigmund Freud, Vol. XVIII*. London: Hogarth.

Freud, S. (1929) *Civilization and Its Discontents*. In J. Strachey (Ed.), *The Standard Edition of the Complete Psychological Works of Sigmund Freud, Vol. XXI*. London: Hogarth.

Giddens, A. (2009) *The Politics of Climate Change*. Cambridge, UK: Polity.

Hinshelwood, R. T. (2002) Psychological defence and nuclear war. In C. Covington, P. Williams, J. Arundale and J. Knox (Eds.), *Terrorism and War: Unconscious Dynamics of Political Violence*. London: Karnac (orig. in *Medicine and War*, 2 (1986): 29–38).

Hirsch, F. (1977) *Social Limits to Growth*. Routledge and Kegan Paul.

Hopkins, J. (2000) Evolution, consciousness, and the internality of mind. In P. Carruthers and P. Smith (Eds.), *Evolving the Mind*. Cambridge, UK: Cambridge University Press.

Horkheimer, M. (1944) The concept of Enlightenment. In T. Adorno and M. Horkheimer, *The Dialectic of Enlightenment*. London: Allen Lane, 1973.

Hrdy, S. B. (1999) *Mother Nature: A History of Mothers, Infants and Natural Selection*. New York: Vintage.

Klein, M. (1935) The psychogenesis of manic-depressive states. In *Love Guilt and Reparation and Other Works 1921–1925*. London: Hogarth Press.

Klein, N. (2010) Gulf oil spill: A hole in the world. *Guardian*, 19 June.

Latour, B. (1993) *We Have Never Been Modern*. London: Harvester Wheatsheaf.

Latour, B. (2004) *Politics of Nature*. Harvard University Press.

Lovelock, J. E. (1979) *Gaia, a New Look at Life on Earth*. Oxford, UK: Oxford University Press.

Marx, K. (1859) Preface to *A Contribution to the Critique of Political Economy*. Moscow: Progress Publishers.

Rustin, M. J. (2010) Looking for the unexpected: Psychoanalytic understanding and politics. *British Journal of Psychotherapy*, 26: 4.

Rustin, M. E., and Rustin, M. J. (2010) States of narcissism. In E. McGinley and A. Varchevker (Eds.), *Mourning, Depression and Narcissism Throughout the Life Cycle*. London: Karnac.

Segal, H. (1987) Silence is the real crime. *International Review of Psychoanalysis* 14 (3): 3–11. Reprinted with postscript 'Perestroika, The Gulf War and 11 September 2002', in C. Covington, P. Williams, J. Arundale and J. Knox (Eds.), *Terrorism and War: Unconscious Dynamics of Political Violence*. London: Karnac.

Segal, H. (1995) From Hiroshima to the Gulf War and after: A psychoanalytic perspective. In A. Elliott and S. Frosh (Eds.), *Psychoanalysis in Contexts* (pp. 191–204). London: Routledge.

Steiner, J. (1993) *Psychic Retreats*. London: Routledge.

Stern, N. (2006) *The Stern Review: The Economics of Climate Change*. Cambridge, UK: Cambridge University Press. Also available at: www.hm-treasury.gov.uk/stern_review_report.htm/

Szerszynscki, B., and Urry, J. (2010) *Theory Culture and Society* (*Special Issue on Changing Climates*), 27: 2–3.

Thomas, K. (1983) *Man and the Natural World: Changing Attitudes in England 1500–1800*. London: Allen Lane.

Urry, J. (2010) Consuming the planet to excess. *Theory and Society*, 27 (2–3): 191–212.

Williams, R. (1958) *Culture and Society*. London: Chatto and Windus.

Williams, R. (1980) Ideas of Nature, in *Problems in Materialism and Culture*. London: Verso.

Williams, R. (1978) *Marxism and Literature*. Oxford, UK: Oxford University Press.

Williams, R. (1985) *The Country and the City*. London: Hogarth Press.

Wolff, G. (2011) *Clean Power from Deserts and Adaptation to Climate Change*. Available at: www.ourplanet.com/climate-adaptation/Wolff_Deserts.pdf

Discussion

How is climate change an issue for psychoanalysis?

Jon Alexander

Thomas Berry, Catholic priest and self-proclaimed 'Earth scholar' who died in 2010, famously wrote that 'The universe is a communion of subjects not a collection of objects' (Berry 2009). Man in this view is one subject among many in the natural world, and all subjects are interdependent. We are not *the* unique subject acting on a range of disconnected objects around us. If you start from there, Berry believed, you could not go far wrong, regardless of the specifics of your theology. This adds what I think is a crucial extra dimension to Michael Rustin's central point, that we are part of nature.

My background is in the advertising industry, which I left in 2010 because of concern about the role my work was playing in promoting consumerism. But as a result of those years I bring to this discussion a slightly different, perhaps more applied, perspective. I am a communicator, not a psychoanalyst. I have freed myself at least temporarily from the pre-determined agenda of clients, because I want to understand what, if anything, I should be 'selling' today in order to try to make a better world.

I suggest that the idea Thomas Berry and Michael Rustin share needs to be sold. It is that we as humankind cannot continue to consider ourselves as the unique subject, separate from an object that is called Nature, whether we do so in a protective or destructive manner. Rather, we must recognize that we *are* Nature, or at least part of Nature, and that that gives us a responsibility to the rest of nature as well.

It is from here that I have some disagreement with Rustin, who seems in his chapter to see the idea of man as nature as an important framing for understanding some of the psychology at play – an academic curiosity, as it were – but then seems to step away from his insight on the apparent view that we are doing all we can.

I disagree. I think there is more here than a new theoretical critique of capitalism and environmentalism, which Rustin characterizes as the Industrialist and Conservationist mind-sets, respectively. Indeed, I believe that working from a new mind-set offers the only practical and viable path to solving the problems we face.

We can see both Conservationists and Industrialists at play in the Royal Society for the Protection of Birds' (RSPB 2010) latest report *In the Red*, their response published to DEFRA's (2010) consultation for a new Natural Environment White Paper. Characterizing Nature as a pure object to be protected, their aim is to 'save' at least some places from the impact of man; characterizing Her as a resource, they latch onto the market mechanism of Conservation Credits, which will effectively require businesses to offset damage done in their area of operation by investing in the restoration of another ecosystem elsewhere. The problem is that, because this takes man to be separate from Nature, it fails to recognize that Nature is everywhere and must function healthily everywhere to function healthily at all. Berry's formulation makes the point clearly: the interconnections in the communion of subjects are such that we cannot just allocate areas to care about and areas to forget.

By contrast, other political approaches to Nature are being taken around the world that do originate from this new, or rather, very old worldview. Many of these are based on Latour's idea of representation. Growing from Latin America outward, there is an increasingly global movement behind the idea of rights for Nature, championed by the South African lawyer Cormac Cullinan (2003). Under the Ecuadorian constitution, for example, citizens can bring a lawsuit on behalf of Pachamama – Mother Earth – for damage done to Her. This might seem a little way off for us, but the Hungarians show what is perhaps a more acceptable way forward – they have a Parliamentary Commissioner for Future Generations, whose representational rights are much the same.

As a second example, consider the Sahara solar installation that Michael touched on. Just as with Conservation Credits, this is a useful interim damage limitation exercise from within the current worldview, but no more. We can source our energy needs differently, but what will this do to our impact on the simultaneous crises of biodiversity, ocean acidification, or water shortage that will follow hot on the heels of climate change (if you will forgive the pun)? These issues are all interlinked because Nature is one whole of which we are part. If we stand separate from Her, we work against Her grain, and we will fail.

I would like to contrast this with the nascent thinking of Michael Braungart and Bill McDonough (2002), among others in the United States, and of Gunther Pauli (2010) and his growing band of disciples from Devon to Namibia. All these people use different names for what they do, but 'Cradle-to-Cradle' thinking is perhaps a good catch-all. Essentially, they look at Nature and design their activity on Her models, working in harmony with the system – the first principle being that in Nature, all waste from one system is the raw material for the next system. By way of example, Pauli has used this principle to create a zero-impact brewery in Namibia, which also hosts a mushroom farm, a bakery and a water purification plant, a process that – and here is the vital point – also generates its own localized energy from the reactions taking place.

Put simply, when you embrace the system of which we are part, the world starts to look a lot more exciting. You start thinking about how we can generate energy from waste and partner this with efforts to raise our energy consciousness, all at a localized level, instead of just accepting the rampant increase of our energy needs as inevitable and seeking an alternative mass source to satisfy them. You start to look at how we can localize supply chains, building resilience and increasing quality of life in doing so, instead of accepting the status quo and seeking incrementally to reduce the carbon intensity of air travel. The list goes on.

But how do you sell a worldview? It is not easy. This is not an argument that will be won rationally or quickly, and so to some extent I do agree with Rustin that interim solutions will be needed, and they will require acceptance of many worldviews. But where I differ is that I maintain that these must be seen as interim solutions – we must keep in mind that without the worldview shift, action will not be commensurate with the scale of the challenge.

So, to repeat the question, how do you sell a worldview? The simple answer is that I am not sure you can, but I do think you can create the conditions necessary for that worldview to emerge.

The first condition currently lacking is the social oxygen, as it were, for a new worldview to breathe. Two aspects of our culture today partner to choke off this opportunity: our overly intense work culture and consumerism. The former is described in full Technicolor by Madeleine Bunting (2004) in her book *Willing Slaves*: in hours worked as well as in what she calls 'emotional labour', our careers occupy ever more of our energy and passion. It is no secret that our jobs define us; the invariable first question on making a new acquaintance is, 'So what do you do'?

Consumerism, though, is a far more troubling, though closely related issue. With 36% of us too tired at the end of a working day to do anything other than slump on the sofa, is it any wonder that the average Briton watches upwards of 3 hours television a day, according to Ofcom (2010)? Is it any wonder, then, that she also sees 1,600 adverts every day, each of them telling her, fundamentally, that her primary role in society is as a consumer? Is it any wonder, then, that a new, more participative worldview is finding it hard to take hold?

If the first part of my prescription is to find ways to loosen the grip of our consumerist culture, with the work culture as its possible cause, the second is more positive. We must get ourselves out into nature and allow experience to work its magic, for, as David Attenborough (2010) put it, 'no one is going to care about what they have never experienced'. This may seem obvious, but we are in serious danger of losing touch as a result of what American author Louv (2005) called the extinction of experience. The average 12-year-old in America, as Louv famously found, can recognize 1,000 corporate brands or logos and fewer than 10 species of flora or fauna. We are not much better: a recent study showed such shocking statistics as 64% of 8–12-year-olds playing outdoors less than once a week.

Most of my current work is in this area, with the National Trust. We are working to take the organization back to its Victorian roots in providing common land for common people; the next five years will see the Trust firmly establish itself as an outdoors organization and see us putting significant effort into getting kids in particular out into nature. We are not the only ones. Louv's Children and Nature

Network now reaches into more than 30 countries. This is a major and vital movement, so watch this space.

To conclude: I celebrate the fact that Rustin has gone right to the nub of the issue, pinpointing an unhealthy distortion of our relationship with Nature that stems back many years, perhaps even as far as Plato. My criticism is that he then backs away from his own insight, when following it through fully could have brought us to some truly exciting propositions.

References

Attenborough, D. (2010) Speech to Communicate conference, November.

Berry, T. (2009) *The Sacred Universe: Earth, Spirituality, and Religion in the Twenty First Century*. New York: Columbia University Press.

Braungart, M., and McDonough, B. (2002) *Cradle to Cradle*. New York: Northpoint Press.

Bunting, M. (2004) *Willing Slaves*. London: Harper Collins.

Cullinan, C. (2003) *Wild Law: A Manifesto for Earth Justice*. Burlington, VT: Chelsea Green Publishing.

DEFRA (2010) The Natural Environment White Paper (20.07.10). Available at: www.defra.gov.uk/news/2010/07/26/new-environment-policy

Louv, R. (2005) *The Last Child in the Woods*. Chapel Hill, NC: Algonquin Books.

Ofcom (2010) TV, phones and internet take up almost half our waking hours. Available at: http://consumers.ofcom.org.uk/2010/08/tv-phones-and-internet-take-up-almost-half-our-waking-hours/

Pauli, G. (2010) *The Blue Economy*. Boulder, CO: Paradigm Publishers.

RSPB (2010) Financing nature in an age of austerity, October. Available at: www.rspb.org.uk/Images/Financingnature_tcm9-262166.pdf

Discussion

How is climate change an issue for psychoanalysis?

Ted Benton

My response to Michael Rustin's chapter is in three parts. First, I offer some thoughts about his mode of argument, including his way of characterizing positions other than his own, and relate this to some further questions about the sort of illumination that psychoanalytic modes of thought might offer. Second, I have some questions about the alternative perspective that he derives from Latour. Third, and most important, I express some reservations about the conclusions Rustin draws for the issue of climate change and possible or desirable ways of addressing it.

First, Rustin's mode of argument: at the outset I should declare myself as a moderate sceptic in relation to psychoanalytic modes of social analysis. Reports on therapeutic practice, together with reflection on much that happens in everyday personal interaction, provide strong evidence for thinking that much of our mental activity is unconscious, and that unconscious emotional dynamics can and do have consequences for the way we think and act in our conscious lives. However, so far I have not been convinced by attempts to impose clear-cut 'symptomatologies' onto these effects and to generalize them as explanatory schemes for interpreting major social and historical processes. The analyses that Rustin draws on early in his contribution, for example, seem singularly unconvincing. Segal's expectation that the end of the Cold War would give way to new objects of hostility to replace the Soviet Union was widely shared. But does the confirmation of the prediction demonstrate the 'insight' of the psychodynamic account, or 'reveal the potency of unconscious structures of mind'? Alternative explanatory frames are possible and can be assessed on the basis of accessible evidence: dominant elites promote hostility to external enemies as a means of sustaining their internal hegemony; massive economic and military complexes of vested interest came to acquire political influence in the United States, especially, during the Cold War: their quite consciously recognized interests required a replacement enemy. Which story do you prefer, and why? Similarly with Hinshelwood's suggestion that the peace movement helped to sustain a destructive system by 'assuaging the conscience' of the majority. But maybe the majority felt guilty because they did nothing to oppose nuclear militarism, and that is why there was no pressure to attack the Soviet Union when its system started to crumble? Any psychological story seems to be as good as any other in the absence of any serious and evidence-based theory of the relationships between individual and collective psychodynamics and between them and the social, economic and political processes of complex societies.

Given the opposition between unthinking modernization and nature-loving conservationism, Rustin sees it as tempting, but mistaken to think that the conservationists have 'the most enlightened and mature psychological orientation'. For him, both states of mind may have paranoid-schizoid characteristics. Since paranoid-schizoid states of mind bring about 'the destruction and inhibition of mental function', this seems to imply a pretty severe pathology on the part of the environmental movement.

Luckily, he has identified a tradition of thought that overcomes the 'cul-de-sac' of competing pathologies and may lead us to the 'depressive' ability to think rationally and recognize there is good and bad mixed up together in what we previously hated as wholly bad.

I have two main objections to Rustin's mode of argument here. The first is his use of psychoanalytic diagnoses to reduce and stereotype supposedly all-pervasive ways of thinking and then pathologize them. This is a very useful argumentative strategy. It means you do not have to provide systematic evidence and argument, but simply present your own view as the only healthy option. It has the extra advantage that you do not have to address in terms of evidence or consistency the arguments of any specific exemplar of the proposed mental pathology. Clearly the two examples of pathological environmentalism that he gives do not fit his stereotype. It would be difficult to make a case that Kennedy ascribes 'all value to nature and withholds it from man'. Why, if so, would Kennedy be attacking the company's anti-unionism and destruction of jobs? In the case of Naomi Klein, it would be a tall order to present her as an opponent of rights of the poor in the rest of the world to greater life expectancy, lower rates of infant mortality and access to education!

My second objection is related. It is the use of the word 'some'. Rustin's analysis of the 'cul-de-sac' of the contending 'structures of feeling', and his own mentally healthy proposal, only work if the 'some environmentalists' he stereotypes really do represent the environmental movement as a whole. Rustin has news for the conservationist who mistakenly thinks she is fighting to protect 'pristine nature' against 'destructive modernity': very little of what she values really is 'pristine'. Downland, fens, brecks and broads are all products of the past interaction of humans and nature. This is the sort of thing sociologists who had just discovered 'the environment' used to present as the one great insight offered by their discipline. Unfortunately it was no new insight then and most certainly is not one now! I spend quite a lot of my time working with other environmentalists, and I cannot think of a single one who comes close to Rustin's stereotype. I do not say they do not exist, but, like ghosts, all I can say is, I have never met one.

This takes us directly to Latour. The work of Latour and other 'actor network' theorists offered a way back towards reality for science-studies academics who

had got themselves into the metaphysical cul de sac of extreme social constructionism: 'there is no such thing as nature', they used to claim. Actor-network
approaches made a crucial break with this sort of rhetoric by analysing practices
as always involving 'networks' of what they called 'actants', which could be
human or non-human – such as scallops, in one classic study. The actor-network
approach was a breakthrough in that it allowed back into analyses of scientific
research and development, technological innovation and such-like a recognition
of the 'agency' of non-human (but also non-natural) artefacts such as expert
systems, psychotropic drugs, gene synthesizers and armaments.

So, to quote Wittgenstein, Latour did show the fly the way out of the fly-bottle,
but that was only necessary for those daft enough to have got into the fly-bottle in
the first place. Aside from the avant-garde posturing of 'some' sociologists, rather
few people took the idea that nature was just a 'social construct' very seriously.

There are several disadvantages to using Latour as a starting point for thinking
about environmental politics. The notion of 'actants' unhelpfully compresses all
ontological complexity, in ways that tend to anthropomorphize non-human entities of all kinds, while collapsing social and economic structures into flat
'networks'. There is also paradox in Latour's (and Rustin's) use of the term
'hybridity' in the attempt to overcome society–nature dualism (Benton and Craib
2010). The concept clearly makes no sense except against the background of
'pure-bred' nature and society. But Latour is even less helpful to Rustin than this:

> We find the myth of reason and science unacceptable, intolerable, even
> immoral. We are no longer, alas, at the end of the nineteenth century, that
> most beautiful of centuries, but at the end of the twentieth, and a major
> source of pathology and morality is reason itself – its works, its pomps and its
> armaments.
>
> (Latour 1988: 149)

Is this a case of paranoid-schizoid thinking? It does look to me rather like the
sort of belief system that Rustin seemed to want to distance himself from.

Now to the most important questions. Notwithstanding the problems I find with
Rustin's way of arguing and his use of Latour, are his broad conclusions about
climate change helpful?

On Rustin's account, the current debate is dominated by the antagonism
between rationalist, modernizing perspectives that advocate expansion of the
human domain as if nature were unlimited, on the one hand, and environmentalist
defences of 'pristine nature' against the predations of modernizing economic
development, on the other. There is too little space here to do much more than
state that this is mistaken. Since the international impact of the Brundtland report
of 1987 and the Rio 'Earth Summit' of 1992, the environmentalist case for the
necessity of respect for nature has become inseparably intertwined with the
demand for global social and economic justice. The concept of 'sustainable development' carries a twin demand. Almost no serious participant in the debate strays

outside the challenge posed by the urgent demand for global justice and the unavoidable requirement to achieve it by means that do not degrade planetary life-support systems that will be required by future generations.

However, the concept of sustainable development is sufficiently elastic to allow within its scope a vast array of analyses and proposals from political left to right and to positions that consider themselves to be neither. Instead of Rustin's imagined dispute between those who seek to defend 'nature' at the expense of life expectancy and infant mortality in the poor countries, or pursue ruthless economic expansion at any cost to exploited nature, we have a much more nuanced set of debates around the concept of 'need', the carrying capacity of the earth, the difficulties of predicting future populations and their ecological needs, the extent to which 'natural capital' may be degraded in favour of 'human capital', the prospects of technological innovation, the design of the institutions that might regulate the distribution of knowledge and resources between global communities, and the respective roles of governments and corporations in defining and achieving solutions.

More substantively, Rustin takes the view that a global economy based directly or indirectly on solar energy, together with drastically reduced energy consumption, is technically possible, given conceptions of human well-being that are responsible in their use of finite material resources. We could, in short, see a technological revolution away from fossil fuel consumption and unsustainable material 'metabolism' with the rest of nature.

I agree with this, but the problems only start here. Rustin opposes 'catastrophist' accounts of the present situation (indicative, presumably, of the paranoid-schizoid mind-set) by suggesting that problems of climate change might have a contingent origin, might be 'unforeseen and unintended effect(s) of developments, which, while they can cause great damage, have also achieved much good.' He contrasts this with the alternative view that the source of the problem is 'innate destructiveness, or its embodiment in capitalism'. I'm not sure whether he means this to include only those who think humans are innately destructive, and that is why we have capitalism, or whether it is meant to refer, more broadly, to those of us who think that causal dynamics endemic to capitalism are a principal source of the problem of climate change. This is, indeed, the view I hold, but I hold it consistently with at least part of what Rustin takes to be the alternative: that is, I think climate change is, indeed, an unintended and unforeseen consequence of capitalist development. And, given a certain understanding of what capitalism is, I can even agree that it has achieved much that is good. However, no matter what the balance of good and bad in capitalism's past, there can be little doubt that its future looks deeply problematic for both people and the nature they live with and from. (For good examples of opposed views on this question, see Porritt 2007 and Kovel 2007.)

This is not the place for a detailed discussion of the social and ecological dynamics of capitalism, but it is generally agreed that growth in both material and energy flows and the transformative powers of technology have so far been endemic, long-term features. These features of capitalist development have been accompanied by a tendency to degrade the environmental, naturally given, conditions of both production and life-quality. This is understood, by 'mainstream' as well as ecological economics, to be a consequence of the fact that these conditions (fresh air, favourable climates, biodiversity, ecosystem services, etc.) are un-priced and so do not enter into economic calculation. I would argue that much of what Rustin presents as the 'good' achieved under capitalist development is a product of the pressure brought to bear by popular movements. Environmentalists have fought to prevent, ameliorate or repair environmental damage, while socialist, feminist and anti-racist movements have fought against exploitation, exclusion and stigmatization. Thus far, this process, uneven and incomplete as it has been, has kept the inequalities, social disintegration and ecological damage that would otherwise have occurred within bounds – at least in the 'developed' liberal-democratic states. However, very few of these 'goods' have been in evidence outside this narrow circle of nation-states, and indeed there is sound evidence that the capacity to deliver these goods has been won at profound cost to human and non-human life and the ecological conditions for life over much of the rest of the world (Global Footprint Network 2010).

These considerations tell against Rustin's view that the problems of climate change have a 'contingent' origin. The history of capitalist development over two centuries has been both enabled and driven by fossil fuel energy-sources. His vision of a thorough-going technological transition on a global scale, which at the same time is 'inclusive of the interests of all human beings', is, as he recognizes, a tall order! But it is a taller order than he allows. First, the neo-liberal transition that has been under way for the past three or four decades has given us a world in which nation states have lost economic sovereignty (many of course never had it!), in which transnational corporations have greatly enhanced power, and in which international capital and financial flows have reached unprecedented levels. This accelerated globalization of capital accumulation has, indeed, taken millions of humans out of poverty, but at the same time it has achieved this good in ways that pose a dire challenge to global futures. The growth dynamic in the demands made by this new phase of capitalist development on its material, energetic and life-support base adds to myriad local and regional ecological problems, a multi-dimensional crisis of social dislocation, inequality, geo-strategic conflict and ecological crisis now evident on a global scale – beyond the reach of national governments, even that of the remaining global superpower.

Second, there is growing evidence that the consequences of this escalation in global socio-economic metabolism with the rest of nature go beyond the single matter of greenhouse gases and climate change – massively important though this is. There is now overwhelming evidence of human-induced extinction of other life-forms comparable to those of past geological epochs, and growing evidence of actual and likely crises in access to fresh water and food (e.g. Foster, Clark, and York 2010; Rockström et al. 2009). These other dimensions of ecological crisis have their own independent drivers, as well as interacting in many complex ways with the consequences of climate change. It is crucially important that this is understood, since attempts to find a 'technical fix' for climate change in abstraction from an understanding of the wider context are likely to exacerbate other aspects of a much deeper socio-ecological predicament. Though Rustin is careful to avoid them, nuclear power and bio-fuels are now standard elements in most governmental recipes for a low-carbon economy. The health and military risks associated with the former and the threats to both food and biodiversity inherent in the latter are clear.

Third, the prospects for the necessary transformation of energy technology, let alone the required socio-technical changes in other domains, are constrained by patterns of entrenched economic, military and geo-political interests in conflict both with one another and with the social movements pressing for those changes. When Rustin says: '. . . in the face of acute anxieties about material or social survival, regression from more inclusive to more divisive and exclusionary modes of thought and action is liable to occur', it seems to me he really does point to a very valuable contribution that psychoanalytic modes of thought can make. My only reservation is that we should be wary of placing too much emphasis on the psychodynamic element in the breakdown and failure of so many attempts at reaching international agreement to resolve these deep and far-reaching issues. Unquestionably there is a psychodynamic element, but as I have tried to indicate above, there are profound socio-ecological, military, political-economic and cultural dynamics, too. It will not be possible to resolve these issues in ways that satisfy the '*interests*' of all, but it may, just, be possible to resolve them in ways that meet the '*needs*' of all: but a society that organizes its activities around the meeting of need rather than the competitive scramble for more will differ from the present in more ways than its methods of generating energy.

References

Benton, T., and Craib, I. (2010) *Philosophy of Social Science*. Basingstoke & New York: Palgrave.

Foster, J. B., Clark, B., and York, R. (2010) *The Ecological Rift*. New York: Monthly Review.

Global Footprint Network (2010) *Living Planet Report*. Available at: www.footprintnet-work.org

Kovel, J. (2007) *The Enemy of Nature*. London & New York: Zed.

Latour, B. (1988) *The Pasteurization of France*. Cambridge, MA: Harvard University.

Porritt, J. (2007) *Capitalism as if the Earth Matters*. London: Earthscan.

Rockström, J. et al. (2009) *Planetary Boundaries: Exploring the Safe Operating Space for Humanity*. Available at: www.ecologyandsociety.orgwww.footprintnetwork.org

Reply
How is climate change an issue for psychoanalysis?

Michael Rustin

My chapter, and indeed most of this book, seeks to address one principal perspective on the problems of climate change, which is that provided by psychoanalytic thinking. It is not proposed that this dimension of explanation should have priority over others, merely that it may add something further to our understanding.

I agree with much of what both Ted Benton and Jon Alexander have to say about the political economy of these issues. Changing the direction of a political and economic system dedicated above all to the expansion of material production is formidably difficult, and also without doubt necessary. The question is whether some part of the explanation of how these systems function can be provided by reference to unconscious structures of mind.

By unconscious structures of mind one is referring to the irrational, to elements of what Slavoj Zizek (1990) calls 'excess'. The conception is that structures of unconscious feeling have a causal role within structures of power, shaping opinion, sharply defining friends and enemies, and often driving the capacity for rational discrimination out of mind. The mentalities evoked in the 'war on terror' are such an instance. Benton claims that 'Segal's expectation that the end of the Cold War would give way to new objects of hostility to replace the Soviet Union was widely shared.' Was it, at the time of the first Gulf War in 1990? It was because Segal had such a clear grasp of the paranoid-schizoid structures of mind in which the Cold War had been framed that she could see so quickly that what was really happening under the cover of protecting Kuwait was the redirection of these same mentalities.

I agree that the grounding of such conceptions of unconscious states of mind is difficult. But if an effect is very powerful, it is better to seek an approximate understanding of it than none at all. Benton acknowledges that elites 'promote hostility to external enemies' – this indeed is one way in which irrational emotions become mobilized as powerful social forces.

Such structures of feeling are also relevant in the context of the environmental crisis. How would this not be so, given the enormity of what is at stake? One way of approaching this issue would have been to focus attention merely on the irrational ways of thinking of those most blind to, or even culpable for, damage to the environment. In his 1938 text on Nazi propaganda, Theodor Adorno (1951) gave a brilliant example of a psychoanalytic analysis of the methods of his undoubted foes which was at the same time a profound political critique of fascist mentalities. But I wanted to pursue a different approach, to consider the possible relevance of these perspectives to those on different sides of these arguments, rather than seek to deploy them as aspect of political polemic. Benton's description of my approach as 'a very useful argumentative strategy' conveys that he thought I was doing this anyway, though this was not my intention. I outlined opposed 'ideal typical' definitions of this issue, citing various sources for these, but this is because I believe that these traditions are historically and culturally important and provide resources for thinking about these issues. It is not a matter of taking sides between them. I was glad to see that at the end of his piece Benton noted, despite his earlier reservations about psychoanalytic thinking, that this perspective could make a valuable contribution to understanding the extreme states of anxiety that we may well encounter as the environmental crisis evolves.

The point about paranoid-schizoid and depressive states of mind is that they are universal dispositions, as likely to have relevance to understanding our own ways of thinking as those of others. It is not a matter of pathologizing one's opponents.

Naomi Klein is an indispensable writer and campaigner, but nevertheless, what the newspaper article of hers that I quoted was doing, through its metaphor of a rape of the sea bed, was to mobilize emotions. This was also the style of the fierce reported debate in the United States about opencast mining. To make this observation does not make one indifferent to the arguments about oil exploration under the sea, or about the excesses of coal-mining companies. The reason I referred to popular polemics is because so far as unconscious states of mind are concerned, I wanted to focus on widely shared public mentalities, not on the well-informed debates of the seminar room.

The idea referred to by Benton that there are structural as well as motivational reasons that make capitalism destructive of environments is an important one. It is indeed a great problem that the calculus of costs and benefits deployed in markets often treats as 'free goods' environmental resources that are of immense value. However, although I would generally be on his side in most arguments about the role of democratic and political constraints on markets, I do not think it is defensible to assign all the benefits that capitalism has brought to those who have resisted the impact of markets and none to the energies and inventiveness of capitalism itself. There are also political risks in formulating the environmentalist case in polemically anti-capitalist terms.

In the wider public world, it seems to me that the polarity of destructive mankind and defenceless nature continues to have purchase, even though we all agree that this does not accurately describe the reality of this relationship. Evidence for this popular state of mind is provided in Jon Alexander's commentary, in his description of the RSPB's (one million plus members, including myself) latest report, which sets 'Nature as a pure object to be protected', with 'at least some places "to be saved" from the impact of man.' I think all three of us probably agree that the point is to see mankind as one element of Nature, but with huge responsibilities for all of it (on this planet, at least). The idea of Nature, and the question of how we should relate to it, is a very complex one, and Alexander argues eloquently for a fully holistic conception. Aspects of Nature that have been shaped by human action can be valued as deeply as those that have hitherto been untouched. The projects for conservation that he describes seem admirable ways of nurturing this feeling of responsibility through practices.

Reference

Adorno, T. (1951) Freudian Theory and the Pattern of Fascist Propaganda. Reprinted in T. Adorno and J. M. Bernstein, *The Culture Industry* (pp. 132–157). London: Routledge, 2001.

Zizek, S. (1990) Eastern Europe's Republics of Gilead. *New Left Review*, 183: 50–62.

Chapter 9

On the love of nature and on human nature

Restoring split internal landscapes

Sally Weintrobe

Introduction

In this chapter I argue that engaging with climate change involves engaging with our loving, caring feelings for nature so that we are more able to be mindful and concerned about our impact on nature in our daily lives in an ongoing way. I look at the way loving nature is an ordinary and natural part of human nature, and I argue that capitalist culture, particularly in its recent neoliberal[1] global phase, actively seeks to erode our loving feelings and to persuade us we are apart from, not part of, nature. It actively fosters in us a sense of entitlement to exploit nature without counting the real cost. Engaging with nature also involves engaging with politics, history and culture, so as to better understand ways in which our thoughts and feelings about nature are profoundly influenced and shaped by cultural and political forces. It involves facing facts about human nature so as better to understand how and why collectively we collude with these influences.

I argue that within Western consumerist societies seductive, coercive and aggressively intrusive techniques are currently used to blunt loving feelings and sap our collective will to think about, care for and protect nature. I give examples of these techniques and suggest that they are used to promote our identities primarily as consumers of nature and to weaken our identities as lovers of nature. I suggest this is a form of colonization of the mind.

What is nature?

Nature is very broadly defined in the environmental literature. Some definitions are very general and include the physical material world as well as all the living creatures – fauna and flora – found within it.[2] Natural landscapes may include pristine wilderness, scrub, the backyard, the city park, the allotment, the window box and the sky. By nature we also mean how we and other life forms naturally are – what is 'our nature'. Within such a general perspective nature might include the mating rituals of young people inside a city nightclub (Jon Alexander, personal communication, 2010) as well as the ways of the lone fox concurrently rifling rubbish bins in the street outside.

Rather than reaching towards a definition of nature, my focus is on exploring aspects of our relationships with nature, suggesting these are complex, permeated with phantasy and with profound resistance to knowledge of nature's unalterable facts. I look at how we represent these relationships within the psyche, what kinds of internal narratives of self guide and inform these relationships and how these are heavily influenced by dominant cultural forces. Narratives of self may be difficult to discern and be mostly unconscious, but they profoundly influence our sense of identity and also our behaviour. I focus on feelings of entitlement as part of our narratives of self, suggesting that we struggle with different and conflicting kinds of entitlement.[3] One is a lively sense of entitlement to get to know, to love and to protect nature, and the other is a more narcissistic sense of entitlement to exploit and disregard nature with the justification that we are special and different from other life forms. In this view we see the Earth as here solely for our benefit and our consumption.

Love of nature

A psychoanalytic view emphasizes that we love not only with heart and mind but also with our bodies, in free movement and with all our senses. Love includes erotic feelings, feelings of attachment, feelings of care and concern and lively curiosity to get to know the loved other. We love nature in all these ways.

We know that loving and engaging with nature can promote states of calm and restoration, resulting from sensual pleasure derived from all our senses. This is true for children and adults. The poet and writer Terry Tempest Williams (1991) described nature as generating a sense of wonder and awe but also 'peace in patterns'. A bodily relationship with nature has been experimentally shown to be beneficial to our well-being. In *The Last Child in the Woods*, Louv (2005) presented research that shows that free play in nature[4] outdoors is linked with mental health and well-being in children. Studies have shown that lack of exposure to nature is linked statistically with an increased likelihood of suffering attention deficit disorder (ADD). For instance, Malone and Tranter (2003) found that children playing on asphalt had play that was more interrupted and they played in shorter segments than children playing on grass or soil. Faber Taylor, Kuo, and Sullivan (2001) found that children exhibit fewer symptoms of ADD after spending time in green surroundings.

Psychoanalysis draws an important distinction between genuine love and idealized love, the latter based on splitting. With splitting, the object of our love, nature in this case, is divided in phantasy into exaggeratedly ideally good parts and exaggeratedly denigrated parts and in a split state of mind one part may gain awareness while the other part is split off and kept out of central awareness. In contrast with idealization, genuine love of nature sees nature as flawed and limited and our capacity to love nature as flawed and limited too. Genuine love includes *moments* of connection rather than idealized notions of a continuous sense of blissful 'oneness' with nature. Our love of nature may, realistically, be lost and re-found.

Genuine love is also based on being able to tolerate very ambivalent feelings. Our ambivalence includes our mixed feelings towards a nature that can fill us with love, awe us with its beauty, terrify us with its power and cause us much discomfort. We can have feelings of hatred as well as love for nature. I suggest the deepest source of our ambivalence towards nature is that it gives us life but also brings death.

Freud (1913a), with his characteristic courage to face that which fills us with dread, noted the problem of feeling grateful towards a Mother Earth that gives us life and then takes it away. He linked our phantasied relationships with nature to the relationship with the mother. In this view we can be seen, like small children, to take Mother Earth for granted, to treat her rather like a breast and toilet mother, there just to fulfil our needs and absorb our waste. Keene makes this point in chapter 7 in this volume. However, I think there are limits to the extent to which nature is linked with the mother. The material reality of Nature has its own specific and unique qualities in the internal world of the psyche. Searles (1972) and Bollas (1992) both argue this.

Our love of nature develops as we ourselves develop. As children, we love nature spontaneously, naturally and fiercely, with our bodies, all our senses and with an engaging curiosity. Nature seems not yet to have lost the quality of a 'there-ness' that greets one, the quality vividly described by Arne Naess (2008), founder of Deep Ecology. We adults delight in this and may pine for our own loss of animistic thinking and freshness of engagement. Ordinary everyday examples that come to mind are little children saying goodnight to the moon and the first star with feeling or down on their hands and knees excitedly finding ants on the pavement. Children have a natural and animistic expectation of a relationship with anybody and anything, including people, animals, machines and inanimate nature.[5]

Children's interest in nature is serious psychic work. Just one example of this work is a small girl on a train that had stopped unexpectedly on the track out in the country, whom I heard say, 'Mummy, why did the train stop? Does it want to do a poo poo?' This reduced the whole carriage to affectionate chuckling. The example conveys the fierce curiosity, the why, why, why, of the small child, the natural identification with the other, and it may also be an illustration of Freud's theory of childhood sexuality. Whereas a baby might want to express 'mouth love' and 'mouth curiosity' of the natural world by taking the world into its mouth and sucking or chewing it, this slightly older child looked to be in a phase of relating to the world in a 'bottom-centred' kind of way.

World literature is full of expression of our mature adult love of nature. It is a love that includes passion, profound ambivalence and concern. It is also a form of erotic love, an Eros of the senses.[6] We all have our favourite writers, and one of mine is William Hudson, of whom Conrad said, 'he writes as the grass grows'. Here is Hudson, writing in 1918:

> I believed that two and two make four and that the world is round in spite
> of its flat appearance; also that it is travelling through space and revolving
> round the sun instead of standing still. . . . These teachings did not touch my

heart as it was touched and thrilled by something nearer, more intimate, in nature, not only in moonlit trees or in a flower or serpent, but, in certain exquisite moments and moods and in certain aspects of nature, in 'every grass' and in all things, animate and inanimate.

(Hudson 1918: 232–233)

When one feels a part of nature, one can more easily derive comfort from nature. This goes beyond aesthetic comfort and includes comfort from knowing one shares commonality in life and also a common fate with other forms of life. In my next quote from Hudson he is working through his ambivalent feelings about personal death. Sitting alone one night near Beaulieu in Hampshire on the Pixie mounds – mounds raised by prehistoric men– he writes of feeling in turn alone, afraid and then grief-stricken at the thought of death. He then says:

I began to grow more and more attracted by the thought of resting on so blessed a spot. To have always about me that wildness which I best loved – the rude incult heath, the beautiful desolation, to have harsh furze and ling and bramble and bracken to grow on me, and only wild creatures for visitors and company . . . the deep-burrowing rabbit to bring down his warmth and familiar smell among my bones; heat-loving adder, rich in colour to find when summer is gone a dry safe shelter and hibernaculum in my empty skull. . . . I thought too, of those . . . I should lie with . . . after my life; and thinking of them I was no longer alone.

(Hudson 1918: 232–233)

Hudson's writing reveals a deep understanding that love of life and feeling alive flowers with awareness of death, and this awareness necessarily includes that time when there is no time, before life and after life. His descriptions come across to me as by someone seeking the conditions to be fully alive and present, *here* and *now*, properly located in time, part of nature and not apart from nature and with the solace and comfort to be found in knowing that one is part of the community of fellow living beings, human, animal and vegetable, that will also die.

We may like to see ourselves as superior to and apart from other life forms, but we share with them the big issues of life and death. And, I suggest, the biggest difference between life forms is whether they are alive or dead. This is beautifully expressed in *Ecclesiastes 9* (King James Version):

For to him that is joined to all the living there is hope. . . . For the living know that they shall die: but the dead know not any thing . . . their love, and their hatred, and their envy, is now perished; neither have they any more a portion for ever in any thing that is done under the sun.

Late in life Freud described nature as 'eternally remote. . . . She destroys us – coldly, cruelly, relentlessly' (1927: 15). Ageing, death and decomposition are indeed relentless natural processes, but Freud's description of them as also cold and cruel brings into the picture our phantasies of a Mother Earth that cruelly and coldly has it in for us, either actively or through an eternal indifference to our fate. In a split state of mind these kinds of more paranoid phantasies will tend unconsciously to accompany phantasies of an idealized all-bountiful Mother Earth.

In the quote above Hudson struggles to find the inner resources to face death as well as life. He works to resolve his ambivalent feelings towards nature through reaffirming his sense of community and commonality with all fellow life forms and reconnecting with his body as a part of nature. This brings him solace. Edward O. Wilson (1984) has termed this 'urge to affiliate with other life forms' biophilia.

For writers such as Hudson, love of nature is strong and openly declared. However, even people in whom loving feelings for nature have apparently been lost or eradicated often have strong feelings about where they want to be buried. They remain deeply attached to landscape, the earth and to nature.

Representing nature in the internal world of the psyche

In a psychoanalytic view, people imaginatively and unconsciously create an internal world within the psyche, one based in part on external reality and 'peopled' with figures that psychoanalysis calls internal objects. The term object is rather impersonal, but psychoanalysis uses it so as not to restrict its scope. An internal object can be a plant or an animal or parents or an abstract idea or classmates or the collective leadership at Copenhagen or the G8. It is anything that the self forms a relationship with, and it has a history in chains of associations of meaning. An internal object can be thought of as like a souvenir. For instance, a little statue of the Eiffel Tower can trigger all the personal memories of that trip to Paris. The self as well as the other is imaginatively constructed as a series of internal objects in relationships with other objects. Self here includes representations of different, sometimes conflicting parts of the self. Internal objects are not simply the inner representation of the figures of external reality but may be subject to considerable distortion by unconscious phantasies.

Internal psychic landscapes

I suggest we locate the internal relationships that we arrange in space and time in imaginary places that I am calling landscapes. By landscape I mean *place* in the internal world of the psyche.[7] The term *landscape* has certain attributes and qualities that are missing in the more abstract term psychic space or place. One can feel attached to a landscape, more grounded in a landscape and have the sense that that ground is shared with other living beings. Internal representations of landscapes have their roots in our physical world. Despite our developed capacity for abstract thinking, we remain and need to remain attached to the physical and the material. In the unconscious we tend to represent our internal world largely as stories taking place in physical landscapes, landscapes that are inhabited by flora and fauna. And landscapes figure prominently in our dreams.

Internal landscapes are not easy to think about and are largely unconscious. They are the series of different sorts of psychic imaginary places in which we relate to our family (perhaps in a house), to our friends (in social settings), to our social groups (more abstract but also spatially and to some extent physically represented), to society, democracy, politics, the marketplace, to nature, and so on. We also relate to different aspects of ourselves within our inner psychic landscapes.

Our landscapes are socially determined to a considerable degree, and we express and also develop different aspects of our identity within the setting of these landscapes. We are already socially placed *within* landscapes, we *find* ourselves placed within landscapes and we also find our *selves* in landscapes. Diversity of inner landscapes is vital to forming an identity sufficiently rich to promote well-being and feeling alive as a person.

Establishing and maintaining internal landscapes

A rich and elaborated sense of self depends on having a diverse range of different types of inner landscape (natural, familial, economic, educational, etc.) and on feeling 'at home' within these different landscapes. By 'at home' I mean with the support of a mindful authority we can identify with and depend on. We feel safe 'at home'. A mindful presence can be parents, or government, or independent public radio, or a national respected figure, or a just and fair legal code. It is also a part of the internal self. A mindful presence tries to imagine how the other feels, thereby including the other, but it also sets limits and boundaries. A mindful presence builds a sense of continuity through which the narratives of self can safely develop. For instance, when Nelson Mandela went on public radio in South Africa to praise Afrikaans culture when Afrikaans ceased to be an official language, he was mindful of how the Afrikaans people would feel anxious and outcast from their homeland, and he sought to include them and restore to them their sense of dignity and belonging at a time of change.

An unmindful presence tends to disregard or denigrate the other, leaving the other vulnerable, frightened, excluded and with no safe homeland. When Margaret Thatcher said there is no such thing as society, British citizens were meant to feel as outcasts in their identity as citizens, without psychic home and location to think of themselves as social beings with civic rights, duties and responsibilities to and for each other. I suggest she was not only attacking a particular internal landscape – the way we imaginatively configure society – but also our very identity as citizens within society. The attack was aimed at undermining the part of the self that cares about others and promoting the part of the self more aggressively out only for self-interest.

Colonization of our love of nature through promoting split and idealized internal landscapes

In a previous paper (Weintrobe 2010a) I discussed runaway consumer greed and its links with a state of mind of narcissistic entitlement, one that says, 'I am entitled to have and to be everything I crave as I am superior and special.' I looked at the way this has become an ordinary everyday kind of thinking in consumerist societies.[8] I suggested it is based on a particular kind of splitting and identification. The splitting is into superior in-groups and inferior out-groups, and the identification is with the superior in-group. When identified with a superior in-group, one may occupy a prejudiced position towards the out-group, and this enables one more easily to cut off feelings of concern at exploiting the out-group. I argued that neoliberal capitalism relentlessly and indifferently appeals to people's wish to feel special and superior, and it does this centrally through encouraging identification with idealized groups and figures, often celebrities. The increased consumerism this is currently leading to, based on fossil fuels, is significantly driving global warming.

Capitalism seeks what advertising calls 'mind share', in effect a form of colonizing the mind. In a colonized state all our relationships in all our various and varied landscapes become narrowed down to just one kind of relationship. This is where we feel superior to the other and entitled to exploit and consume the other. This is entitlement of a narcissistic and narrow-minded kind where the other is seen as there only to service our needs.[9] Narcissistic entitlement also includes feeling entitled not to have to be burdened by the pain of guilt, shame and responsibility about this treatment of the other.

In this chapter my focus is on the way our relationships with nature are colonized. An ordinary everyday example of the effects of 'mind share' here might be on people who love birds and also love walking who may be seduced away from loving birds into seeing themselves as the owners of the most special binoculars, the best new walking poles and with a superior capacity to find the best and most exotic global locations in which to walk and see birds. The net result is an increased carbon footprint that will adversely affect birds as well as the people themselves. I suggest such people have been both willingly and unwillingly colonized. What in particular is colonized, exploited and deformed is their love of nature.

When we become identified with a position of entitlement to exploit the other without concern or apparent cost, the result is a split self and a split in our inner landscapes. One result of the splitting is that in our landscapes the sense of space between self and other/s has been unconsciously rearranged.[10] Concern becomes something we only show for those we assign to our in-groups, *kept near us in our imagination* while those we split off and *assign to being far away from us* we can more easily treat without concern. Spatially, the 'far-away' objects can be experienced as in the shadows, or in a forgotten-about place, or denigrated, inferior and placed on 'the other side of the tracks', or located spatially in a far-off land that may even be called the future. The unconscious aim is to create emotional distance from those we feel guilty towards for our maltreatment.[11] Cohen in his discussion paper in chapter 4, this volume, refers to the 'distant other', which, I suggest, is the internal object when split off in this way.

However, when we split, it is not simply that we love and care about those we keep near us in our imagination and do not care about those we imaginatively assign to being far away from us. Splitting tends to go together with idealization, and the 'caring' we show in split states of mind is often idealized caring that covers over hidden levels of indifference, neglect and, indeed, sometimes great cruelty. In the example I gave, our bird lover ends up eroding his/her concern for birds and thinking him/herself rather special and entitled. Another example of this form of splitting is that when in consumerist societies we see ourselves as ideal parents giving our children inflated amounts of possessions and treats, we may have split off more genuine concern about their long-term welfare in a sustainable world.

When we find pets and wild animals especially 'cute' and mistake this for loving and caring feelings, we may have split off our cruelty and indifference and the violence that lies beneath this. Examples can be found in the burgeoning number of 'cute' animal webcams on YouTube that we watch and send to our friends by e-mail. One very popular webcam showed koala bears in a recent severe drought in Australia begging water from humans on the public highway. Koala bears sucking water bottles and looking like babies were seen as 'cute', and in the 'oh, how cute is that'! state of mind, awareness of the distress that may have led bears to show such atypical behaviour was split off.

Non-split natural landscapes

What might a relatively *non-split natural* landscape look like? I suggest in such a landscape common ground is shared between self and other humans and between self and non-human species. Also, this common ground supports feelings of empathy, humaneness and solidarity with other life forms, particularly in relation to issues of life and death. The common ground may be visualized spatially as a landscape that includes the other rather than the other being imagined in a far-away landscape where they are kept dehumanized, their significance is minimized and they are hermetically sealed off from being able to touch the self emotionally.

With shared landscapes comes awareness of conflict and issues of mourning. When we know, in a feeling way, that we share the Earth with endangered and maltreated species, then we are liable to feel grief.[12]

We can perhaps appreciate the enormity of our difficulty in not splitting our landscapes in which our relationships with nature are set within Western cultures when we realize we have no word for cross-species empathy, that it is clearly highly suspect to claim humaneness as a uniquely human trait and that we regularly project into animals all our undesirable attributes (greedy pig, dirty dog, filthy swine, dishonest fox, stupid sheep and so on). In addition we are taught to disregard our empathic projective imagination about animals' feelings on grounds that we are anthropomorphizing and have no 'scientific evidence'. Instances of prejudice and splitting are embedded in our prevailing scientific discourses, and recognizing this should not undermine but, rather, strengthen scientific method. The recent and growing body of evidence from evolutionary biology is currently successfully challenging a prevailing scientific consensus that our species alone has a capacity for empathy and a moral life (de Waal 2006).

Our sense of entitlement to see ourselves as superior to other life forms and the idea that nature is there to be tamed have become deeply embedded in our culture, religious and philosophical beliefs and political ideologies (see Hamilton, chapter 2, and Rustin, chapter 8, in this volume). It is in essence a colonizing mental outlook that necessitates our natural concern for the other to be split off. We are less consciously troubled by guilt and shame and find it easier to exploit the other, whether other people or other species, if they are seen as denigrated and through a prejudiced eye. In addition, we may treat in a prejudiced and denigrated way the lively parts of ourselves that seek meaning, suffer painful feelings and struggle to face the ongoing conflicts within ourselves. I explored these ideas in a paper on dehumanizing forms of prejudice (Weintrobe 2010b).

A current prevailing culture in the human sciences has it that *only* what is measurable can be studied. This may end up excluding from, or not giving proper weight to, areas of human subjectivity such as our *feelings* about nature and about climate change and our empathic sense of connection with other species. We need to take care lest we split off and throw out the baby under study – ourselves – with the bathwater.

Our very concept of self has been extensively colonized. Rather than recognizing the self to be divided, struggling between different parts and involving competing and sometimes contradictory narratives, some of which may not be fully conscious, the self has tended and still tends to be seen as unitary, conscious and rational.

Also, the concept of self has more recently become identified with selfishness following analyses of the 'me culture' (see Lasch 1978). I suggest that in this particular view self becomes equated with the narcissistically entitled self. But another kind of 'self'ishness is the expression of the part of the self that seeks to be alive and feels entitled in a lively way to express its love of reality, to take feelings seriously and to show concern.

In unitary perspectives what can get lost is knowledge that we are not one thing or another thing by nature but, rather, we are complex, conflicted and ambivalent and that we struggle with our feelings. The part of the self that is narcissistically entitled hates the psychic pain of working through conflict, ambivalence and psychic pain and rather seeks to embrace the wishful phantasy that the self is *either* exploitative *or* solely caring.

In seeking to redress current dominant cultural narratives that say that we are basically exploitative and selfish by nature, the danger might be that we promote the simplistic view that we are basically caring and unexploitative by nature. In reality we are both, and this is the narrative that needs air to breathe.

The human tendency to split into superior and inferior and identify with the superior as a way to avoid difficult feelings such as envy, helplessness, guilt and shame is not just something encouraged or imposed on us by outside forces. These mechanisms are an integral part of our psychic lives, and the psychic work needed to repair a more loving and caring identity within more integrated and non-split inner landscapes is ongoing in life. It is a perspective where we see ourselves as part of the problem as well as part of the solution.

Colonization of our identities involves finding ways not only to encourage but also to *maintain* the splitting, in phantasy, of our internal landscapes. Seeing ourselves as idealized and superior consumers of nature and entitled to consume nature goes together with actively denigrating in an ongoing way the part of ourselves that simply and powerfully loves, needs nature as nature and wants to protect nature. What also gets denigrated is the part of us that loves and is curious about our own human nature.

Ecological debt and gratitude

Randall discusses the subject of indebtedness and gratitude towards nature in this volume in terms of Simms' (2005) concept of the carbon debt that accrues when our activities generate more carbon emissions than is sustainable. The whole area of our relationships of dependence, indebtedness and also flagrant ingratitude to nature is one that could benefit from considerable further exploration and under-standing. In a split state of mind the part of the self that feels narcissistically entitled to exploit nature abhors feeling dependent and grateful as this undermines feeling special and superior. In a non-split state of mind we are better able to mourn our idealized expectations of Mother Earth, tolerate ambivalent feelings, face our dependency and feel grateful for what we receive from nature.

Current nature programmes

Neoliberal capitalist TV and film culture currently uses various techniques not only to promote but to maintain our identities as consumers. Techniques I concentrate on here are: encouraging identification with an attitude of arrogant entitle-ment, a particular use of sound, and visual and auditory 'flash bang' techniques.

I illustrate the 'self-aggrandizing hero' theme and the use of sound by looking at some major changes that have occurred in nature programmes over the past 10 years (excluding programmes like the BBC's Natural World Series and, of course, David Attenborough). These programmes, rather than providing public space in which to encourage curiosity about and love of nature and wild animals, tend increasingly to provide a space for encouraging identification with central narra-tors who use nature in order to generate excitement, or promote themselves as superior through the ability to 'tame' nature, to 'excite' themselves through experience in nature or to bring wild animals under their control. In these sorts of programmes a loving relationship with nature can also become corrupted and subverted through becoming erotized. Erotization is where having power over the object, not love and mutuality, is the turn-on. Sex, aggression and danger tend to dominate as themes. What is meant to be awesome and wonder-full in these programmes is not nature but the programme presenter, and nature is used and exploited to this end.

A recent review of *Lost Land of the Tiger* (BBC1) by Guardian journalist Sam Wollaston makes the point. It is, he says:

> . . . by those people who go on grand-scale expeditions with tonnes of equipment to the remotest parts of the world and then make films which are mainly about themselves. . . . Gordon heads north, high into the Himalayas, to be manly. . . . Ooh, hello, that looks interesting, a beautiful moon moth, I'd like to know a bit more about one of them. . . . But no, we have to go back to see how Gordon is managing with the altitude, and the snow, and how he crosses a river. And how they all cope with a bit of rain one night. . . . right at the end of this we actually get to meet a couple of tigers. But then of course we cut to the team, watching the tigers on the laptop. Except for Gordon who's up his flipping mountain.
>
> (Wollaston 2010)

Music and sound in these kinds of nature programmes tends to be pumped up in volume, suggesting that there is nothing much of interest in nature itself – including its silences.[13] In this way of thinking the sounds of nature are boring, need sexing up and to be made, in current phrasing, more 'edgy'. But unless 'mood' music in nature programmes is chosen with sensitivity and based on knowledge of how little we do understand about our fellow sentient non-human beings, it can tend to superimpose an anthropomorphic view. The result is reduction of space in which to tolerate our state of not knowing and for granting respect due to other species of their otherness. Appreciation of otherness also provides checks to our more greedy and possessive tendencies. It checks our sense of omniscience. Until we know that we do not know the other and that the other moves in its own ways, not dictated by us, we do not begin to know the other.

Pumped-up loud music can be jarring and as such be actively corrosive and assaulting of our capacity to think and feel.[14] In more extreme cases it is reminiscent of the way in which soldiers may go into battle with pop music blaring in order to spread confusion and promote 'shock and awe'.

Loud sudden flash/bang noises are more frequent right across the range of current films and TV programmes. An absence of flash/bang is becoming the exception, not the rule. It is a cutting *whoosh* sound that we do not have a word for. Aware I am being highly speculative, I nevertheless see some of these flash-bangs as potentially promoting splitting with a wall of sound.[15] The splitting may result in the viewer reacting by keeping genuine experience of contact with the other in a far-away place.

Sudden, *whooshed-in*, unannounced visual material is also more common and, because unannounced, may be experienced as an intrusion and at times shocking. Increasingly younger audiences are exposed to these techniques. The *whooshes* can operate as visual assaults, placing the viewer wanting to preserve the integrity of their inner psychic home in a no-win situation. Either they protect themselves by numbing their feelings or they may experience feelings of helplessness that may be traumatic to the meaning and continuity-seeking part of the self. Either way they disrupt the narrative of relating and they undermine the human will to connect.[16]

Justification for these kinds of recent changes, changes that have appeared across a wide range of subjects in TV and cinema, particularly within the Hollywood tradition, is that they just provide people with what they want. However I suggest the situation is far more complex and involves industry-driven ways to promote identification with idealized cruelly indifferent and exploiting human 'hero' figures and to attack, assault and maltreat the lively parts of the self that resist this. The result may be a vicious cycle of seduction and assault, followed by further identification with a blank state as a means to defend against being assaulted. Where resistance is explicitly part of the narrative of adventure films, resistance is often from an idealized superhero figure, winning against the cruel powerful exploiting enemy in magical ways against frankly impossible odds. While this is meant to create hope, I suggest it reinforces an underlying more reality-based sense of hopelessness. When feeling up against impossible odds, idealization and splitting can be more readily resorted to as a 'quick-fix solution'.[17]

Film messages that promote identification with the narcissistic part of the self and break up the continuity of being psychically at home in a mindful way are destructive to a sense of coherence as a person, where coherence comes from the struggle to remember about and own the *different parts* of the self.[18]

The increased use of loud pumped-up music and intrusive disruptions of narrative with possibly traumatizing auditory and visual material may well constitute the 'trickle down' into general culture in diluted form of the 'shock and awe' strategy explicitly described by neo-con strategists and used under the Bush administration. There is nothing new about shock and awe as a potent form of persuasion. Naomi Klein (2007) recently outlined its key elements. An event – either natural (tsunami, Katrina) or engineered (Iraq) – that traumatizes people is used to push through measures that, ordinarily, people would resist. We know that when people feel traumatized, they are less able to think, and their will for action is sapped. They are also more likely to identify with the aggressor. The measures I have described are particularly effective in deadening more concerned, caring and sad feelings about nature and blocking our capacity to grieve for the damage that has been done to nature. Instead, they promote a blank state of mind, one that blanks the here-and-now of reality and seeks to replace it with the pumped-up, self-aggrandized 'here-and-now' state of a dream world.

Notes

1 This refers to the phase of US capitalism significantly deregulated under the Regan administration, ideologically led by Milton Friedman and the Chicago school and by now with a global reach.

2 Searles (1960), one of the relatively few psychoanalysts to have written on our relationships with nature, gives a definition of this general kind.

3 For a psychoanalytic exploration of entitlement attitudes, including narcissistic and lively forms of entitlement, see Weintrobe (2004).

4 By nature, Louv means the natural physical environment, and he includes wilderness, local clumps of trees, flora and fauna in the city, the suburban backyard and the grass or earth school playground.

5 Piaget (1929) has pointed out that so do adults. We may like to think we have transcended animism, but it is inscribed into our language. 'Adult language provides the very conditions necessary to foster the child's animism. When speaking in images we are always compelled to draw on forms of expression that we have already outgrown. For example, we say, "the sun is trying to break through the mist" which is an animistic and dynamic way of speaking' (Piaget 1929: 278).

6 The erotic relation to nature is a theme explored by several writers – see, for instance, Terry Tempest Williams (1991, 2001) and Susan Griffin (1981).

7 Freud first wrote of internal place in *Totem and Taboo* in a section on taboo and emotional significance. He described the way internal objects can be 'localized in the subject's mind' (1913b: 29).

8 Consumerism is a social and economic order based on the systematic creation and fostering of the desire to purchase goods and services in ever greater amounts. Consumerism involves influencing identity (see Crompton and Kasser, 2009).

9 The tendency in the United Kingdom to alter our language so that a train is renamed a service and a passenger a customer, a school is renamed a business college and a pupil a client, is part of mind share.

10 The psychoanalyst Henri Rey (1994) made for me a profoundly helpful point about space. He said we tend to think of space as deep space, outer space. But he meant space as the psychic distance between oneself and the other in a relationship.

11 Freud *in Totem and Taboo* described the way internal objects can be 'localized in the subject's mind in such a manner that they cannot come up against each other (1913b: 29). He was describing what I am calling split landscapes.

12 As Leopold said, one of the penalties of an ecological education is that one lives alone in a world of wounds (1993: 165).

13 The wildlife filmmaker Amanda Barrett, when asked in an interview on the radio what music she took with her into the wild, said she did not listen to music in the wild; she listened to the sounds that are there.

14 It reminds me of a clinical situation described by Britton (1989), where he suggested that the way the patient was talking was motivated by an underlying wish for the analyst to 'stop that fucking thinking!'

15 It resonates for me with certain clinical situations where the patient may rapidly defend against a moment of genuine contact by suddenly and abruptly changing the subject, or swiftly taking the material in another direction, to another field of meaning altogether, this often appearing to be accompanied by a rapid identification with arrogance.

16 The use of a sudden disruption of narrative through an attack on the background feeling of safety is an explicit and common device of torturers aiming to weaken the will and soften people up; see, for instance, Jacobo Timerman (2002) tortured in Argentina, who described how he found defended himself against the helplessness of never knowing when the next body invasion and shock was coming by cutting off from all feeling and all meaning.

17 There are, of course, many exceptions to my analysis. In the film *Avatar*, for instance, the whole oppressed group bands together to defeat the violent corporate giant. The solution there is not one superhero armed with omnipotent powers.
18 As clinicians, we recognize the pattern. Manic patients may be mindful one day but have no memory of this the next day, or indeed later in the same session. The seductive pull is away from the here-and-now of reality. The manic patient brings the predicament of the destruction of narrative to the psychoanalytic setting where hopefully it can be taken in, contained and thought about by a mindful other – the analyst.

References

Bollas, C. (1992) *Being a Character*. Routledge: London.

Britton, R. (1989) The missing link: Parental sexuality in the Oedipus complex. In J. Steiner (Ed.), *The Oedipus Complex Today: Clinical Implications* (pp. 83–101). London: Karnac.

Crompton, T., and Kasser, T. (2009) *Meeting Environmental Challenges: The Role of Human Identity*. Godalming, UK: WWF-UK.

De Waal, F. (2006) *Primates and Philosophers*. Princeton, NJ: Princeton University Press.

Faber Taylor, A., Kuo, F., and Sullivan, W. (2001) Coping with ADD: The surprising connection to green play settings. *Journal of Environmental Psychology*, 1: 54–77.

Freud, S. (1913a) The theme of the three caskets. In J. Strachey (Ed.), *The Standard Edition of the Complete Psychological Works of Sigmund Freud, Vol. XII*. London: Hogarth Press.

Freud, S. (1913b) *Totem and Taboo*. In J. Strachey (Ed.), *The Standard Edition of the Complete Psychological Works of Sigmund Freud, Vol. XIII*. London: Hogarth Press.

Freud, S. (1927) *The Future of an Illusion*. In J. Strachey (Ed.), *The Standard Edition of the Complete Psychological Works of Sigmund Freud, Vol. XXI*. London: Hogarth Press.

Griffin, S. (1981) *Pornography and Silence*. New York: Harper & Row.

Hudson, W. (1918) *Far Away and Long Ago*. London: Eland Press, 1982.

Klein, N. (2007) *The Shock Doctrine*. Audio, CD, audiobook, MacMillan audio.

Lasch, C. (1978) *The Culture of Narcissism: American Life in an Age of Diminishing Expectations*. New York: Norton.

Leopold, A. (1993) *Round River*. New York: Oxford University Press.

Louv, R. (2005) *Last Child in the Woods* (revised and updated in 2009). London: Grove Atlantic.

Malone, K., and Tranter, P. (2003) School grounds as sites for learning: Making the most of environmental opportunities. *Environmental Education Research*, 9 (3): 283–303.

Naess, A. (2008) *The Ecology of Wisdom*. Berkeley, CA: Counterpoint.

Piaget, J. (1929) *The Child's Conception of the World*. London: Routledge and Kegan Paul.

Rey, H. (1994) *Universals of Psychoanalysis in the Treatment of Psychotic and Borderline States: Factors of Space-Time and Language*, ed. J. Magagna. London: Free Association Books.

Searles, H. F. (1960) *The Nonhuman Environment in Normal Development and in Schizophrenia*. New York: International Universities Press.

Searles, H. (1972) Unconscious processes in relation to the environmental crisis. *Psychoanalytic Review*, 59 (3): 361–374.

Simms, A. (2005) *Ecological Debt: The Health of the Planet and the Wealth of Nations.* London: Pluto Press.

Tempest Williams, T. (1991) *Refuge: An Unnatural History of Family and Place.* New York: Vintage Books.

Tempest Williams, T. (2001) *Red: Passion and Patience in the Desert.* New York: Vintage Books.

Timerman, J. (2002) *Prisoner without a Name, Cell without a Number.* Madison, WI: University of Wisconsin Press.

Weintrobe, S. (2004) Links between grievance, complaint and different forms of entitlement. *International Journal of Psychoanalysis*, 85: 83–96.

Weintrobe, S. (2010a) On links between runaway consumer greed and climate change denial: A psychoanalytic perspective. *Bulletin Annual of the British Psychoanalytical Society*, 1: 63–75. London: Institute of Psychoanalysis.

Weintrobe, S. (2010b) A dehumanising form of prejudice as part of a narcissistic pathological organization. In E. McGinley and A. Varchevker (Eds.), *Enduring Loss: Mourning, Depression and Narcissism through the Life Cycle.* London: Karnac.

Wilson, E. O. (1984) *Biophilia.* Cambridge, MA: Harvard University Press.

Wollaston, S. (2010) Lost land of the tiger. *The Guardian*, 22 Sept. Availble on: www.guardian.co.uk/tv-and-radio/2010/sep/22/excluded-lost-land-tiger-review

Discussion

On the love of nature and on human nature: restoring split internal landscapes

Mike Hannis

Nature, consumption and human flourishing

Questions about the relationship between human beings and the rest of the world require an interdisciplinary approach. It is therefore a pleasure to offer a brief philosophical response to Sally Weintrobe's vivid psychoanalytic diagnosis of how modern capitalist society influences us into being consumers of nature, rather than lovers of nature. This psychoanalytic account argues that an appropriate relationship with the nonhuman world is important for our psychological health. Philosophers interested in environmental virtue ethics would say that it is important for a flourishing life. I attempt here to explore some parallels between the two perspectives.

Greed and flourishing

Weintrobe describes how individuals are encouraged to identify at an unconscious level with the 'runaway corporate greed' by which Western societies are led, and in so doing to become destructively greedy themselves. She defines destructive greed as arrogant unlimited consumption and describes how this is encouraged by inculcating a sense of narcissistic entitlement through membership of an in-group. This drive towards unlimited consumption may well prove ecologically disastrous.

Yet even if resources were unlimited and the climate unthreatened, greed would still be bad for us, and consumerism would still have a corrosive effect on our minds and hearts. This is not only because of the well-documented empirical findings about the tenuousness of the connections between affluence and happiness. Social scientists know that, beyond a certain point, increases in consumption do not correlate well with increases in reported 'life-satisfaction' (Layard 2005).[1] But many philosophers, going back at least as far as Aristotle, would go further than this and say that a greedy person will never be a fully flourishing person, no matter what their level of material consumption.

What would an 'ungreedy' person be like? Virtue ethics approaches this question by identifying greed as a vice, to be contrasted with the relevant virtues or excellences of character, which we might in this context identify as proper relationships with possessions, consumption or affluence. Understanding what constitutes a proper relationship with possessions or consumption requires, in turn, working out just how these things contribute to a flourishing human life. Clearly, such reflection will not necessarily result in an endorsement of asceticism. From a virtue ethics perspective, a balanced or virtuous character would exhibit not just the opposite or absence of greed, but a virtuous mean between two opposing vices, of self-denial on the one hand and greed on the other.

The language of character, virtue and vice may seem quaint and old-fashioned today. This is partly because colloquial usage now tends to apply the words 'virtue' and 'virtuous' to practices (such as recycling or volunteering), rather than to dispositions or character traits. However, another reason such talk sounds anachronistic is that the implicit value structures of modern consumerist societies encourage us to see as virtues many character traits previously thought of as vices. Wenz (2005) quoted Lewis Mumford, who already understood this transformation in 1956:

> Observe what has happened to the seven deadly sins of Christian theology. All but one of these sins, sloth, was transformed into a positive virtue. Greed, avarice, envy, gluttony, luxury and pride were the driving forces of the new economy: if once they were mainly the vices of the rich, they now under the doctrine of expanding wants embrace every class in (industrial) society.
>
> (Mumford 1956, quoted by Wenz 2005: 205–6)

Wenz argued that consumerist society, not least through advertising, fosters and relies upon traditional vices such as pride, envy, greed, selfishness and indifference (see also Cafaro 2005). Given the 'baleful' effects of consumerism both on the environment and on people, he went on to say that these traits should still be considered vices – specifically, though not exclusively, they should be considered environmental vices. By contrast, traditional virtues such as humility, frugality, generosity, empathy and benevolence tend to 'inhibit the consumerism that impairs human flourishing and degrades the environment'. Thus 'people in industrial consumer-oriented societies should cultivate traditional virtues to benefit themselves, other human beings, and the nonhuman environment'. Similarly, Sandler (2007) wrote:

> Consumptive dispositions are bad for people. Greed, intemperance, profligacy and envy are vices. They tend to be detrimental to their possessor's well-being, and they favour practices that compromise the environment's ability to provide environmental goods. Moderation, self-control, simplicity, frugality and other character traits that oppose materialism and consumerism are environmental virtues, inasmuch as

they favour practices and lifestyles that promote the availability of environmental goods.

(Sandler 2007: 47)

While, as Cafaro (2001: 60) noted, 'the exhortation to avoid materialism and subordinate economic activities to higher values was already old in Athens and Jerusalem 2,500 years ago', this remains a recurring theme in environmental virtue ethics.

Right orientation to nature

This kind of analysis can also be applied in a more overarching way, going beyond examining the relevance of traditional virtues to explore others more directly concerned with human relationships with the nonhuman world. Hursthouse (2007: 162–4), for instance, sought to identify and encourage what she called 'the virtue of right orientation to nature'. Such an orientation requires understanding and appreciation of nature and of the human place(s) within it. It is marked by an appropriate, though not excessive, level of humility, described by Barry (1999: 33–35) as 'a mean between a timid ecocentrism and an arrogant anthropocentrism'. For Barry, this humility is the key to 'the cultivation of those modes of character and acting in the world that encourage social-environmental relations that are symbiotic rather than parasitic'.

A right orientation to nature is also marked by respect for the non-human world. Hursthouse claimed that respect for nature should be seen as 'a character trait rather than an attitude', and hence as something that cannot simply be adopted but requires inculcation and continued practice. Her emphasis on 'moral habituation and training, beginning in childhood and continued through self-improvement' closely echoes MacIntyre's descriptions of the ongoing familial and social processes by which we learn and practise what he terms 'the virtues of acknowledged dependence' (MacIntyre 1999: 9). Following MacIntyre, I have argued elsewhere (Hannis 2009) that developing the virtues of acknowledged *ecological* dependence is both a part and a consequence of developing a well-grounded sense of one's own identity. Such virtues help build healthy human/nonhuman relationships, which contribute both to human flourishing and to ecological sustainability.

I would say that the conditioning we undergo in capitalist society pushes us in exactly the opposite direction. It promotes simplistic ideas of entitlement and free-floating autonomous identity, expressed through endless consumption. In so doing it discourages understanding of the self as constituted by interdependent relationships within social and ecological networks. As Weintrobe reminds us, it encourages us to split our inner landscapes, and hence ourselves, into distinct and non-communicating parts.

Loving nature as other

Once split, Weintrobe tells us, we have to protect ourselves from truly loving the nonhuman, which would be painful because we have now become unconsciously identified with the arrogant aggressor who destroys 'nature'. By contrast, genuine love accepts both lover and beloved as flawed, rather than idealizing the other. Capitalism seeks to warp our loving feelings towards nature into idealization, and then to colonize and coopt them. Of course consumer capitalism relies on many kinds of idealization. The consumer is encouraged to seek eternal youth, to accept no limits to personal wealth or economic growth, to claim their 'right' to live life as an endless fantasy. An idealized 'nature', cleanly repackaged into a standardized consumable product, fits perfectly into this virtual (hyper) reality. This inert product is loved like a chocolate bar, not like a lover. This seems wrong, but is there a right way? How *should* we love nature?

There is a long-running debate in environmental philosophy about which stance best allows us to appreciate and value the nonhuman world, seeing ourselves as *part* of nature or as *apart* from it. Deep ecologists (e.g. Naess 1973) and holists stress the continuity of human and nonhuman and seek to overthrow the post-Enlightenment separation of rational human agents from passive inert nature. Other writers (such as Hailwood 2004) argue, however, that it is essential to respect nature's otherness, its 'not-us-ness', if we are to appreciate the nonhuman world for what it really is. Expanding our circle of ethical concern beyond the human does not make it reasonable to project human characteristics or values onto the nonhuman.

The psychoanalytic perspective sheds a helpful new light on this debate by making clear that we do indeed need to relate to nature as other, not as an extension of ourselves – but in so doing we also need to beware of idealizing or reifying it, thereby losing the fine grain of its imperfections, its agency, its reality.

Ethicists and aestheticians have also discussed how, and indeed whether, environmental science helps us to appreciate nature. Does understanding the other always help us to love, or can it sometimes get in the way? Is there a loss of immediacy, of visceral engagement, when for instance we 'understand' a forest as an ecosystem and express this understanding in terms of complex equations? As Weintrobe notes, children and adults love nature in different ways: but maybe part of this is simply that children are better at feeling unmediated emotions. One such emotion, much discussed in environmental aesthetics, is wonder.[2]

Of course not all experiences of nature are wonderful, or even pleasant. Weintrobe discusses how experiences of nature, and perhaps particularly of 'extreme' – or, as aestheticians used to say, 'sublime' – nature, can help us to cope with death and grieving. More generally, such experiences can help us to acknowledge our own finite physicality and mortality. On the other hand, experiences of loved familiar places can enrich life by enhancing our sense of connectedness and belonging. People also report intense experiences of sadness at the loss of such places, a syndrome recently christened 'solastalgia' (Albrecht 2005). One reason why these more complex emotional responses to nature are particularly valuable is that they are less easily warped into simplistic idealizations.

Marketing and nature

We are witnessing not only the marketing of nature but also its marketization. Nature is becoming an idealized product, and human relationships with nature are being transformed into market relationships. The insights of psychology and psychoanalysis have long been applied to marketing, not least by members of the Freud dynasty (Curtis 2002): they are now being enthusiastically applied to the marketing of nature. Perhaps the 'shock and awe' techniques of desensitization Weintrobe describes, whose effectiveness has been well proven in military contexts, are simply the current cutting edge of the science of persuasion. Like other effective forms of psychological manipulation, the reason they are effective is that they distort how we relate to the world.

Yet there is a simple positive point to make here. If policymakers were looking for an effective place to intervene in the destructive cycle of overproduction, overconsumption and ecological damage, this is probably it. Restrictions on marketing, broadly construed, would surely be among the most effective climate change mitigation measures available. They would, of course, also be good for our own mental and physical health.

Politics

Finally, all this leads into debates about the political legitimacy of such interventions. The variety of liberal politics that legitimizes consumer capitalism does so largely by appealing to a false ideal of neutrality between conceptions of the good life. The role of the state is seen as simply ensuring that all are 'free' to pursue happiness in their chosen way. But in fact this conception of politics inevitably imposes unexamined and problematic conceptions both of the good life and of freedom.[3] Furthermore, as discussed above, in modern capitalist society we do not in practice choose our conceptions of the good life freely: we are aggressively conditioned into the idea that fulfilment comes through consumption.

Escaping our ecological predicament thus requires not only changes in our physical practices but also a reconfiguration of politics, around a core commitment to honest reflection and debate about just what a flourishing human life consists of. Such a politics might even achieve what Weintrobe calls 'mindful government'.

Notes

1   For a far-reaching discussion of the implications of such findings, see O'Neill 2008.
2   On ethical aspects of this question, see O'Neill 1993. On aesthetic aspects, see Rolston 1995. On the importance of wonder in environmental virtue ethics, see Hursthouse

2007; in environmental aesthetics, see Hepburn 1984. For an overview of environmental aesthetics, see Brady 2003.
3   Influential versions of this general communitarian critique of liberalism are expressed
in MacIntyre 1985, Sandel 1998, Walzer 1983, and Taylor 1991. For a more specific
discussion of the problematic environmental implications of liberal neutrality, see
Hannis 2005.

References

Albrecht, G. (2005) 'Solastalgia': A new concept in health and identity. *Philosophy,
Activism, Nature*, 3: 41–55.
Barry, J. (1999) *Rethinking Green Politics*. London: Sage.
Brady, E. (2003) *Aesthetics of the Natural Environment*. Edinburgh, UK: Edinburgh
University Press.
Cafaro, P. (2001) Less is more. *Global Bioethics*, 14 (1): 45–59.
Cafaro, P. (2005) Gluttony, arrogance, greed and apathy: An exploration of environmental
vice. In R. Sandler and P. Cafaro (Eds.), *Environmental Virtue Ethics*. Lanham, MD:
Rowman and Littlefield.
Curtis, A. (2002) *The Century of the Self*. BBC TV documentary series.
Hailwood, S. (2004) *How to be a Green Liberal*. Montreal: McGill-Queens University
Press.
Hannis, M. (2005) Public provision of environmental goods: Neutrality or sustainability?
A reply to Miller. *Environmental Politics*, 14 (5): 577–595.
Hannis, M. (2009) *Reconciling Freedom and Sustainability: A Human Flourishing
Approach*. PhD thesis, Keele University.
Hepburn, R. (1984) *Wonder and Other Essays*. Edinburgh, UK: Edinburgh University
Press.
Hursthouse, R. (2007) Environmental virtue ethics. In R. Walker and P. Ivanhoe (Eds.),
Working Virtue: Virtue Ethics and Contemporary Moral Problems. Oxford, UK:
Clarendon Press.
Layard, R. (2005) *Happiness: Lessons for a New Science*. London: Allen Lane.
MacIntyre A. (1985) *After Virtue* (2nd ed.). London: Duckworth.
MacIntyre, A. (1999) *Dependent Rational Animals*. London: Duckworth.
Mumford, L. (1956) *The Transformation of Man*. New York: Harper and Row.
Naess, A. (1973) The shallow and the deep, long range ecology movement: A summary.
Enquiry, 16: 95–100.
O'Neill, J. (1993) *Ecology, Policy and Politics*. London: Routledge.
O'Neill, J. (2008) Sustainability, well-being and consumption: The limits of hedonic
approaches. In K. Soper and F. Trentmann (Eds.), *Citizenship and Consumption*.
London: Palgrave Macmillan.
Rolston III, H. (1995) Does aesthetic appreciation of landscapes need to be science-based?
British Journal of Aesthetics, 35 (4): 374–386.
Sandel, M. (1998) *Liberalism and the Limits of Justice* (2nd ed.). Cambridge, UK:
Cambridge University Press.
Sandler, R. (2007) *Character and the Environment*. New York: Columbia University
Press.
Sandler, R., and Cafaro, P. (Eds.) (2005) *Environmental Virtue Ethics*. Lanham, MD:
Rowman and Littlefield.

Taylor, C. (1991) What's wrong with negative liberty? In D. Miller (Ed.), *Liberty*. Oxford, UK: Oxford University Press.

Walzer, M. (1983) *Spheres of Justice*. New York: Basic Books.

Wenz, P. (2005) Synergistic environmental virtues: Consumerism and human flourishing. In R. Sandler and P. Cafaro (Eds.), *Environmental Virtue Ethics*. Lanham, MD: Rowman and Littlefield.

Discussion

On the love of nature and on human nature: restoring split internal landscapes

Tom Crompton

On love of nature and the nature of love

There can be little hope of building adequate responses to today's environmental challenges unless we begin, collectively, to re-examine our relationship with nature. In exploring the ways in which this relationship develops, Sally Weintrobe's chapter echoes, from a psychoanalytical perspective, themes about which I am more familiar from a social psychological perspective: what shapes our relationship with nature, and how does this, in turn, shape our attitudes towards the despoilment of nature? That there are some strong parallels between the conclusions that Weintrobe draws and the results of empirical work in social psychology makes her chapter all the more compelling.

Social psychologists have developed approaches to assessing people's sense of connection to nature. The 'inclusion of nature in self' scale asks subjects to assess the extent to which they incorporate nature into their sense of self. People who score more highly on this scale have been found to express greater concern for environmental problems. They are also more likely to report engaging in a range of pro-environmental behaviours (see Frantz, Mayer, Norton, and Rock 2005; Mayer and Frantz 2004; Schultz 2001; Schultz, Shriver, Tabanico, and Khazian 2004). Other approaches have been used to assess a subject's implicit, or nonconscious, connection to nature, and this is also found to correlate positively with pro-environmental attitudes and behaviours.[1] It seems that the more connected a person feels to the natural environment, the more his or her concerns move away from self-interest and towards broader-based concerns about environment and life on the planet. The social psychologist Wesley Schultz, who has for many years researched the behavioural implications of people's conscious and nonconscious connection to nature, suggests that most people have a deep-seated connection, which motivates pro-environmental attitudes and behaviour. However, it seems that this is overridden by social and contextual factors that impinge on our everyday behaviours. He suggests that if we were to move these deep-seated identities closer to the surface (for example, by making them more explicit), we could anticipate that motivation for pro-environmental behaviour would increase (Wesley Schultz, personal communication, 12 October 2008).

But if these things are to be of any practical help to those who are working to motivate greater pro-environmental concern, then we must ask harder questions about what 'nature' – the thing to which we feel a greater or lesser sense of connection – actually is. Weintrobe herself is ambiguous on this point. She sets out by rejecting attempts to circumscribe the 'natural' as distinct from the 'human'. She suggests that we should include within our concept of nature 'a group of people in a city nightclub or bar'. Is this really 'nature'? That is to ask, more practically and specifically, is it 'nature' in the sense of something that, once incorporated more strongly into our identity, is likely to promote more pro-environmental behaviour? In the rest of her chapter, Weintrobe implies not. She suggests that 'loud pumped-up music' – which surely characterizes nightclubs – is the antithesis of nature. She also draws on, for example, Louv's (2006) work highlighting the mental health benefits of time spent in nature, but here she is writing of nature circumscribed more narrowly to mean (a little tautologically) 'the natural physical environment', which includes 'wilderness, local clumps of trees, flora, fauna in the city, the suburban backyard and the grass or earth school playground'. Louv casts his definition wide, but it does not seem to include people in nightclubs and bars.

This is not a pedantic discussion, because what I think Weintrobe is really writing about is not what is commonly understood as 'nature' at all but, rather, 'the other'.

Social psychologists have also characterized a set of 'self-transcendence' values. These values include 'understanding, appreciation, tolerance and protection for the welfare of all people and for nature', and 'preservation and enhancement of people with whom one is in frequent personal contact'. These are Schwartz's definitions of 'universalism' and 'benevolence' values, respectively (see, for example, Schwartz, 1992). These values are held in opposition to 'self-enhancement' values, which include concern for 'social status and prestige, control or dominance over people and resources', and concern for 'personal success through demonstrating competence *according to social standards*'.[2]

A large body of research in social psychology reveals several important points. First, as might be anticipated, self-transcendence values are found to be associated with greater concern about environmental problems and with higher motivation to act in ways that will help to address these problems. But these values are *also* associated with greater levels of concern about social problems – and greater motivation to help address these. That is, studies find that there is 'bleed-over' between social and environmental concern.

Second, it is found that self-transcendence values can be activated, for example, by encouraging people to think about being helpful. But they can also be 'deactivated' by activating opposing self-enhancement values. Thus, for example, experiments show that by encouraging a person to think about financial concerns, their motivation to address environmental problems is actually diminished.

In one experiment, the social psychologist Tim Kasser and colleagues (Sheldon 2011) prompted American subjects to reflect on a 'self-enhancement' national identity (thinking about America as the land of opportunity and fortune) or a 'self-transcendent' national identity (thinking about their country as one that has a long history of helping others).[3] Note, here, that subjects were not prompted to think about either of these identities in relation to the environment. Kasser then asked participants to imagine that they were advising the US President on policy interventions to help reduce Americans' ecological footprint. By comparison to subjects in a control group, those individuals who were prompted to think about the 'self-transcendent' identity were likely to recommend significantly lower ecological footprints, whereas – most interestingly – those prompted to reflect on the 'self-enhancement' national identity were found to recommend significantly higher ecological footprints as targets for government policy.

Experiments such as this corroborate the suggestion that we at times transcend a more narrowly circumscribed sense of self, perhaps through activation of self-transcendence values, and that this leads to an increase in motivation to behave in pro-environmental ways. At other times, through the activation of self-enhancement values, our sense of self may be more restricted and more narrowly focused on our own material desires, and our concern about environmental problems seems therefore to be diminished. Although social psychologists may rarely express it in these terms, such work seems to underscore the importance of love – not just for nature, but for people as well.

Such understanding has profound implications (see Crompton, 2010).

First, it suggests that anyone concerned about social or environmental issues would do well to work to strengthen self-transcendence values and to tackle those influences that currently serve to strengthen self-enhancement values (e.g. a celebrity culture or commercial advertising).

Second, it implies that it will be counterproductive to work to motivate concern for nature (e.g. biodiversity) while simultaneously trampling concern for other humans (e.g. disregarding human rights).

Third, it cautions against promoting environmental concerns while simultaneously activating self-enhancement values. Many environmental campaigns may serve, inadvertently, to activate such values. Campaigns that focus on the financial savings that attend some pro-environmental behaviours (e.g. taking simple steps to improve domestic energy efficiency) or on the social status that may be successfully associated with other pro-environmental behaviours (e.g. buying the latest hybrid car) are likely to have this effect. Similarly, at a political level, attempts to assess the economic value of biodiversity may facilitate dialogue with some decision-makers, at least in instances where economic signals happen to be supportive of the need to conserve a natural resource. But such valuations are likely, simultaneously, to be damaging at a more systemic level: they will help to normalize the perception that the value of natural resources is to be assessed primarily in economic terms. As such, they will risk helping to undermine the self-transcendence values upon which a more systemic and durable commitment to nature conservation might otherwise be built.

There is one other important aspect of the social psychology of values: it seems probable that we all express all these values at different times; it is not the case that people can be narrowly assigned to particular value sets. This, too, echoes Weintrobe's perspective. She writes: 'In seeking to redress current dominant cultural narratives that say we are basically exploitative and selfish by nature, the danger might be that we promote the simplistic view that we are basically caring and unexploitative by nature. In reality we are both, and this is the narrative that needs air to breathe.'

Recognizing that we each hold each of these values, in dynamic tension, enables us (as Weintrobe writes) to 'see ourselves as part of the problem as well as part of the solution'. Again, Weintrobe's insight here is corroborated by social psychology. We all (irrespective of our concern about social and environmental problems) both inadvertently, and at times consciously, work to strengthen social norms that promote self-enhancement values. We therefore each contribute, at a systemic level, to undermining public concern about both environmental and social problems.

Weintrobe's analysis does the environment and conservation movements a great service by underscoring the dangers of anthropocentrism. But it does not go far enough in situating its analysis on a broader canvas: one that rejects prejudice towards the other, whoever – or whatever – that other might be. I do not believe, contrary to the rhetoric of many opponents of environmentalism, that there are many bunny-hugging misanthropes: people who would trample on the needs of their fellow humans in pursuit of the interests of other species. My conviction that such people are occasionally conspicuous because of their scarcity is one that is supported by the evidence from social psychology. Yet exhortations for us to 'love nature' (where it remains at best ambiguous as to whether or not 'nature' includes other people) can only embolden those who would argue that the conservation and environment movements struggle to remain empathetic towards humans.

It may be because Weintrobe does not consistently see nature as including people (or, put differently, because she tends to focus on non-human nature rather than 'the other') that she takes nature documentary soundtracks as her primary example of how 'neoliberal capitalism seeks not only to seduce us away from loving nature, but also tries to damage and intimidate the reality-based mindful part of us that does love nature'. A more integrated perspective on the cultural influences that strengthen self-enhancement values (and therefore undermine public concern about both social and environmental issues) might have led to other, more significant examples. These could include public policy that primes citizens to adopt self-interested values; national progress indicators that emphasize economic growth (rather than social or environmental improvement); a great deal of commercial advertising; the control of large parts of the media by individuals whose interest is to promote self-enhancement values; or many aspects of celebrity culture. Among TV programming, it seems likely that *The Apprentice* or the *X-Factor*, in modelling self-enhancement values of achievement and power, will wreak far greater social and environmental harm than nature documentaries – irrespective of the soundtracks used in the latter.[4]

Nonetheless, the arguments that Weintrobe advances resonate with accumulating evidence from social psychology. They serve to underscore the critical importance of establishing common purpose across *both* the social *and* the environmental movements – that is, the importance of working to strengthen self-transcendence values and to identify and tackle the factors that work to promote opposing self-enhancement values.

Notes

1 Implicit connection to nature is assessed through 'implicit association tests', which are based on subjects' reaction times, rather than conscious deliberation. Readers can assess their own implicit connection to nature at: www.conservationpsychology.org/game/ (accessed 4 Apr. 2011). For further discussion, see Bruni and Schultz 2010; Schultz and Tabanico 2007; Schultz et al. 2004.
2 Emphasis added. These are Schwartz's definitions of 'power' and 'achievement' values, respectively (see Schwartz 1992).
3 In fact, Kasser primed subjects with 'intrinsic' and 'extrinsic' identities. Although significantly different from 'self-transcendence' and 'self-enhancement' identities, this distinction is not of central importance for the purposes of the current discussion (see Grouzet et al. 2005).
4 Indeed, there is evidence that viewing nature documentaries increases people's environmental concern, although I am not aware of studies that control for the effects of the music used in the soundtracks (see Holbert, Kwak and Shah 2003).

References

Bruni, C. M., and Schultz, P. W. (2010) Implicit beliefs about self and nature: Evidence from an IAT game. *Journal of Environmental Psychology*, 30: 95–102.
Crompton, T. (2010) *Common Cause: The Case for Working with Our Cultural Values*. Godalming, UK: WWF-UK.
Frantz, C. M., Mayer, F. S., Norton, C., and Rock, M. (2005) There is no 'I' in nature: the influence of self awareness on connectedness to nature. *Journal of Environmental Psychology*, 25 (4): 427–436.
Grouzet, F. M. E., Kasser, T., Ahuvia, A., Fernandez-Dols, J. M., Kim, Y., Lau, S., Ryan, R. M., Saunders, S., Schmuck, P., and Sheldon, K. M. (2005) The structure of goal contents across fifteen cultures. *Journal of Personality and Social Psychology*, 89: 800–816.
Holbert, R. L., Kwak, N., and Shah, D. V. (2003) Environmental concern, patterns of television viewing, and pro-environmental behaviors: Integrating models of media consumption and effects. *Journal of Broadcasting and Electronic Media*, 47: 177–196.
Louv, R. (2006) *Last Child in the Woods*. Chapel Hill, NC: Algonquin Books of Chapel Hill.
Mayer, F. S., and Frantz, C. M. (2004) The connectedness to nature scale: A measure of individuals' feeling in community with nature. *Journal of Environmental Psychology*, 26: 503–515.

Schultz, P. W. (2001) The structure of environmental concern: concern for self, other people, and the biosphere. *Journal of Environmental Psychology*, 21: 327–339.

Schultz, P. W., Shriver, C., Tabanico, J. J., and Khazian, A. M. (2004) Implicit connections with nature. *Journal of Environmental Psychology*, 24: 31–42.

Schultz, P. W., and Tabanico, J. J. (2007) Self, identity, and the natural environment: Exploring implicit connections with nature. *Journal of Applied Social Psychology*, 37 (6): 1219–1247.

Schwartz, S. H. (1992) Universals in the content and structure of values: Theoretical advances and empirical tests in 20 countries. In M. Zanna (Ed.), *Advances in Experimental Social Psychology, Vol. 25* (pp. 1–65). Orlando, FL: Academic Press.

Sheldon, K. M., Nichols, C. P., and Kasser, T. (2011). Americans recommend smaller ecological footprints when reminded of intrinsic American values of self-expression, family, and generosity. *Ecopsychology*, 3: 97–104.

Chapter 10

Climate change, uncertainty and risk

Stephan Harrison

Introduction

The issue of Anthropogenic Global Warming (AGW)[1] should be purely scientific and the questions clear: can we detect warming, and to what can it be attributed? However, because AGW has considerable implications for governmental, economic, social and environmental policies, arguments against AGW have been developed based largely on politics and ideology rather than science. In this chapter, I outline the elements of climate science generally accepted by informed scientists with a high level of certainty, and I then discuss where some of the remaining uncertainties exist. By doing this, I aim to shed some light on some of the complexities in climate science and on the potential risks that we face.

The first point to consider is that the climate is naturally variable on a range of different timescales. For example, over millennial timescales the climate has gone through cycles of glaciation and deglaciation. Over shorter timescales such as the last thousand years, the climate has shown periods of regional warming (e.g. the Medieval Warm Period largely restricted to parts of the Northern hemisphere, and periods of cooling during the sixteenth- to nineteenth centuries, which have been loosely termed the Little Ice Age). Given this, how do we know that recent warming is largely caused by human activity? The arguments supporting this proposition mainly come from our understanding of the physics of the greenhouse effect. We have known for nearly two centuries that the earth's temperature is artificially raised by the composition of the atmosphere, and this has been called the greenhouse effect. A number of atmospheric gases play a role in the greenhouse effect, and one of the most important of these is CO_2. Basic radiative physics shows that increasing greenhouse gases (GHG) in the atmosphere (such as CO_2) must have a warming effect, and the pattern and rate of warming that we see is consistent with the increase in atmospheric CO_2 that we have measured.

As a result, there is a scientific consensus (Oreskes 2004) that the mean surface temperature of the Earth has warmed in recent decades and that the warming amounts to around 0.8 C since the beginning of the twentieth century (IPCC 2007). From this, the Goddard Institute for Space Studies estimates that 2005 and 2010 are tied for the warmest year since reliable instrumental measurements become available, although the UK Hadley Centre-Climatic Research Unit places these just behind 1998. Detection and attribution studies show that there is high probability (at least 90%) that this warming is largely the result of anthropogenic emissions of greenhouse gases, mainly CO_2, in the troposphere and that the amount and rate of warming are outside the range of natural variation and unprecedented for the past 11,000 years of the Holocene.[2]

Continued warming is expected to have important consequences for a range of Earth systems. These include the atmosphere, cryosphere, oceans, hydrological systems and the biosphere. There are compelling reasons to expect increases in the magnitude and frequency of some natural hazards such as floods (Huntington 2006), droughts (Mason and Goddard 2001) and landslides (e.g. Fischer, Kaab, Huggel and Noetzli 2006) and increases in the intensity of tropical cyclones (Emanuel 2005). There are also concerns about the stability of several of the large ice sheets on Earth (e.g. Overpeck et al. 2006; Rahmstorf 2010), as these have the ability to impact upon global sea levels and regulate ocean currents.

With concern about future climate change building through the 1960s and 1970s, the Intergovernmental Panel on Climate Change (IPCC) was set up by the World Meteorological Office and United Nations Environment Programme in 1988 to deliver assessments of the current state of climate science and projections for the future. To date, four reports have been produced by the IPCC – in 1991, 1995, 2001 and 2007. The latter is known as AR4 (Assessment Report 4). Each of these at the time constituted probably the most in-depth review of any science in history, understandable given the enormous implications that future climate change will have for environmental, economic and social systems on Earth. As a consequence, there is very wide scientific consensus on the broad conclusions of the reports. For instance, the conclusions of AR4 have been supported by all of the National Academies of Science of all the leading industrial nations, and all major professional scientific bodies (such as the American Geological Union, American Meteorological Society and UK Royal Society).

Such consensus suggests that there is considerable certainty about the science. While this is true, there is also considerable uncertainty. This chapter reviews what is known about climate change and what remains uncertain and, to various extents, controversial. It is important to say that all suggestions of certainty come with an important caveat: all scientific statements can be falsified and beliefs overturned if new evidence is put forward and confirmed. Consensus exists when, despite repeated attempts at testing data or theories, the original theory remains unfalsified.

Certainty

We have a high level of certainty about a number of key issues in climate science. These include: the basic radiative properties of certain atmospheric gases, the changing composition of the atmosphere, the detection of recent warming and the attribution of large amounts of that warming (IPCC AR4 WG1, 2007).

In climate science, we have high confidence that the basic understanding of the workings of the atmosphere is generally correct. This understanding is based upon nearly 200 years of research in atmospheric physics, the radiative properties of atmospheric gases and atmospheric chemistry. Pioneers in these fields include Joseph Fourier (1824), John Tyndall (1859), Svante Arrhenius (1896) and Callendar (1938). We also know from the ice core record that the basic composition of the atmosphere has changed over time. For instance, during the Last Glacial Maximum around 20–25 thousand years ago, CO_2 levels in the atmosphere were low (around 200 ppm), as CO_2 and other greenhouse gases remained sequestered in permafrost and in the deep oceans. Following deglaciation around 20–15 thousand years ago, CO_2 levels in the atmosphere rose as permafrost (permanently frozen ground) melted, releasing methane, and the oceans degassed CO_2 as they warmed. This rapid increase in GHGs helped to drive the climate out of glaciation, forming a powerful positive feedback that operated to reinforce the warming imposed by long-term changes in earth's orbit around the sun.

Following the melting of the mid-latitude ice sheets by the early part of the Holocene, CO_2 levels rose to around 280 ppm, and this figure remained relatively stable until the rapid rise of the last few centuries imposed by humans. Since then, CO_2 levels have risen from 280 ppm to current levels of 390 ppm. From the changing isotopic composition of the atmosphere and from other evidence, we know that all of this increase in CO_2 was caused by human activity and very largely by the burning of fossil fuels. This has imposed a radiative forcing on the top of the atmosphere, which currently overwhelms all natural changes in radiative forcing during the recent past (such as changes in solar activity and volcanic eruptions). It means that the atmosphere has warmed by around 0.8°C since the beginning of the twentieth century.

This warming is not distributed evenly across the earth's surface. The oceans have tended to warm least because of their large thermal mass, the northern hemisphere has warmed more than the southern hemisphere, and northern land masses have warmed most, with large parts of the Arctic having warmed more quickly and rapidly than anywhere else on earth. Climate models have predicted this spatial pattern and Arctic amplification (where the Arctic warms quickly as positive feedback mechanisms start to operate) was predicted by early attempts at modelling the earth's response to rising GHG and warming (Manabe and Stoufer 1980).

We therefore have high confidence that increasing atmospheric concentrations of GHG will cause the atmosphere to warm, in the absence of any countervailing cooling trend. We can also detect this warming in the instrumental record from a number of sources. Meteorological stations show warming, as do measurements from radiosonds, satellites and data from ocean temperatures. Proxy measures of warming are also compelling. For instance, ice on earth is responding to warming; the vast majority of mountain glaciers on earth are undergoing recession, and permafrost temperatures are rising. The largest ice sheets, the Greenland Ice Sheet and West Antarctic Ice Sheet, are losing mass and contributing significantly to sea level rise. Other proxy records that demonstrate recent warming are available from biological systems where earlier spring temperatures are producing phenological change[3] in plants and animals.

Overall, these converging lines of evidence build up to show that human activities such as the burning of fossil fuels have significantly increased the levels of GHG in the atmosphere, notably CO_2, over the last few centuries (and from perhaps the last 6–7,000 years) and that current levels of atmospheric CO_2 are higher than for at least the last 650,000 years, and probably much longer (Siegenthaler et al. 2006). It is also clear that the rise of the GHG is happening faster than past periods of rising GHG concentrations. This GHG forcing is driving climate change and will continue to do so in the future.

In conclusion, we can see that there is a high level of certainty concerning the warming that elevated atmospheric GHG are causing, their attribution and the physical processes that are causing this warming. It is also clear that other forcings (e.g. internal variability, stochastic events, variations in galactic cosmic ray flux and variations in solar irradiance) cannot explain either the pattern or the rate and timing of recent warming.

Lower levels of certainty

There are, however, areas in climate science where considerable uncertainty exists, and these can be discussed under four main headings.

How much warming will we see?

As the mainstream sceptics have, over time, come to accept the reality of AGW, this remains the main area of contention and can be viewed within the lens of climate sensitivity. This is defined as the equilibrium global mean temperature response to a doubling of atmospheric CO_2 levels over pre-industrial levels (Dessler and Parson 2006): in other words, what is the temperature response associated with atmospheric CO_2 levels of 550 ppm?

Global climate models have been used to demonstrate that the increase in global-average outgoing radiative flux (essentially the amount of energy lost from the atmosphere to space) when the climate is perturbed from a steady state is proportional to the global-average surface temperature change. With climate change, the imbalance between radiative forcing and the radiative response is mainly absorbed by the heat capacity of the oceans (Levitus, Antonov, and Boyer 2005).

With an increased radiative forcing (caused by reduced outgoing radiation from greenhouse gases or changes in solar activity), heat flux into the oceans rises, and temperature rises. With a constant radiative forcing, the climate reaches a new equilibrium, and heat flux into the oceans eventually reaches zero. The equilibrium climate sensitivity is defined as the changed temperature in response to a doubling of CO_2 (Gregory, Stouffer, Raper, Stott and Rayner 2002).

While the general concept of climate sensitivity has been discussed since at least the end of the nineteenth century – Arrhenius (1896) calculated the likely rise in global temperature following a doubling of atmospheric CO_2 using simple energy balance equations – the standard modern estimate of sensitivity (of around 3°C) comes from the work of Jule Charney and colleagues in 1979, and this figure has remained essentially static. The 'consensus' scientific view is outlined by IPCC AR4, which says:

> The equilibrium climate sensitivity is a measure of the climate system response to sustained radiative forcing. It is not a projection but is defined as the global average surface warming following a doubling of carbon dioxide concentrations. It is likely to be in the range 2°C to 4.5°C with a best estimate of about 3°C, and is very unlikely to be less than 1.5°C. Values substantially higher than 4.5°C cannot be excluded, but agreement of models with observations is not as good for those values.
>
> (IPCC AR4 2007: 12)

However, this estimate includes only the fast-acting parts of the climate system, not the longer-term feedbacks. It is not possible to assess equilibrium climate sensitivity directly from current observations of warming in response to current CO_2 forcing due to the lag between increased CO_2 levels and global temperatures (Annan and Hargreaves 2005, 2006; Gregory et al. 2002). All this shows is the transient sensitivity. As a result, Charney (1979) makes the unrealistic assumption that over time the atmospheric composition, land surface, ice cover and other important variables remain constant. What this actually means is that climate sensitivity is a measure of the response of a *model* of part of the climate system to a simulation of sustained radiative forcing. Here it has been assumed implicitly that the best estimate of the model is the best estimate for the full climate system. However, the present generation of global climate models generally exclude long-term feedbacks, either because they are difficult to model or because the physical processes are not sufficiently understood. These longer-term effects include albedo effects from changes in ice sheet extent and vegetation. Therefore the explicit assumption in deriving a climate sensitivity of 3°C is that ice sheet extent and volume cannot respond quickly to greenhouse gas forcing. The palaeoclimate record suggests that this view is erroneous.

We can then see the uncertainties in climate sensitivity as having arisen from the methodology employed in assessing the temperature response. There are two distinct ways in which climate sensitivity has been estimated (Harrison 2009; Schneider von Deimling, Held, Ganopolski and Rahmstorf 2006). The bottom-up approach uses empirical, quantitative understandings of the physical processes forcing climate such as changes in radiation balance, feedbacks and lapse rates (changes in the way that air cools with altitude) to drive climate models. Owing to the uncertainties in the strength of the feedbacks (especially those concerned with the behaviour of clouds), it has not been possible to reduce the climate sensitivity uncertainty beyond that which was derived in the late 1970s (Charney 1979).

A more robust approach uses a top-down assessment whereby palaeoclimate reconstructions have assessed the covariance of past temperature changes in response to changing CO_2 forcings. Palaeoclimate estimates of sensitivity to carbon dioxide have the advantage that all feedback processes, known and unknown, are included in the estimate, apart from those relating to the carbon cycle itself. Such approaches have tended to use the term 'Earth system sensitivity' rather than 'Climate sensitivity', given the presumed totality of feedbacks incorporated in the estimate. Earth system sensitivity is defined as the long-term equilibrium surface temperature change given an increase in CO_2, including all Earth system feedbacks, but neglecting processes associated with the carbon cycle (Lunt et al. 2010). Recent estimates using palaeoclimate data suggest that Earth system sensitivity is around 30% to over 100% higher than Climate sensitivity.

However, one important caveat remains: it is not always possible to isolate the temperature response to changes in CO_2 as variations in other forcings often occur at the same time. Additionally, during past glaciations the climate was colder than it is now, and the feedbacks partly responsible for this were probably also different (Schneider von Deimling et al. 2006).

Future climate change at the local or regional scale – problems with modelling

The pattern and extent of future warming has enormously important policy implications for governments and business, and the methodology employed to understand and predict future climate change is to construct computer models that model the evolution and dynamics of the climate system. These are called general circulation models and were originally designed for short-term weather forecasting. For understanding climate change, global climate models were developed to include atmospheric and oceanic processes and the influence of land-use change, vegetation and ice sheets, and these models have been further extended to form Earth system models. These contain sub-models within them to describe the operation of carbon fluxes and other processes. The models are constructed on a grid structure so that the Earth's surface is covered by a grid with spacing of around $1°$ of latitude and longitude and 20 to 40 atmosphere layers. Processes that occur at smaller spatial scales are parameterized, and these include land-use change, hydrological and albedo variables and processes such as those forming clouds.

Global climate model projections are generally robust for global temperature in that they mostly agree that Northern Hemisphere land masses will warm more than the global average, that the Southern Hemisphere oceans will warm least, and that the Arctic will undergo rapid and enhanced warming. However, there are a number of uncertainties associated with modelling the climate system, and these relate to uncertainties in understanding and modelling processes governing climate dynamics, uncertainties in future forcings and model limitations. Over the last couple of years, there has been greater recognition of the nature and policy implications that follow from these uncertainties and limitations, and these issues have been explored in a number of papers (e.g. Stainforth, Downing, Washington, Lopez and New 2007).

The uncertainties that do exist are magnified at the regional scale to the extent that different models will produce different regional climates, even when forced by identical emissions scenarios. This is partly because of the operation of regional feedbacks and partly a consequence of model inadequacy. This is clearly a problem for policymakers who wish to have credible climate projections for specific locations. The problem is exacerbated by the poor ability of global climate models to resolve large-scale elements of the climate system, such as El Niño Southern Oscillation. This is important because such large-scale characteristics of the climate system are those that play a central role in determining the nature, location, amount and timing of precipitation and therefore water availability. In addition, future trends in precipitation are more uncertain than those for tempera-ture since precipitation is affected by features such as the position of frontal zones and wind fields whose future behaviour is not easily modelled, and projections from regional modelling show wide variance. For example, projections for central and tropical South America range from increases in precipitation for 2020 of 5% to decreases of 5%. By 2050, projections are still more uncertain, ranging from around 10% increases and decreases. Such uncertainties are a feature of projec-tions from global climate models, and Magrin et al. (2007: 594) caution that 'the current (global climate models) do not produce projections of changes in the hydrological cycle at regional scales with confidence. In particular the uncertainty of projections of precipitation remain high.'

Such uncertainty in future precipitation is a characteristic of many attempts to model the climate evolution in low-latitude regions (e.g. Allan and Soden 2007; Lin 2007). For instance, Giannini et al. (2008) argue that there has been a shift in focus with regard to the causes of recent drought in African rainfall in the Sahel region of Africa, from those that stress land-use change, over-grazing and defor-estation to those recognizing the role of global climate change, driven by anthro-pogenic greenhouse gas emissions. In trying to model such changes, researchers have used global climate models to simulate twentieth-century climate change in the region in an attempt to demonstrate their usefulness for future predictions. In one study, Lau, Shen, Kim and Wang (2006) used 19 coupled global climate models to examine the 1970s–90s Sahel drought (which caused considerable loss of life, migration and conflict). Of these models, only eight produced a reasonable simulation of the drought, while seven produced excessive rainfall over these time periods. Clearly, if many of the models have failed to simulate this long-lasting regional drought, then their usefulness in predicting future water shortages in other regions may be questioned. As Douville, Salas-Mélia and Tyteca (2006) caution, uncertainties in precipitation change are, like precipitation itself, very unevenly distributed over the globe, the most vulnerable countries sometimes being those where the anticipated precipitation changes are the most uncertain.

Earth system responses

Following on from the uncertainties discussed above, we also have limited information on the likely response of important earth surface systems to continued warming. Perhaps the most important of these for policymakers is the timing and magnitude of future sea level rise. By the middle of the century, this will be largely dependent on the dynamical evolution of the two large ice sheets most at risk from global warming: the Greenland Ice Sheet and the West Antarctic Ice Sheet.

Over the past decade our understanding of the dynamic evolution of the ice sheets under conditions of present and future AGW has been limited by the low level of sophistication of numerical ice sheet models (Alley, Clark, Huybrechts and Joughlin 2005). These models are inadequate largely because the empirical data with which to tune them are limited, and our physical understanding of ice sheet processes such as those operating at the junction between ice sheets and the ocean (the grounding line) are low (Vieli and Payne 2005). We also have limited understanding of basal conditions under large parts of the ice sheets and under the outlet glaciers and ice streams that drain them (e.g. De Angelis and Skvarca 2003). More research on subglacial processes and characteristics (such as rheology, debris concentrations and basal temperature gradients) are required as these affect basal shear stresses at the base of the ice, sliding processes, water availability and the likelihood of rapid sediment deformation. All of these variables have the potential to affect the dynamic response of the ice sheets to warming.

Prediction of future sea level rise is therefore severely compromised by the inability of climate models to incorporate the dynamic behaviour of ice sheets. IPCC AR4 projections were based upon coupled atmosphere–ocean global climate models and suggested that sea levels could rise by up to 59 cm higher than present by the end of this century. This figure was based upon the 'worst-case' emissions scenario (A1F1) where rapid economic growth occurs, population growth reaches 9 billion by 2050 and then gradually declines and fossil fuel use is intensive.

However, it is clear that this figure for future sea level change forms a likely lower bound as it only accounts for sea level rises in response to thermal expansion of the oceans and the melting of glaciers and ice caps; both of the latter make up only a very small proportion of the ice on earth. This projection specifically excluded the rapid increase in calving (when ice loss from ice sheets and glaciers occurs through the rapid disintegration of the ice terminus in water) and melting from ice sheets as the scientific data from these was largely incomplete and partial.

Available data from satellite altimetry show that sea level rise is currently not uniform, with some regions of the world experiencing higher-than-average sea level increases. For instance, in parts of the Western Pacific sea level rises are around 3 times the globally averaged rate. Although the contribution of the West

Antarctic Ice Sheet and the Greenland Ice Sheet to overall sea level rises is expected to increase markedly over this century, present rises are the result largely of thermal expansion of the oceans, and this is spatially variable. In addition, other factors influence regional sea level rise, including isostatic adjustment of the crust (often associated with unloading following the melting of Pleistocene mid-latitude ice sheets) and changes in water salinity. Such regional variations also change over time in response to decadal and shorter fluctuations in ocean and wind currents such as the El Niño Southern Oscillation, the Pacific Decadal Oscillation and the North Atlantic Oscillation. Consequently, decadal variations in sea levels are not modelled well in coupled global climate models. IPCC AR4 used 16 global climate models running on one emissions scenario to produce a regional sea level map for 2090–2100, and this predicted higher-than-average sea level rises in the Arctic Ocean and parts of the South Indian and Atlantic Oceans. However, there is considerable inter-model variability in these projections, and the uncertainties remain high.

We can use analysis of the past behaviour of ice sheets during episodes of global warming to help us to constrain and estimate their future dynamic behaviour, and thanks to recent advances in Quaternary science we have detailed information on the nature and timing of deglacial events at the end of the Pleistocene. From palaeoglaciological investigations, we can show that the ice sheets with major terrestrial margins (such as large parts of the Laurentide and Fenno-Scandian ice sheet) were largely stable and melted slowly following the Last Glacial Maximum. Those ice margins that were significantly coupled to the ocean (such as that which drained through the Hudson Strait) disintegrated rapidly, and this resulted in rapid discharge of icebergs and significant sea level rise from displacement by ice.

During the deglaciation between the Last Glacial Maximum and the early Holocene, large sections of the Northern Hemisphere ice sheets underwent periods of dynamic change, and at this time sea levels rose rapidly by over 100 m. Two elements of this change were Dansgaard-Oeschger events and Heinrich events. Dansgaard-Oeschger events were periods of repeated regional rapid warming and gradual cooling, which occurred with an underlying periodicity of 1,500 years or so (Rahmstorf 2003). At least 20 Dansgaard-Oeschger events occurred during the last glaciation, and, although evidence for these is found in many regions of the world (Voelker 2002), their strongest effect is seen in the Greenland ice cores, where at times temperatures rose abruptly by between 10° and 15°C. While these events are therefore more rapid and of higher magnitude than anything predicted by global climate models over the next century, Rial et al. (2004) ask,

> Could present global warming be just the beginning of one of those natural, abrupt warming episodes, perhaps exacerbated (or triggered) by anthropogenic CO_2 emissions? Since there is no reliable mechanism that explains or predicts the Dansgaard-Oeschger, it is not clear whether the warming events

occur only during an ice age or can also occur during an interglacial, such as the present.

(Rial et al. 2004: 28)

Heinrich events are rapid cooling events that tended to occur during deglaciation. Several have been identified in the Northern Hemisphere following the Last Glacial Maximum, where large numbers of icebergs broke off from ice sheets.

It is clear that the amount of sea level rise expected from the melting of these ice masses is currently uncertain. Early assessments suggest that if the GIS were to melt, it would raise the global sea surface by circa 7 m and the West Antarctic Ice Sheet by circa 5 m. More recent work by Bamber, Riva, Vermeersen and LeBrocq (2009) used elevation and topographic data to estimate the amount of ice below sea level under the West Antarctic Ice Sheet and its likely vulnerability to rapid collapse. They used these assessments to obtain a revised global figure of around 3.3 m of sea level rise if the West Antarctic Ice Sheet collapsed. Further assessments of the likely sea level rise associated with rapid deglaciation have attempted to quantify the physical constraints on the amount of ice that could be discharged into the oceans given current understanding of glacier flow and the topography of Antarctica and Greenland (Pfeffer, Harper and O'Neel, 2008). Although this view is contested, they argue that the maximum sea level rise expected by the end of the twenty-first century is less than 2 m.

The prospects for global sea level changes in the future are thus for, at the least, a rapid rise on a decadal timescale of up to ten times the rate that obtained a century ago, and very likely much greater if the changes feared for both the Greenland and Antarctic ice sheets take place. Taken with known crustal movements, the prospects for some coastal communities, especially in the developing world, are a legitimate concern for the global community.

Human responses to this – cultural, economic, political and social

The final, and ultimately most important, uncertainty is the human response to global climate change. Understanding this is crucial, for it holds the key to whether we will be able to maintain earth's temperature at a level where catastrophic damage to biodiversity and human societies are largely avoided. Given the known lags and response times of the climate system to external perturbations such as elevated GHG concentrations and the likelihood of future rapid climate change as has been seen in the past, it is probable that human societies will have to deal with a climate system out of control. How this could be managed and the implications of this remain unknown.

Conclusions

While the science of climate change is robust and well established, communicating this to the public and policymakers in the face of a vigorous misinformation campaign by sceptics is difficult, yet of overriding importance. Issues concerning the meaning of 'certainty' and 'uncertainty' are difficult for scientists to discuss in public arenas, as the concepts are often highly nuanced. No scientist would say that any part of science is 'certain', but admissions of 'uncertainty' are also misunderstood and misused, with sceptics arguing that such uncertainties must be eradicated before policy changes are made. Clearly, this is a delaying tactic. Public and health policy is made all the time in the face of uncertain science. For instance, the precise mechanisms by which smoking causes cancer have uncertainties attached to them. Similarly, epidemiologists have incomplete knowledge of how vaccines work in populations. Despite these uncertainties, meaningful public policy is possible and desirable.

One way I have found of communicating such uncertainties in the field of climate change is by using metaphors and analogues to clarify the issues. Two examples will suffice. The first tries to show that we can predict the future climate while not knowing what the weather will be like. The way to do this is to point out that even though we are not able to predict the weather for any one specific day, we do know that summer months are always warmer on average than winter months. But what about predicting the climatic effects of increased greenhouse gas concentrations? Here we have to imagine standing at the top of a steep, bumpy hillside with a rugby ball. The potential energy represented by the hillside represents the greenhouse gas forcing. The rugby ball represents the current weather. If the ball were dropped so that it rolled down the hill, the exact path it would take would be essentially unknowable. No computer programme that could plausibly be built would be able to predict *exactly* how the ball would respond when it hit one undulation or another. This seems to be a reasonable analogy for the intrinsic uncertainty involved when trying to predict the weather in response to a forced climate. However, despite these intractable uncertainties, we do know that the ball will eventually reach the bottom, and this eventual predictability of the ball's path is analogous to the idea that with increased greenhouse gas forcing, the climate *must* warm over the long term. If the hillside is very bumpy, this can be used to describe the effects of 'climatic shocks' to the system. For instance, if the ball hits a rock on the way down, its trajectory could momentarily be uphill. Within a few seconds, the ball would then resume its downhill travel. The climate system can also show anomalous behaviour within a general warming trend, in response to short-term perturbations such as volcanic eruptions, which tend to cool the climate for a few years. For instance, the volcanic eruption of Pinatubo in 1991 caused about 0.3°C cooling, which lasted for two years until the general warming trend was resumed.

Overall, then, our understanding of the climate system, while incomplete, is enough for policymakers and the public to take the decisions to reduce greenhouse gas forcing. The sceptics have mounted a well-funded and vigorous campaign to halt or delay policy change, but their arguments are transparently ideological. Eventually climate change will be so obvious that such arguments will fail.

Notes

1 AGW is the term used to describe the consensus view that most of the observed warming seen towards the end of the twentieth century and into the twenty-first is caused by the emission of CO_2 by human activities.
2 The current interglacial following the Pleistocene. The Pleistocene is the period of time covering the last 2.5 million years, when the Earth experienced repeated glaciations. The Holocene is the interglacial of the last 11,000 years, by which time the mid-latitude continental ice sheets had largely melted.
3 Phenological change is the study of the life cycles of plant and animals that are influenced by cyclic variations in climate.

References

Allan, R. P., and Soden, B. J. (2007) Large discrepancy between observed and simulated precipitation trends in the ascending and descending branches of the tropical circulation. *Geophysical Research Letters*, 34, L18705. doi: 10.1029/2007GL031460

Alley, R. B., Clark, P. U., Huybrechts, P., and Joughlin, I. (2005) Ice-sheet and sea-level changes. *Science*, 310: 456–460.

Annan, J. D., and Hargreaves, J. C. (2006) Using multiple observationally-based constraints to estimate climate sensitivity. *Geophysical Research Letters*, 33, L06704. doi: 10.1029/2005GL025259

Annan, J. D., Hargreaves, J. C. Ohgaito, R., Abe-Ouchi, A., and Emori, S. (2005) Efficiently constraining climate sensitivity with paleoclimate simulations. *SOLA*, 1: 181–184.

Arrhenius, Svante (1896). On the influence of carbonic acid in the air upon the temperature of the ground. *Philosophical Magazine*, 41, 237–276.

Bamber, J., Riva, R. E. M., Vermeersen, B. L. A., and LeBrocq, A. M. (2009) Reassessment of the potential sea-level rise from a collapse of the West Antarctic Ice Sheet. *Science*, 324: 901–903.

Callendar, G. S. (1938) The artificial production of carbon dioxide and its influence on climate. *Quarterly J. Royal Meteorological Society*, 64: 223–240.

Charney, J. G. (1979) *Carbon Dioxide and Climate: A Scientific Assessment*. Climate Research Board, National Academy. Washington, DC: NAS Press.

De Angelis, H., and Skvarca, P. (2003) Glacier surge after ice shelf collapse. *Science*, 299: 1560–1562.

Dessler, A. E., and Parson, E. A. (2006) *The Science and Politics of Global Climate Change: A Guide to the Debate*. Cambridge, UK: Cambridge University Press.

Douville, H., Salas-Mélia D., and Tyteca, S. (2006) On the tropical origin of uncertainties in the global land precipitation response to global warming. *Climate Dynamics*, 26: 367–385.

Emanuel, K. A. (2005) Increasing destructiveness of tropical cyclones over the past 30 years. *Nature*, 436: 686–688.

Fischer, L., Kaab, A., Huggel, C., and Noetzli, J. (2006) Geology, glacier retreat and permafrost degradation as controlling factors of slope instabilities in a high-mountain rock wall: The Monte Rosa east face. *Natural Hazards and Earth System Sciences*, 6: 761–772.

Fourier, J. (1824) Remarques generales sur les temperatures du globe terrestre et des espaces planétaires. *Annales de Chimie et de Physique*, 27, 136–167.

Giannini, A., Biasutti, M., Held, I. M., and Sobel, A. H., (2008) A global perspective on African climate. *Climatic Change*, 90: 359–383.

Gregory, J. M., Stouffer, R. J., Raper, S. C. B., Stott, P. A., and Rayner, N. A. (2002) An observationally based estimate of the climate sensitivity. *Journal of Climate*, 15 (22): 3117–3121.

Harrison, S. (2009) Climate sensitivity: Implications for the response of mountain geomorphological systems to future climate change. *Geological Society, London, Special Publications*, 320: 257–265.

Huntington, T. G. (2006) Evidence for intensification of the global water cycle: Review and synthesis. *Journal of Hydrology* 319 (2006): 83–95.

IPCC (2007) *Climate Change 2007: The Physical Science Basis. Contribution of Working Group I to the Fourth Assessment Report of the Intergovernmental Panel on Climate Change* ed. S. Solomon, D. Qin, M. Manning, Z. Chen, M. Marquis, K. B. Averyt, M. Tignor and H. L. Miller. Cambridge, UK: Cambridge University Press.

Lau, K. M., Shen, S. S. P., Kim, K. M., and Wang, H. A. (2006) Multimodel study of the twentieth-century simulations of Sahel drought from the 1970s to 1990s. *Journal of Geophysical Research*, 111, D07111. doi: 10.1029/2005JD006281

Levitus, S., Antonov, J., and Boyer, T. (2005) Warming of the world ocean, 1955–2003. *Geophysical Research Letters*, 32, L02604. doi: 10.1029/2004GL021592

Lin, J-L. (2007) The double-ICTZ problem in IPCC AR4 coupled GCMs: Ocean-atmosphere feedback analysis. *Journal of Climate*, 20: 4497–4525.

Lunt, D. J., Haywood, A. M., Schmidt, G. A., Salzmann, U., Valdes, P. J., and Dowsett, H. (2010) Earth system sensitivity inferred from Pliocene modelling and data. *Nature Geoscience*, 3: 60–64.

Magrin, G. C., García, G., Cruz, D., Choque, D., Giménez, J. C., Moreno, A. R., Nagy, G. J., Nobre, C., and Villamizar, A. (2007) *Latin America. Climate Change 2007: Impacts, Adaptation and Vulnerability. Contribution of Working Group II to the Fourth Assessment Report of the Intergovernmental Panel on Climate Change*, ed. M. L. Parry, O. F. Canziani, J. P. Palutikof, P. J. van der Linden and C. E. Hanson. Cambridge, UK: Cambridge University Press.

Manabe, S., and Stouffer, R. J. (1980) Sensitivity of a global climate model to an increase of CO_2 concentration in the atmosphere. *Journal of Geophysical Research*, 85: 5529–5554.

Mason, S. J., and Goddard, L. (2001) Probabilistic precipitation anomalies associated with ENSO. *Bulletin of the American Meteorological Society*, 82: 619–638.

Oreskes, N. (2004) Beyond the ivory tower: The scientific consensus on climate change. *Science*, 306: 1686.

Overpeck, J. T., Otto-Bliesner, B. L., Miller, G. H., Muhs, D. R., Alley, R. B., and Kiehl, J. T. (2006) Paleoclimatic evidence for future ice-sheet instability and rapid sea-level rise. *Science*, 311: 1747–1750.

Pfeffer, W. T., Harper, J. T., and O'Neel, S. (2008) Kinematic constraints on glacier contributions to 21st-century sea-level rise. *Science*, 321 (5894): 1340–1343. doi: 10.1126/science.1159099

Rahmstorf, S. (2003) Timing of abrupt climate change: A precise clock. *Geophysical Research Letters*, 30, No. 101510. doi: 10.1029/2003GL017115

Rahmstorf, S. (2010) A new view on sea level rise. *Nature Reports Climate Change*. doi: 10.1038/climate.2010.29

Rial, A., Pielke Sr., R. A., Beniston, M., Claussen, M., Canadell, J., Cox, P., Held, H., De Noblet-Ducoudré, N., Prinn, R., Reynolds, J. F., and Salas, J. D. (2004) Nonlinearities, feedbacks and critical thresholds within the Earth's climate system. *Climatic Change*, 65: 11–38.

Schneider von Deimling, T., Held, H., Ganopolski, A, and Rahmstorf, S. (2006) Climate sensitivity estimated from ensemble simulations of glacial climate *Climate Dynamics*. doi: 10.1007/s00382–006–0126–8

Siegenthaler, U., Stocker, T. F. Monnin, E., Lüthi, D., Schwander, J. Stauffer, B., et al. (2005) Stable carbon cycle–climate relationship during the late Pleistocene. *Science*, 310: 1313–1317.

Stainforth, D. A., Downing, T. E., Washington, R., Lopez, A., and New, M. (2007) Issues in the interpretation of climate model ensembles to inform decisions. *Philosophical Transactions of the Royal Society A: Mathematical, Physical and Engineering Sciences*, 365: 2163–2177.

Tyndall, J. (1861) On the absorption and radiation of heat by gases and vapours. *Philosophical Magazine*, ser. 4, 22: 169–194, 273–285.

Vieli, A., and Payne, A. J. (2005) Modelling the grounding line migration of marine ice sheets. *Journal of Geophysical Research*, 110: F01003.

Voelker, A. H. L. (2002) Global distribution of centennial-scale records for Marine Isotope Stage (MIS): 3: A database. *Quaternary Science Reviews*, 21: 1185–1212.

Index

Descartes, R. 176
Dessler, A. E. 229
destruction of civility 58
destructive drive 81
destructive forces, inevitability and
   universality of 81, 85
destructive narcissism 38
destructive rapaciousness 135
destructiveness 8, 9, 160, 162; of
   capitalism 181, 193, 197; of civility, 58;
   disavowal of 8, 9; dynamic of 172;
   facing 11–13; human 8, 9, 12, 42, 53,
   85, 167; narrative of, modernization as
   178; taking responsibility for 136;
   unconscious 172 [pathologies of 173]
de Waal, F. 5, 207
Diamond, J. 145, 151, 155, 162
Dickens, C.: Great Expectations 11,
   87–100, 103, 104, 109; Oliver Twist 105
Dilling, L. 99
disavowal: concept of 7, 49; culture of 9,
   43 [and irrationality 40; perverse 8]; as
   defence 59; denial as 6–12, 36–46, 50,
   53; as knowing and not-knowing at the
   same time 7; of needs of future
   generations 173; and negation,
   distinction between 7, 38; as part of
   pathological organization 39;
   psychoanalytic concept of 7; and
   triumph of arrogant omnipotent part of
   self 39
'disembedding' 65
Disney 166, 167, 168
Disneyfication 64
'distant other' 8, 75, 206
'Doctors' Tea Party' 24
doubts, about global warming 7, 19, 62,
   63, 110, 111, 114; children's 104;
   defences against facing 147, 155
Douville, H. 233
Downing, T. E. 233
Dresher, M. 153
Dreyfus affair 21
drought(s) 1, 111, 161, 206; increases in
   magnitude and frequency of 228; in
   Sahel region 233
Dunlap, R. E. 21

Earth: as 'breast-and-toilet' mother 12, 42;
   dependency on, as modern neurosis 12
Earth system models 232
'Earth system sensitivity' vs. 'Climate
   sensitivity' 232

earthquakes 167
Ecclesiastes 9 202
ecocentrism 85; vs. anthropocentrism 216
ecological damage, destructive cycle of
   218
ecological debt 87–100, 103, 109, 112,
   114; and guilt 93–5; psychodynamics of
   87–101; and reparation 93–5; and sense
   of proportionality 12, 94; struggle to
   come to terms with 95
ecological dependence 216
ecological deterioration 117, 134
economic growth 8, 53, 112, 217, 224, 234
Einstein, A., theory of relativity of,
   campaign against 20–5
El Niño Southern Oscillation 233, 235
Elias, N. 176, 177
Eliot, T. S. 148
Emanuel, K. A. 228
emissions reductions 67, 68
empathic civilization 78
empathy: capacity to feel, humans sharing
   with animals 5; cross-species 206
'empire of mankind' 176
energy consumption, reduction in 193
Enlightenment 28, 29, 144; fragility of
   17–18
Enron, psycho-social analysis of 58, 60,
   65, 84
entitlement 90; arrogant, encouraging
   identification with 60, 208; conflicting
   kinds of 200; human, to take/dominate
   5, 89; narcissistic 38, 205, 214; sense of
   42, 146, 162, 199, 200, 207, 216
environment, 'structures of feeling'
   towards 174–7
environmental activism and 'analytic
   attitude' 119
environmental aesthetics 217
environmental communications 120, 130
environmental crisis 12, 45, 172–7, 194,
   196, 197
environmental degradation, apathy about
   9, 118
environmental destruction 177
environmental ethics 119
environmental issues, public apathy about,
   apparent 45
Environmental Justice Foundation 89
environmental melancholia 9, 124
environmental movement 77, 191
environmental neurosis 41; and illusion of
   autonomy 48–51